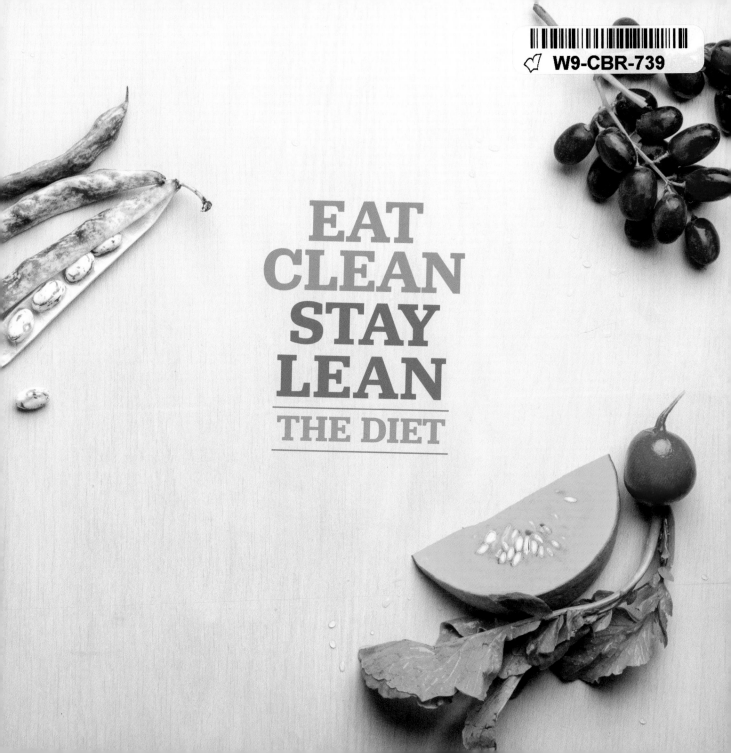

EAT
CLEAN
STAY
LEAN

THE DIET

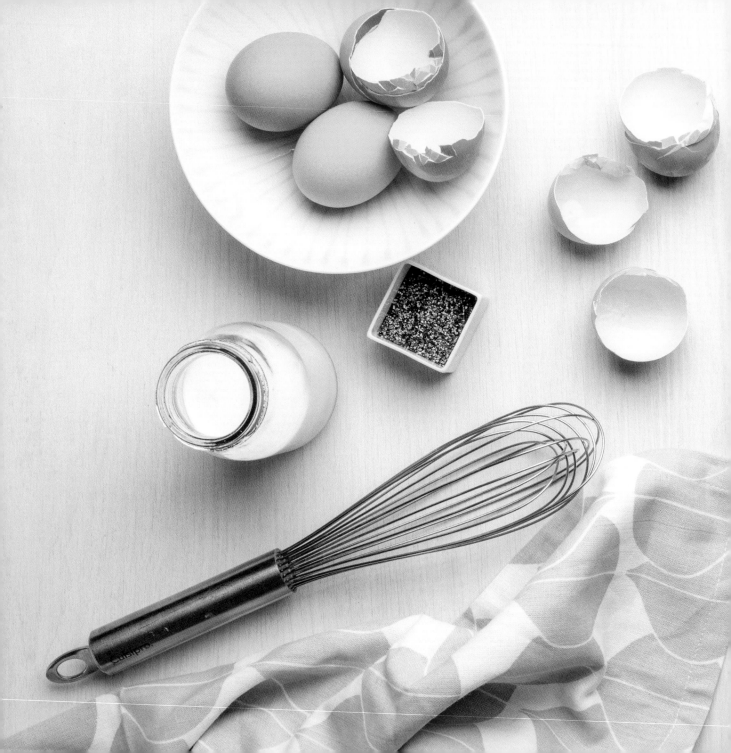

EAT CLEAN STAY LEAN

THE DIET

Real Foods for Real Weight Loss

THE EDITORS OF **Prevention**®
AND **WENDY BAZILIAN**, DrPH, RD
WITH **MARYGRACE TAYLOR**

RECIPES DEVELOPED AND TESTED BY
THE RODALE TEST KITCHEN

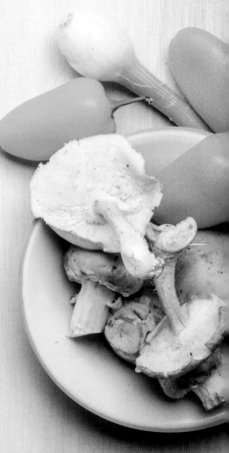

RODALE.

RODALE
wellness

Live happy. Be healthy. Get inspired.

Sign up today to get exclusive access to our authors, exclusive bonuses,
and the most authoritative, useful, and cutting-edge information on health,
wellness, fitness, and living your life to the fullest.

Visit us online at RodaleWellness.com
Join us at RodaleWellness.com/Join

Library of Congress Cataloging-in-Publication Data is on file with the publisher

ISBN 978-1-62336-789-3   paperback

Distributed to the trade by Macmillan

2   4   6   8   10   9   7   5   3   1   paperback

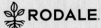 RODALE.

Follow us @RodaleBooks on

We inspire health, healing, happiness, and love in the world.
Starting with you.

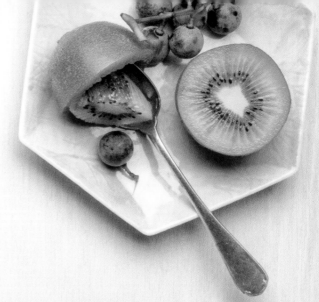

Dedicated to everyone who loves food
and is committed to taking steps toward better health and
healthy weight loss through wholesome, delicious fare.
Clean eaters, this one's for you!

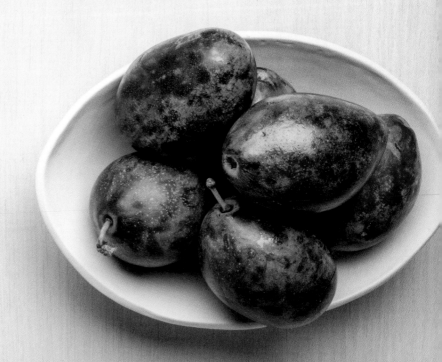

Contents

Preface

Welcome to your own personal weight-loss journey. The decision to begin eating cleaner and getting leaner is *yours*, and yours alone—and you should be proud and excited to take this step toward better health. There are many different paths you can try taking to reach your destination, and maybe you've started down one (or more) of those roads before. But this time, you'll see: Things are different.

If you are fed up with gimmicky eating plans, tasteless and hard-to-follow recipes, and complex rules with zero flexibility (No bread! No fat! No fun!), you've opened the right book. Chances are, you've tried time and again to lose weight by dieting. And you know what? There's absolutely nothing wrong with that. Like finding the perfect pair of jeans or the most flattering pair of glasses, most of us have to try on many sizes and styles before we find our *right fit*.

Hopefully that's just what you'll find here: your right fit—in a setting of complete support and zero judgment.

There's no question that achieving a healthy weight for your own best self is highly individual. All of the turns, hills, loose pebbles, and smooth walkways you'll find on your route are unique. And it's up to you to determine how best to deal with the hurdles and course changes you may encounter. Wouldn't it be great if there was a plan, a program, and an approach that actually *admits* that this journey isn't always easy? And better yet—one that then helps you navigate the sometimes confusing road map, and offers up strategies for coping with the inevitable obstacles, so you can achieve *lasting* success? Best of all, wouldn't it be wonderful if, all along the way, you actually felt good—like you are doing something that's positive for your body?

That's what *Eat Clean, Stay Lean: The Diet* is all about. It's really not a *diet* in the trendy, and ultimately temporary, way to lose weight that most of us have come to despise. **This is a simple, no-nonsense plan designed to teach you how to eat in a way that supports your own best weight and energy for your own best body.** And it all starts—and continues—with eating clean. Of course, healthy weight loss also involves regular movement (in other words, exercise, though it doesn't have to *feel* that way). It also involves employing strategies that enhance your overall health, happiness, and well-being—like rest, stress management, and having fun.

You'll find all of that—and more—in the chapters

ahead. With the guidance of the trusted Editors of *Prevention* magazine, *Eat Clean, Stay Lean: The Diet* offers small steps and simple yet effective tools designed to help you make lasting, sustainable shifts in the way you eat. The end goal isn't simply that you lose unneeded weight (though that will certainly happen). It's that eating to support your best body simply becomes your normal—and more importantly, your *favorite*—way to stay fueled. Because there's absolutely nothing easier to maintain than a style of eating that you love.

In these pages, you'll learn how to achieve those goals. Much of the information you'll find will surprise you, and some may reinforce what you already know. In both cases, you'll learn how to eat clean with our easy-to-follow program and delicious menus. Just as important, you'll find out why eating clean is the best path for lasting weight loss. Best of all? You'll do it with the support of experts who fully understand the challenges you may face.

When I developed this effective, research-backed weight-loss plan, I had you—as I would a new client and friend—in mind. When I wrote the menus and worked with *Prevention*'s test kitchen to develop more than 70 delicious, tested, and Clean Eater–approved recipes, I had you—a health-inspired but also busy individual—in mind. As a doctor of public health, registered dietitian, and exercise physiologist who has helped thousands of individuals work toward their weight-related health goals, I have listened, talked, strategized, planned,

advised, laughed, and occasionally even shared tears around the challenges and opportunities my clients, perhaps like you, have faced when it comes to pursuing a healthier weight while still living a rich and happy life. I know that it's not always easy, but I promise you that it *is* worth it. Especially when your path is marked with simple strategies and delicious recipes that can help you stay lean for life.

Want proof that this plan works? Take a look at the stories of our amazing test panelists, who graciously allowed us to share their 6-week journeys on the Eat Clean, Stay Lean plan. You'll be inspired, as I was, by their challenges, successes, and valuable lessons learned. And their impressive results, observations, and experiences will reinforce *your* motivation as you step forward on your own Eat Clean, Stay Lean path.

Be kind to yourself, put in the effort, and enjoy the ride—and rewards!—of getting lean by eating clean!

—Wendy Bazilian, DrPH, RD

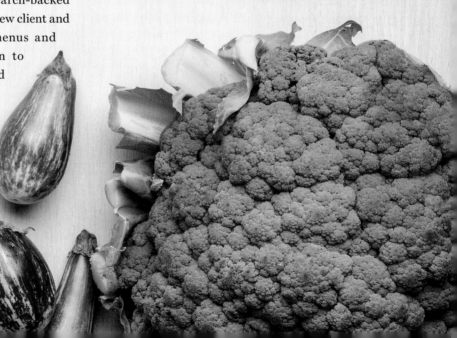

Acknowledgments

Thanks to our smart, mighty editor Marisa Vigilante and her equally wonderful editorial assistant Isabelle Hughes for their commitment to the project, manageable but aggressive deadlines, and active and instructive communication throughout the development of this book. Thank you to Sarah Toland, *Prevention* magazine's food and nutrition director, for her direction, confidence in, and support of the project from inception. We are grateful to the vision and oversight of *Prevention*'s editor in chief Barbara O'Dair and editorial director Michael Lafavore for their vision and confidence in the strength of the weight-loss plan and the entire book.

Many thanks to the members of Rodale's Test Kitchen, including Juli Roberts, Jennifer Kushnier, Amy Fritch, and Melanie Hansche, for their creative culinary ideas and for bringing this plan to life with delicious, nutritious, easy-to-make recipes.

To our photographers Mitch Mandel, Matt Rainey, and Ryan Hulvat and designer Amy King for the mouthwatering recipe and cover photos and for making this book look so beautiful.

A gigantic thank-you to Michele Stanten for organizing and managing our test panelists. And we are so appreciative of our Clean Eater panelists themselves for their tireless dedication to eating clean and getting lean over our 6-week—and ongoing—journey together. You inspire us!

Thanks to our writer, Marygrace Taylor. Her thoughtful and collaborative approach, attention to detail, and knack for making words flow helped bring these pages to life.

Finally, thanks to our guiding force and health expert, Dr. Wendy Bazilian. Her infectious positivity, thorough research, dedication to detail, willingness to solve problems, and commitment to this project—and to our test panelists and readers—were essential in creating this plan and developing a book designed to truly serve those who want to achieve sustainable weight loss.

Thanks from Wendy Bazilian

To my chief partner in life and business and best friend Jason Bazilian, for his unflappable calm and balanced ways; my creative and driven assistant, Jen Ratanapratum; and my incredibly artistic professional photographer and dear friend, Pearl Preis. My utmost thanks to the incredible Rodale Test Kitchen team; our fabulous

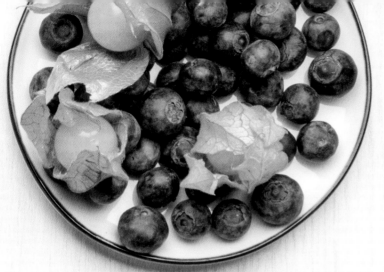

editor, Marisa Vigilante, her editorial assistant, Isabelle Hughes; and also to Sarah Toland for her support and encouragement. So much gratitude is extended to Marygrace, whose talent with words and spirit of professional teamwork and timely collaboration were unparalleled. And of course, tremendous thanks to our Clean Eater panelists, who graciously shared their personal journeys—and a peek into their lives—with us all.

Thanks from Marygrace Taylor

To my husband, Sam Taylor, for his unwavering support, encouragement, and patience. To Amy Beal, who first invited me to write for *Prevention*; to Sarah Toland, for her continued guidance and for bringing me on to this project; and to Marisa Vigilante and Isabelle Hughes. Thanks also to our test panelists, who generously shared their inspiring stories. Finally, thank you to Wendy Bazilian for her guidance, collaboration, enthusiasm, and total dedication to this project.

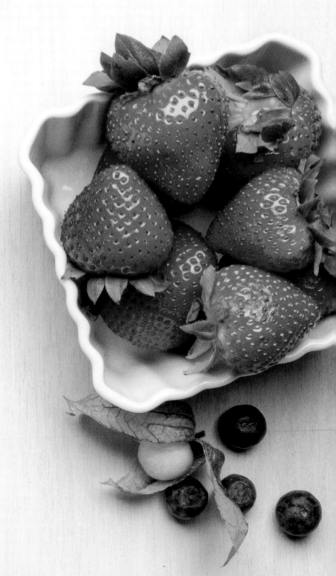

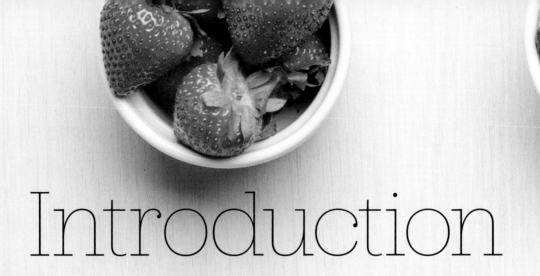

Introduction

Get ready for a radically simple way to lose weight.

In case you haven't noticed, weight has become a major problem for a lot of Americans. In the not-so-distant past, most people were lean—and they didn't spend much time thinking about how to eat right or fit into a smaller pair of jeans. These days, many of us devote countless hours to thinking about diets (Paleo or vegan?), carbs (good or bad?), calories (to count or not?), and more in the name of trying to lose weight.

But it doesn't seem to be doing us much good, because obesity rates are higher than ever. Yes, it's a great thing to be conscious of our food choices and to try to make smart ones as often as possible. But if the scale continues to creep a little bit higher each year, and if you notice that you seem to be feeling *less* vibrant and energized instead of more, is all that effort really paying off?

Complicated, gimmick-filled, and ultimately useless diet plans are a dime a dozen. So if you've tried to slim down before—or have never actually *stopped* trying—

another trendy weight-loss plan might sound like the last thing you need. And it is. You don't need another fad diet that can't teach you anything other than how to eat according to its weird, impossible-to-stick-with rules. That isn't going to help you take control of your health, and it definitely isn't going to help you get lean for the long haul.

But thankfully, what this book offers is not a trend, and not a fad. *This* is eating clean. It's getting back to the basics of what people were eating for hundreds and hundreds of years before highly processed, packaged foods became the norm. These are the same foods that most people who maintain a healthy weight eat today: whole foods such as fresh fruits and vegetables; simple nuts, seeds, and beans; clean meats and fish; unrefined grains; and simple dairy products. You know—stuff that your grandma probably ate. In short, foods that are free (or mostly free) of added chemicals, pesticides, flavors, sweeteners, or preservatives.

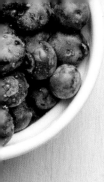
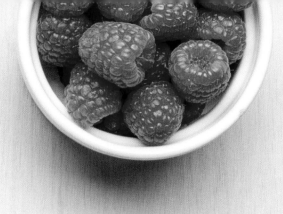

Right now you're probably thinking, "Wait. That's it? *That's* what I need to do to lose weight and keep it off for good?" Like we said, it's a radically simple idea. But it works. Diets rich in clean, unprocessed foods deliver loads of the vitamins, nutrients, minerals, and phytochemicals that your body needs to be healthy—and less of the unhealthy fats, sugars, and other junk that it doesn't. Clean foods also satisfy your hunger, keep cravings at bay, and boost your mood and energy levels. Plus, they're delicious, so they don't leave you feeling deprived.

This book might reinforce some of the things you already know about eating to support your health and weight loss. But we guarantee that it will also surprise you with plenty of new information and smart advice that you can actually use. Most importantly, it lays out a practical 3-week meal plan and gives you tools, strategies, and motivation to help you achieve your goal: A lighter, stronger, leaner, and *cleaner* you, for life!

Once you start, there's no stopping. Because when you begin eating clean, your body will actually start craving those nutritious, delicious foods instead of the ones you might have dreamt about before. You'll be eating for the healthy size you are meant to be—once and for all.

Yes, You Can

How do we know for sure that the Eat Clean, Stay Lean plan will help you lose weight? Because we've watched people just like you succeed on it already. Our Clean Eater Test Panel tried following the menus, making the recipes, and sticking with our eat-clean guidelines out in the real world for 6 weeks. And every single one of them lost weight (as much as 22 pounds!), improved their health, ramped up their energy, and came away with the knowledge they needed to *keep* eating clean even after we said our farewells. Best of all, you'll find their inspiring transformations, smart tips, insightful advice, and motivating experiences throughout this book. Keep your eyes peeled—and prepare to be seriously impressed by their achievements.

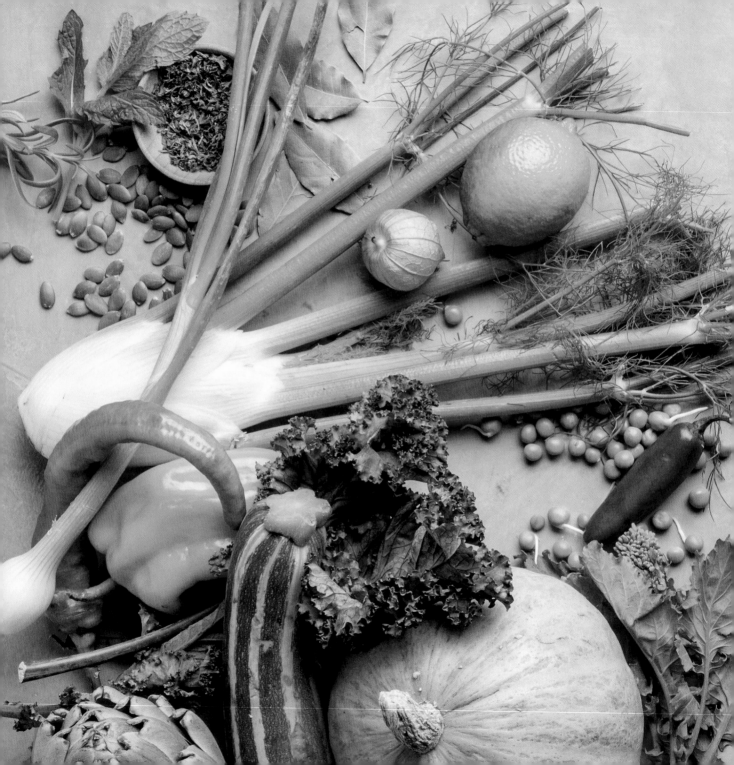

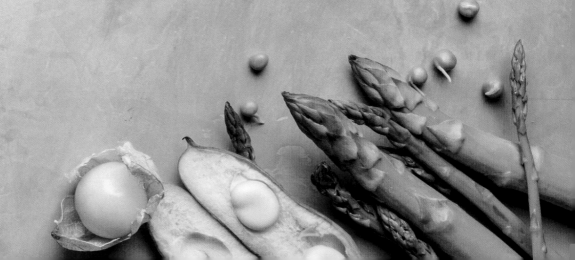

PART

I

Why You Should Be Eating Clean

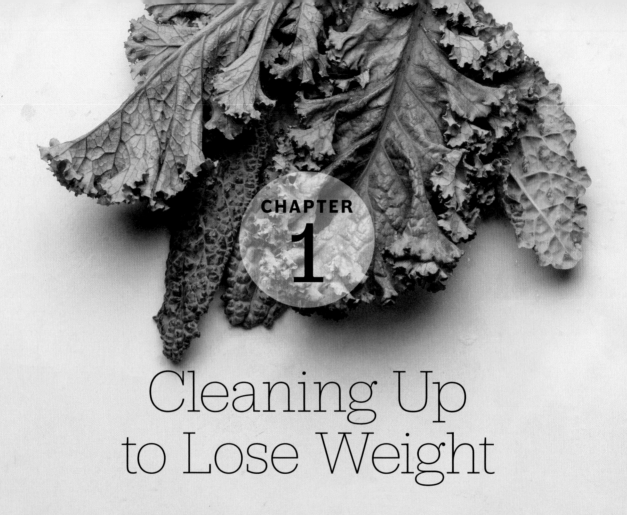

Cleaning Up to Lose Weight

Let's get straight to the point: Most diets are really only designed to be temporary. Sure, they might promise that you can stick with them forever. But in reality, all those crazy rules and restrictions practically guarantee that they'll be impossible to stick with long-term. If you've dieted before, you're used to hearing endless nos and barely any yeses. You're used to eating in a way that's inconvenient instead of a way that actually fits into your real life. You're used to tons of hard work that always ends in disappointment. Aren't you tired of that?

If you picked up this book, we're willing to bet that the answer is yes. It's time to try a new way to lose weight—that *really* works—and makes you feel good for life. It's time to eat clean.

What *Is* Clean Eating?

You've probably heard the term plenty of times before, but what exactly does it mean? Clean eating is a way of life that can help you lose the weight and keep it off for good—plain and simple. When you eat clean, you choose whole or minimally processed foods that are made from real ingredients, rather than choosing their highly processed counterparts. These clean foods look (and taste) like they came from the ground, or the farm, or the ocean, or maybe even someone's kitchen—not from a factory or a science lab. Think fresh fruit and nuts instead of a sugary granola bar. Organic roast chicken instead of frozen, breaded, chickenlike strips. A whole egg-and-vegetable omelet instead of a fast-food breakfast sandwich. Even homemade chocolate chip cookies instead of the kind that come in a box. You get the idea!

If you're used to eating the standard American diet, the idea of giving your diet a clean makeover might feel a little overwhelming. But it's actually pretty easy to get the hang of. And once you do, it doesn't feel like you're doing anything weird or different or difficult. It's just *how you eat*. When you choose to eat clean, you're giving your body the fuel it needs and the nutrients it craves. You're *not* constantly scrutinizing calorie counts, not cutting out food groups, and not depriving yourself of the things that you love. Clean eating allows you to feel your best. And it's the most effective way to get lean—and stay that way for life.

Meet the *Non*diet Diet

If you've tried other diets before, you might be wondering whether clean eating is truly all that different. It is. In fact, it's the complete and total opposite of every restrictive, gimmicky, run-of-the-mill diet out there. That's because eating clean doesn't just help you achieve a healthy weight—it also makes you *feel* good, so keeping it up to keep the pounds off is easy. Instead of trying to follow a hundred different rules, you follow just one basic principle: Choose real foods over their packaged, processed counterparts whenever possible.

Of course, you have to keep your portions in check. And of course, you have to enjoy things like clean desserts *in moderation*. In order to lose weight, both of those things are absolute musts. But eating clean, whole foods makes doing those things a lot easier, because *clean foods are what your body was designed to run on*. They're designed to fill you up, so you don't want to keep eating and eating and eating. They're designed to help your blood sugar stay steady, so you're less susceptible to sugary cravings. They're designed to help you feel your best, so you have the energy to be active and keep on making smart choices. It sounds pretty great, right?

No Restrictions, No Guilt

Most traditional diets work by doing one of two things. Some force you to limit the *types* of foods that you're allowed to eat, such as by cutting out carbs or only eating raw fruits and veggies. Others say that it's completely fine to eat anything you want—from doughnuts to Doritos—as long as you stay within your allotted (read: stingy) calorie budget. Both of these methods might work for a couple of weeks, or maybe even for a couple of months. But eventually you get tired of, say, never getting to eat bread or constantly feeling hungry because you're stuck eating too-tiny portions. At that point, it's totally natural to start dreaming about all of the delicious food that's been off-limits. Eventually, your cravings get the best of you—and you find yourself at the table with a half-eaten pepperoni pizza and an empty pint of chocolate fudge ice cream thinking, *I messed up* big *time. Now what?* By then, you feel so guilty that you end up abandoning your diet altogether and going back to your old ways. You regain the weight that you lost and maybe pile on a few extra pounds. Sound familiar?

Here's how eating clean is different. When you commit to eating real food, *nothing* is off-limits. You don't have to cut out any category of food. You don't have to

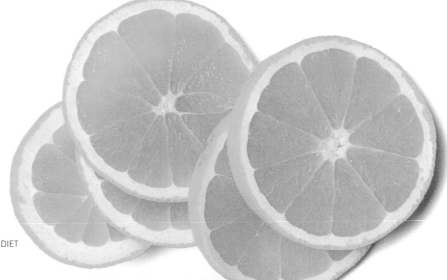

say no when you're invited to a restaurant or party because you're worried that the stuff on the menu won't work with your eating plan. With clean eating, there's almost always an option—even when the food being served isn't under your control. You don't have to subject yourself to eating pre-portioned diet meals or weighing and measuring every bite of food that goes into your mouth for the rest of your life. It's *really* freeing!

Naturally, we need to face the fact that portion sizes still matter. Food has calories whether it's clean or not, and there's no way around it: **You have to eat less—and therefore take in fewer calories—in order to lose weight.** But trimming portion sizes is much easier when you take the clean route. Clean foods deliver nutrients that help you stay full longer, so you're not hungry and cranky all the time. Plus, they make you feel like you're eating a lot, so you're less likely to feel deprived. Think about a sweet, crunchy apple. It has around 100 calories, which is similar to the calories you'll find in a tiny granola bar. But the apple makes you *feel* like you're eating more because it's bigger, and also because you have to spend more time chewing each bite. By the time you're done eating an apple, you feel like you're done eating, period. When you're done eating that snack bar? Chances are, you just want to grab another one.

Delicious Satisfaction-Guaranteed

One of the biggest reasons that people abandon their diets is because the food just doesn't taste that good. And to make matters worse, it isn't very filling. After all, how many times can you eat a bunless, low-cal turkey burger or fat-free mac and cheese for dinner before you start dreaming about something better? Clean foods are fresh, vibrant, and unadulterated, so they naturally pack more flavor than their bland, processed counterparts. After

Dr. Wendy Says . . .

Can you really eat *anything*? If it's made from real ingredients, yes. But let's exercise some common sense: There are some clean foods that are great to eat all the time and some that you need to save for once in a while in order to lose weight. For instance, it's better to make buttery steak and warm, homemade apple crisp for dinner the exception, rather than the rule—even if the steak is grass-fed and the apple crisp is made with rolled oats and unrefined sugar. (Though deep down you already knew that, right?)

But here's the thing: **When you stop looking at food in terms of *good things I can have* and *bad things* that are never allowed—especially if you're in weight-loss mode—you might find that you actually start daydreaming about those formerly forbidden foods less often.** This might seem hard to believe now. But trust me, it can—and most likely will—happen! In fact, among people actively trying to lose weight, studies show that even the *thought* of having to restrict certain foods can trigger overeating. And when it comes to not feeling deprived and achieving a healthier weight, that means *everything*.

eating them, you're satisfied and you no longer feel hungry. So when you get up from the table, you aren't hit with an overpowering urge to raid the pantry for a snack. (Not so sure yet? Check out the mouthwatering recipes and meal ideas in Part III.) In all, a delicious approach to eating is one that's easy to stick with.

And it's more than just a nice-sounding theory. Science shows that when you eat foods that are bursting with flavor, you'll probably eat less overall. In one *Flavour* journal study, researchers measured subjects' hunger and fullness levels while they ate a basic bowl of tomato soup.[1] On another day, researchers measured the subjects' hunger and fullness levels again while the subjects ate a more flavorful tomato soup made with chile peppers. Unsurprisingly, the subjects said they liked the more flavorful soup better. But that didn't lead them to want to eat more of it. Instead, they decided that they were satisfied sooner.

Of course, the takeaway isn't that you need to add chile peppers to everything you eat. (Unless you want to, of course.) It's that foods with more flavor—like fresh, clean fare—leave you genuinely more content with your meal, so you're less likely to want to keep noshing and noshing and noshing. While portion control is always key to losing weight, eating clean will likely lead you to eat less without even realizing it—and you'll manage to enjoy your food even *more*.

Notes from a Clean Eater

"Every day, I've had the opportunity to sit down to eat fresh, delicious food. The recipes are easy to follow, and I love all of the new whole grains I've been introduced to. In the evenings, I have a gourmet dinner to sit down to—and I'm the cook!"—**Almarie K.**

A Way of Life That Works

When you're on a diet, you're constantly in a fight. You're fighting to maintain crazy food restrictions that don't fit your real day-to-day life. You're fighting the urge to scarf down a chocolate chip muffin instead of a yucky packet of artificially sweetened instant oatmeal. (Two *equally* poor options.) And you're fighting the urge to eat, period, because you're hungry *all the time*. No wonder diets don't work—after a while, most of us give up out of sheer exhaustion.

There's no fighting in eating clean, which is why it's so easy. Instead of food and your appetite being the enemy, food becomes the thing that nourishes your body and satisfies your hunger. Instead of living in a vacuum of prepackaged meals and diet snacks that force you to eat differently than everyone around you, you can make eating clean work anytime, anywhere. You're just eating the way that you were designed to eat—and reaping the benefits of feeling strong, energized, and lean. Which is pretty easy to do, well, forever!

(continued on page 10)

Learn How to Love Healthy Foods

If you're used to the addictive, over-the-top flavors of processed foods, the idea of black bean soup or an apple with peanut butter might seem sort of . . . blah. That'll change as your taste buds adjust to fresh foods that aren't loaded with sugar, salt, and unhealthy fats—promise. But if you're not quite there yet, here are some tips to help get you hooked on clean fare faster.

1 Forget how you felt as a kid. Maybe you haven't let a certain vegetable slip past your lips since elementary school but you've repeatedly heard that it delivers multiple benefits and could help you lose weight. Though it can sometimes be tough to reconcile your feelings with the facts, now might be the time to give long-hated foods another try. Your taste buds are more sensitive to bitter flavors when you're young, so even though Brussels sprouts might have tasted like lawn clippings when you were 10, your adult self might actually like them. Preparation is so important, too. The broccoli of your childhood might have been mushy and bland—but cooking it differently today might yield a completely different result. (Ready to give it a go? Try the Roasted Broccoli with Chile and Lemon on page 277.)

2 Surround yourself with healthy stuff. French people aren't born loving snails, and Japanese people don't come into this world craving sushi. Instead, they may come to like those foods because they're a regular part of the environment, according to findings published in the journal *Appetite*.[2] Instead of buying more boxed mac and cheese or chicken fingers, get into the habit of stocking your kitchen with whole wheat pasta and organic chicken breasts. As you get used to having the clean stuff around, you might find yourself wanting it more often.

3 Take small steps. If the thought of eating plain raw carrots grosses you out, don't do it. Start by pairing them with something outrageously delicious, like homemade ranch dressing. After a while, you might decide to start dunking them in something a little more nutrient-dense, like hummus or the Lemony Rosemary White Bean Dip on page 286. And if that's where you decide to stay? No problem. If you still don't like plain raw carrots, you don't have to eat them.

4 Appeal to your sweet tooth. Take advantage of the fact that humans are hardwired to crave sugar. Instead of trying to choke down raw or steamed vegetables, try roasting them to bring out their natural sweetness and make them more palatable. You might not think a cauliflower floret could ever truly taste like candy, but when it gets caramelized and crispy, it really can.

5 Go for the fancy stuff. Research published in the *Journal of Sensory Studies* found that people who paid $8 for a buffet lunch reported being more satisfied with their meals than those who only paid $4, even though both groups ate the same exact fare.[3] Why? Because sometimes we're shallow, and we automatically think that cheaper food is going to be lower quality. When possible, spend the extra couple of bucks on organic kale from the farmers' market instead of that so-so bunch at the corner store. Chances are it's a fresher, overall better choice than the droopy bunch flown in from who-knows-where. Thanks to your built-in selectivity, you might trick yourself into thinking the pricy stuff is pretty delicious.

6 Make sure you're actually hungry. Before you bother sitting down to that beet and quinoa salad, check in with your appetite. Why? Because when your stomach's really rumbling, you'll be way more willing to eat whatever's in front of you—even if it's a big bowl of vegetables. (For much more on how to read your body's hunger cues, check out Chapter 4.)

Clean Eaters

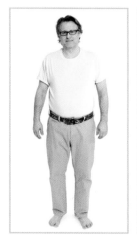 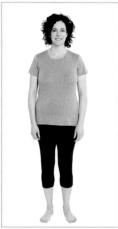

BEFORE

Steve and Jenny were already familiar with eating clean, and they ate that way some of the time. Jenny says, "I didn't have a terrific amount of weight to lose. But I was at my highest weight, and even the fat pants weren't fitting. So it was really more of a shift of focus."

Before they started on the program, the couple would sometimes have nutritious foods like beans or kale. But living in New York City, they also tended to dine out a lot with friends—which meant that their meals were often heavy on the bread, pasta, and wine. Portion control was another big issue. Steve used to eat spoonfuls of peanut butter, treating it like ice cream, without thinking twice. And he'd help himself to some chocolate almost every day.

After committing to eating clean, the couple quickly learned what counted as a reasonable serving size. Now, Steve serves himself a tablespoon of peanut butter and pairs it with an apple. And they figured out how to make the plan work with their social life. Now Jenny orders salmon and lentils with a side of Brussels sprouts for dinner and skips the extras that she realized were making her bloated and puffy. When Steve goes to his friend's house for dinner, he brings ingredients to make a salad that the group can enjoy alongside their spaghetti and meatballs.

It's that kind of flexibility that makes the couple feel like they can eat this way for life. "I don't think I could fall out of this, because I know I can even go to a diner and get two poached eggs, some whole wheat toast, and berries. I don't have to do anything special," Steve says. "You should just call this The Easy Diet."

Dr. Wendy Observes: People often tell me that an active social life makes it harder to make healthy choices, and at times, that can certainly be true. But as Steve and Jenny discovered, having a plan, a partner, and some know-how makes it easier—especially with a bit of practice. Plus, the fact that Steve's itchy skin and chronic heartburn were completely gone within days of starting the program is tremendously motivating and helps him continue to make healthy choices. And the plan's flexibility with guidelines helped both of them succeed individually, as well as together.

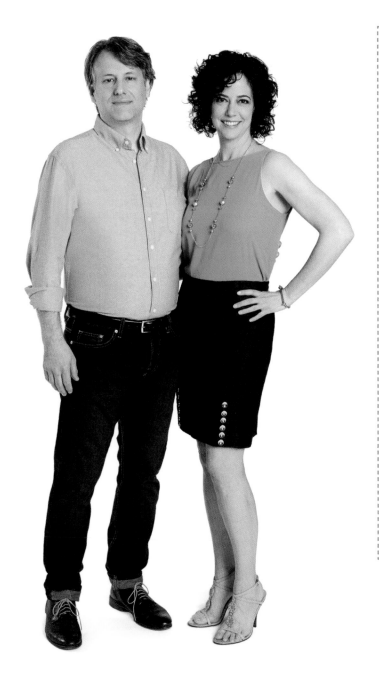

TOTAL POUNDS LOST

STEVE
22 lbs

JENNY
7 lbs

TOTAL INCHES LOST

STEVE
13

JENNY
5

MOST NOTABLE IMPROVEMENTS

Steve: His skin stopped itching and his chronic heartburn went away completely. He noticed he had significantly fewer headaches, too.

Jenny: Her LDL ("bad") cholesterol went from the unhealthy range to the healthy range, while her HDL ("good") cholesterol increased. She also noticed that her sleep was deeper and more restorative.

Clean Foods Do the Work

Trying to fuel your car with pancake syrup instead of gasoline would be insane, and the same is true when it comes to fueling your body. Humans were designed to eat whole, unprocessed foods. They deliver the nutrients that your body needs to carry out its daily functions. Unlike your car—which wouldn't even turn on—you might be able to get by on pancake syrup for a while. But without the right nutrition, your body's functions—including your metabolism—would eventually grind to a halt. You'd feel exhausted, sick, and weak. Who would want to live like that?

Of course, no one would actually try to survive on syrup alone. But the refined, processed foods most Americans scarf down at breakfast, lunch, and dinner (and during all the hours in between) aren't actually that much different. Aside from the fact that they're loaded with sugar, they're virtually devoid of the vitamins and minerals that your system was built to run on. Take iron, for instance: It's essential for helping you feel energized so you can be active instead of sitting around on the couch feeling tired all day. You'll find it in lean poul-

try, fish, meat, lentils, and leafy greens—but it's not exactly abundant in doughnuts or crackers. Or how about magnesium? It's needed for more than 300 bodily functions, including helping your body turn protein into calorie-torching muscle tissue. You'll find it in almonds, black beans, and brown rice—but it's tough to get enough of it if the foods you eat most often are French fries and sugary cereals. As for fortified packaged foods? Don't rely on those to get the vitamins and minerals you need. What makes whole foods so powerful is the fact that they contain an entire suite of good-for-you stuff acting harmoniously together—and not just single nutrients.

When you think about the fact that eating a diet high in processed foods actually deprives your body of the nutrients it needs to work efficiently, you understand why your ability to burn calories starts to decrease. Your body is, in effect, starving for nutrition. And as a result, it goes into conservation mode and starts to cling desperately to any source of energy that it can get. By eating clean, you stop feeding your body empty calories and

Clean Foods = Weight-Loss Foods

Eating clean lets you abandon the diet mentality, but that isn't the only way it leads to lower numbers on your scale. Processed foods are brimming with ingredients like sugar, refined carbs, and weird chemicals that can actually make it easier to pack on the pounds. But clean foods? They do the opposite by keeping you full for longer and by staving off junky cravings so you're less tempted to raid the vending machine for a candy bar or polish off a bag of pretzels the minute you get home from work. And believe it or not, they actually rev your metabolism and turn you into a lean, fat-burning machine.

Bottoms Up!

When it comes to filling up faster and steering clear of junky snacks, plain old water might be your secret weapon. Research published in the journal *Obesity* found that dieters who downed 16 ounces of water before each meal for 12 weeks lost 3 more pounds than those who skipped the extra sips.[4] The reason why is brilliantly simple: Having all that liquid in your belly means that you need less food to feel full.

start giving it the nutrient-dense foods it craves. Once it's fueled with the right stuff, it can get out of this vicious and unsatisfying cycle—and start kicking your metabolism into high gear.

They Keep You Full

You probably don't need us to remind you that it's tough to lose weight if you're hungry all the time. The louder your stomach rumbles, the more likely you are to want to gobble down anything that'll fill you up, pronto—such as a giant bag of chips or the leftover birthday cake staring at you from the fridge. To make matters worse, these sorts of refined carbohydrate-heavy foods have almost zero staying power, so in an hour or two you end up feeling ravenous again. Can you guess what might happen next?

When you eat a meal or snack consisting of clean foods, you get full. And because these foods deliver the nutrients that are essential for satiety, you stay that way for a while. Which nutrients will help you make the most of your snacks? Well, let's take a look.

- **Fiber.** The fiber in complex carbohydrates (such as fruits and vegetables, beans, and whole grains) is bulky but can't be digested, which means that it takes up space in your digestive tract and helps you feel fuller on fewer calories. Plus, since fiber takes a while to move through your system, high-fiber foods literally stay in your stomach for longer than low-fiber ones do. (Though high-fiber foods can help slow down your digestion of low-fiber ones, too, when you pair them together. Talk about teamwork!) With all of that in mind, it makes perfect sense that people who eat more fiber tend to be leaner than those who eat less.

- **Protein.** Like fiber-rich foods, foods that are high in protein take longer to digest than foods that consist mainly of refined carbohydrates. What's more, research also suggests that protein may make you more sensitive to fullness hormones that signal to your brain that it's time to stop eating. In fact, one study from the *American*

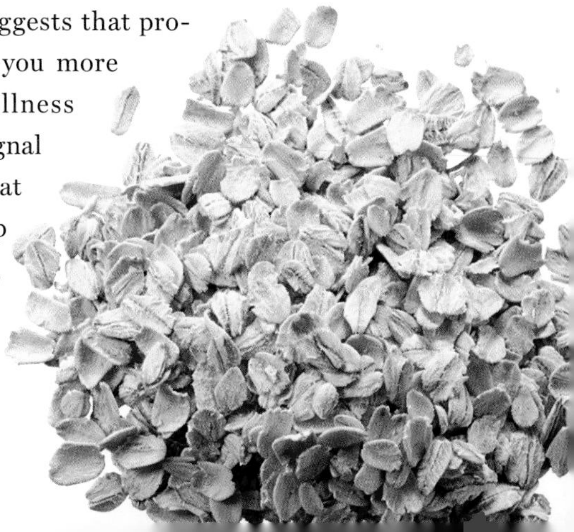

Journal of Clinical Nutrition found that dieters who consumed 30 percent of their calories from protein for 12 weeks ate almost 450 fewer calories per day and lost nearly 11 pounds—without making *any* other changes to their diets.[5]

✽ **Healthy fats.** These delicious foods work a lot like protein to keep you full. They take a while to digest and seem to release hormones that make you feel fuller, faster. Creamy Chicken, Green Grape, and Farro Salad (page 237), anyone?

They Crush Cravings

Ever plucked a single cookie from a box, eaten it, and thought, *I'm so satisfied! I definitely don't want another one of these*? Didn't think so. The refined carbohydrates found in processed foods don't just do a poor job of squashing your hunger. They also cause your blood sugar to spike and quickly come crashing down, which sets you up to crave more junk food. To make matters worse, processed foods are engineered to be addictive to our sugar-, salt-, and fat-loving brains. That's why stopping at just one cookie can be so tough.

Instead of working against your body to make you crave more sugar, clean foods do the opposite. The fact that they allow you to stay fuller for longer helps, but it isn't the only factor at play. By slowing down the rate at which your food is digested, protein, fiber, and healthy fats minimize the blood sugar spikes that send you on a mad hunt for candy bars or cupcakes. In fact, one study published in the *American Journal of Clinical Nutrition* found that women who ate 35 grams of protein at breakfast experienced fewer junk food cravings throughout the day than those who ate 13 grams of protein or no protein at all.[6]

There's more. A growing number of experts are starting to suspect that the bacteria in your gut could also affect your urge to consume poor-quality, sugar-laden foods. According to a review published in the journal *BioEssays*, not having enough diversity in your microbiome—the bacteria population in your gut—could actually drive you to crave sweets and other unhealthy fare.[7] The idea, researchers say, is that only having a few types of bacteria in your belly makes each type more powerful, so the bacteria are better able to organize and send signals to your brain that prompt you to eat the unhealthy foods *they* want. (Weird, right?) But when your gut has a high level of bacterial diversity, no one type of bug is strong enough to exert its sugar-loving influence.

And the best way to make your microbiome more

diverse is by eating clean foods. Processed, sugary fare seems to discourage bacterial variety in your gut. But whole, unprocessed foods, particularly those that are high in probiotic "good" bacteria (such as plain yogurt, raw sauerkraut, kimchi, tempeh, and miso) contribute to more variety. Foods like whole grains, artichokes, asparagus, onions, and bananas are important, too. They're high in prebiotics, a type of fiber that feeds probiotic bacteria to keep them happy and thriving. The vast majority of processed, packaged foods don't contain *either* of these belly boosters, which, of course, is just another reason to eat clean.

They Melt More Fat

The energy from refined, sugary foods floods your system lickety-split, which is why you get that quick boost from nibbling on a handful of pretzels or some candy. The instant jolt can be great if you're, say, actually running a marathon. But most of us tend to snack on junk when we're doing things that don't really call for extra fuel, like working at a desk, watching TV, or driving. Still, your body is nothing if not efficient—and it isn't about to let that precious energy go to waste. Instead, it squirrels the calories away by making fat in case food is hard to come by in the future. This was a genius way to help ensure that our cave people ancestors didn't starve to death. But when's the last time you walked into the grocery store and found that it had completely run out of food?

Of course, it's possible to overeat clean foods and have *those* calories get stored as fat, too. But remember how we said that the fuel from clean foods—which tend to be higher in protein, fiber, and healthy fats—enters your system at a slower, more sustained rate? That even-keeled pace means that you have energy that you can use over the course of several hours. Since the energy from clean foods doesn't bombard your bloodstream all at once, your body doesn't have to sock away the leftovers as fat quite as fast.

Clean foods aren't just less likely to get stored as extra fat, though. They can actually help you burn more of it. Part of that has to do with food's thermogenic impact, or how much extra energy your body uses to digest it. Refined, sugary foods aren't very thermogenic, so your body doesn't have to expend very many calories to turn them into energy. But protein-rich foods require more energy for your body to break them down and use them. Your body has to work a little harder to digest them—and in the process, it burns more calories. Think of it like you're deciding between two routes you can ride your bike on to get to a coffee shop downtown. Both routes are about the same distance, but one of them is completely flat and the other is pretty hilly. On the flat route, pedaling is pretty easy and you can coast a little bit. On the hilly one, you have to push a lot harder. Even though both routes take you to the same place, you'll burn more calories taking the hilly route than the flat one.

But protein isn't the only thing that plays a role in revving your metabolism. Clean foods are full of nutrients that can increase your calorie burn and help you lose weight faster. Citrus fruits, along with vegetables like broccoli and bell peppers, are loaded with vitamin C, which research suggests can help your body metabolize fat faster during exercise.[8] Apples, blueberries, and strawberries are brimming with flavonoids, anti-inflammatory plant compounds that have also been shown to help with weight control.[9] Cruciferous vegetables like kale and broccoli contain a beneficial compound called indole-3-carbinol, which can help fight against obesogenic compounds (more on those later!) that can promote fat storage.[10] Healthy fats like vegetable oils, nuts, and seeds seem to target abdominal fat.[11] Even garlic has been shown to boost calorie burn while simultaneously turning down fat production.[12] Think a slice of processed white bread can do any of that stuff? Sorry, not a chance.

They're Free of Weight-Wrecking Additives

You get it: Clean foods are packed with good stuff that can support your weight loss. But what they *don't* contain might be equally important. At the top of the list? Artificial sweeteners. Sure, they deliver sugary flavor for few to no calories—but that flavor comes at a cost. First, these sweeteners set you up to get used to supersweet

The Winning Starch That Helps You Lose

You've heard a lot about how starchy, sugary foods can thwart your weight loss. But resistant starch is different. It acts more like a fiber than a starch—and since it's indigestible, it delivers fewer calories than other types of carbs. But that's not all. One study recently showed that adding resistant starch to participants' diets increased their fat-burning by more than 20 percent.[13] And in another, it prompted the release of fullness-signaling hormones that resulted in the men consuming 320 fewer calories a day—without actually *trying* to eat less.[14] Thankfully, resistant starch is easy to get when you're eating clean. It occurs naturally in foods like lentils, black beans, kidney beans, green peas, barley, and oats. And you can increase the amount of resistant starch in some carbs—like pasta and potatoes—by letting them cool after you cook them. (Reheat them before you eat them, of course!) You can even swap some resistant-starch–rich flours, like green banana flour and some high-fiber non-GMO corn flours, for some of the refined white flour in baked goods.

Slimming Sips

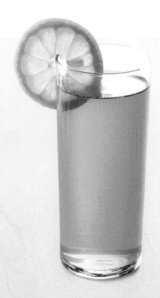

Would you like some coffee or tea? When it comes to losing weight, your answer should be, "Both, please!" The caffeine that occurs naturally in coffee, black tea, and green tea has been shown to dull your appetite,[15] which may help you eat less. (Since herbal "teas" like rooibos and chamomile are naturally caffeine-free, they don't have the hunger-squashing effect.)

Green tea seems to be particularly powerful. Aside from containing a hefty dose of caffeine, it's also rich in epigallocatechin gallate (EGCG), an antioxidant that actually helps your body's fat-burning enzymes and muscle cells work harder, stops new fat cells from forming, and even revs your metabolism. In fact, sipping the stuff regularly was shown to help over-weight men lose nearly a pound and a half in just 6 weeks, according to a study published in the *British Journal of Nutrition*.[16] Both bagged and loose-leaf green tea get the job done, but for the biggest benefit, reach for matcha, a powdered form of green tea. Findings show that you'll get around three times more EGCG, since the powder dissolves in hot water instead of just being steeped, like tea leaves.[17] Add a squirt of fresh lemon juice, and you'll get an even *bigger* boost: Consuming EGCG with something acidic, like citrus, helps your body absorb up to five times more of the fat burner, according to research conducted at Purdue University.[18]

One thing to remember: We're talking about *plain* coffee and tea here—not sugary lattes. A splash of milk or a pinch of a clean sugar (such as raw sugar or honey) is fine if you prefer the taste. But you won't reap any weight-loss benefits by decking out your coffee or tea like an ice cream sundae.

tastes, making it harder to feel satisfied with a food's natural sweetness. Compared to, say, diet soda, a ripe strawberry or crunchy apple tastes almost sour. So you might be more inclined to sprinkle the strawberry with sugar or dunk the apple slices in caramel to achieve the sweetness level you're used to. And consequently, you'll take in more empty calories along the way.

There's more. Our brains evolved to equate sweet tastes with plenty of energizing calories. A diet soda or package of sugar-free cookies still delivers that saccharine flavor, but the calories that your brain is expecting don't come with it. So what happens? You're driven to get the missing energy from somewhere else. In other words, the diet fare you think is helping you take in fewer calories might actually be leading you to take in *more*.

It gets worse, if you can believe it. Artificial sweeteners like aspartame, saccharine, and sucralose seem to mess with your microbiome. Changing the balance of bacteria in your gut can lead to glucose intolerance, where your bloodstream is flooded with more sugar than it can handle and that sugar is more likely to get turned into fat. And you don't have to gorge on the stuff for it to have an effect. Findings published in the journal

Fat-Fighting Foods

Clean foods can help you lose weight, period. But some picks pack an extra powerful punch.
Here's the best stuff to reach for when you want to . . .

Crush Cravings for Salt, Fat, and Sugar

- Apple cider vinegar
- Asparagus
- Avocado
- Barley

- Ground cinnamon
- Coffee
- Eggs
- Kale

- Raw sauerkraut
- Plain Greek yogurt and kefir

Stay Fuller, Longer

- Artichokes
- Chickpeas
- Chile peppers (including crushed red pepper, cayenne, paprika)

- Lentils
- Mushrooms
- Oatmeal
- Pears

- Pine nuts
- Raspberries
- Salmon
- Walnuts

Melt More Fat

- Chile peppers (including crushed red pepper, cayenne, paprika)
- Coconut oil
- Garlic

- Grapefruit
- Sunflower seeds
- Black, green, oolong, or white tea (not herbal tea)

- Boneless, skinless turkey breast
- Plain Greek yogurt

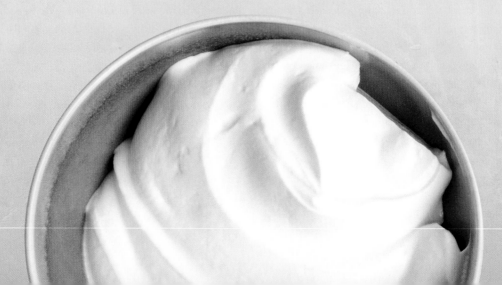

Nature[21] show that eating just an average amount of artificial sweeteners—say, the equivalent of a couple of packets in your coffee—is enough to negatively impact your gut—and, potentially, your weight.

Clean foods aren't just devoid of fattening artificial sweeteners—they're also free of obesogens, a group of toxic chemicals thought to boost fat storage, increase hunger, and slow your metabolism. Yup, these nasties are a triple threat! Many of the compounds used to produce conventional foods—such as artificial hormones and the fungicide triflumizole—seem to trigger the body to store more fat.[22] And animal studies suggest that unnatural additives such as the emulsifiers called polysorbates (often added to jarred mayonnaise and salad dressings) might play a role in throwing your microbiome out of balance and increasing your odds of developing metabolic syndrome.[23]

Even the stuff conventional food is *packaged in* might make it harder to lose weight: The bisphenol A (BPA) and bisphenol S (BPS) found in plastics and canned food linings are endocrine disruptors that promote fat storage and make it harder for your body to build the lean muscle tissue that keeps your metabolism revved. Even perfluorooctanoic acid (PFOA), a chemical used in conventional microwave popcorn bags, appears to be linked to obesity.[24] Who knew that something as simple as a can of chickpeas or your Saturday night movie snack could have such a potentially profound effect on your body? The good news, though, is that you have a choice. By committing to eating clean, you can bypass these questionable ingredients and rest easy knowing that you're picking the best possible foods for your weight and your health.

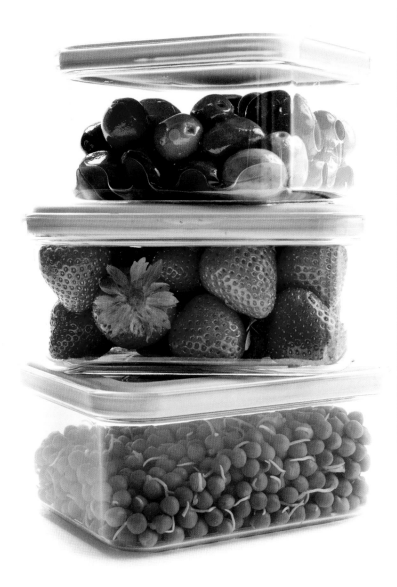

BPA, Begone!

Avoiding BPA altogether might be unrealistic. A whopping 93 percent of us have measurable levels of the stuff in our urine, according to Centers for Disease Control and Prevention (CDC) estimates.[25] But there are plenty of simple ways to drastically downgrade your exposure—and stack the weight-loss cards in your favor. How about . . .

- Buying beans, tomato products, and stocks or broths in BPA-free cans, cartons, or glass jars instead of conventional cans?
- Storing your leftovers in glass containers instead of plastic ones?
- Microwaving food in glass containers or on ceramic plates instead of in plastic containers?
- Using aluminum foil or parchment paper instead of plastic wrap?
- Drinking from a reusable stainless steel water bottle instead of a disposable or reusable plastic one?
- Opting for e-mail receipts instead of paper ones? (Receipt paper is high in BPA.)

Putting It All Together

1 **Eating clean is not a diet.** It's just the way you were designed to eat! It's enjoyable, it makes you feel great, and it's something you can do for life.

2 **Clean foods make losing weight easier.** They keep you feeling full for longer, help fight sugar cravings, and even boast properties that can rev your metabolism and melt more fat.

3 **Clean foods are free of additives that can mess with your weight.** When you choose whole or minimally processed foods, you're automatically steering clear of artificial sweeteners, BPA, and other chemicals that could cause the pounds to pile on.

4 **Remember, portions still matter.** No whole foods or foods made from real ingredients are off-limits. But in order to lose weight, you have to eat less—and commit to eating certain clean foods more often than others.

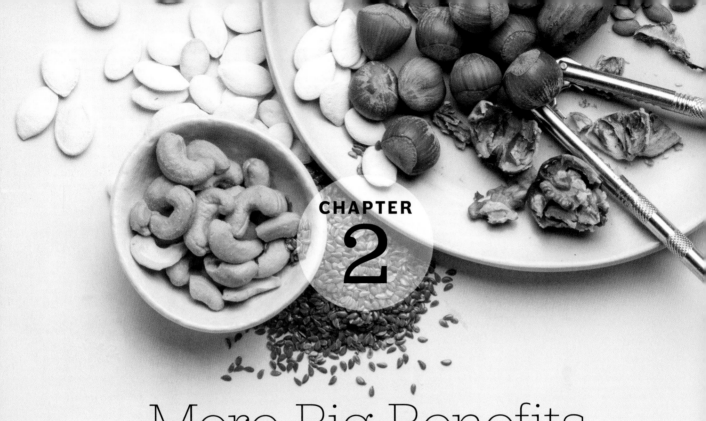

More Big Benefits of Eating Clean

Are you convinced that clean eating is essential for real, sustainable weight loss? Good, because there's a lot more to learn! Clean foods don't just help you lose weight by keeping you full, crushing your cravings, and delivering key nutrients that keep your metabolism running like a well-oiled machine. They can also give you more energy, slash your stress, boost your mood, and help you sleep better. And believe it or not, *all* of these things can significantly impact the number you see on the scale.

Food for Total Wellness

Let's take a minute to check in and see how you're feeling while you read this. Are you wide awake or kind of tired? Relaxed or tense? Content or cranky? No matter your answers, chances are they have a lot to do with whatever you've eaten today. Enjoyed a bowl of oatmeal with chopped nuts and fresh fruit? You might be bright-eyed, bushy-tailed, and ready to tackle whatever comes your way. Went for the giant cinnamon bun instead? Exhausted and frazzled may be your mood *du jour*.

You know that old phrase "You are what you eat"? It's usually used to make the point that you'll have a healthy, lean body if you eat mostly healthy foods and a not-so-healthy, not-so-lean body if you eat mostly unhealthy ones. But the foods that make up the majority of your diet can also help determine your mood, stress level, and overall sense of well-being. In other words, your food affects your external, internal, *and* emotional health.

Physically, you *are* what you eat. But in a way, you also *feel* what you eat. And when you feel good, you're more motivated to make smart choices that support your health and weight loss, like taking the time to cook a clean meal instead of ordering pizza, or heading outside for a walk instead of binge watching your favorite TV show all night. Sure, those might sound like small choices that don't matter much in the grand scheme of things. But it's the little decisions like these that, over time, form the healthy (or not-so-healthy) habits that end up determining your weight.

Of course, no one's saying you have to be perfect. We all have those occasional days where there's zero time to cook dinner and the mere thought of working out is too exhausting to contemplate. As long as those days are the exception instead of the rule, you don't need to worry. Your goal is to focus on making choices that foster wellness—and healthy weight loss—*most* of the time. One of the most effective ways to do that? You guessed it. It's by eating clean.

Notes from a Clean Eater

"I have more energy, less stress, and I'm happy that I'm doing something for *myself*. I'm definitely going to continue eating clean because now I know I can do this."—**Maryann L.**

Eating for Energy

Once you have the right tools (like this book!), you'll find that the principles behind losing weight and keeping it off are pretty simple. But putting them into practice *does* take more effort than you'd expend hanging out on the couch and ordering takeout. You don't have to spend hours in the kitchen, but you do need to devote some time to thinking about what you'll eat, shopping for your ingredients, and prepping clean meals and healthy snacks. You don't have to train to become a marathon runner, but you do need to find ways to move more.

All of that stuff requires energy. And if you're used to eating the standard American diet, you might not feel like you have all that much of it to spare. When it comes to the nutrients that keep your body fueled and your mind focused, processed foods are a veritable wasteland. To make matters worse, they're brimming with the sugar and refined carbs that practically guarantee exhaustion and brain drain. Skeptical? Try subsisting on sugary granola bars for a day or two and see how you feel. Or take science's word for it: Sugar actually inhibits neurons in your brain that promote feelings of wakefulness, according to British findings published in the journal *Neuron*.[1] No wonder that afternoon candy bar always ends up leaving you feeling even fuzzier than you did before you peeled back the wrapper.

With clean foods, it's just the opposite. Fiber-rich complex carbohydrates and lean proteins get digested more slowly than their processed, refined counterparts, so you

Your Get-Energized Rx

Need a boost? Certain nutrients play particularly important roles in staving off sluggishness. Pay attention to these three biggies to increase your focus and fight fatigue.

IRON

Why it matters: Your red blood cells need this mineral to transport oxygen throughout your body, and when you don't get enough, you can end up feeling foggy, weak, and even out of breath.
Aim to get: 18 mg daily for women under age 50, 8 g daily for men and women over age 50
Find it in: Oysters, lean beef, sardines, non-GMO soybeans and tofu, lentils, beans (kidney, lima, black, and pinto), clams, and spinach

MAGNESIUM

Why it matters: Your body relies on magnesium to convert food into energy, as well as for proper muscle function. Fall short, and even basic activities like carrying a bag of groceries can feel harder.
Aim to get: 320 mg daily for women, 420 mg daily for men
Find it in: Halibut; almonds, cashews, and other nuts; peanuts; black beans; spinach; avocado; milk; whole grains; and dark chocolate

VITAMIN B$_{12}$

Why it matters: Vitamin B$_{12}$ plays a role in building the red blood cells that transport oxygen throughout your body, and too little will leave you weak and foggy-headed. Since the vast majority of plant foods don't naturally contain B$_{12}$, vegetarians and vegans should take extra care to meet their needs. Look for fortified foods or consider taking a supplement.
Aim to get: 2.4 mcg daily for women and men
Find it in: Clams, fatty fish, canned light tuna, lean beef, dairy foods, eggs, nutritional yeast, fortified nondairy milks, and fortified cereals

stay revved for longer and don't end up crashing. And whole foods are rich in important nutrients like magnesium, iron, and vitamin B_{12}, all of which are essential for helping you feel energized. The bottom line? When you eat clean, you have more *oomph* to tackle your day—and to put in the work needed to meet your weight-loss goals.

(Real) Happy Meals

There's no doubt that an ice cream cone or a plate of freshly baked chocolate chip cookies will put a smile on your face. But that kind of happiness, while worthwhile, is only temporary. If you were in a crummy mood before you treated yourself to a scoop of rocky road, chances are you'll go back to feeling rocky yourself after the last lick. But sometimes, that can be tough to remember—since in the moment that you're eating it, junk food can make you feel pretty awesome. That's because loading up on sugar or refined carbs activates the reward system in your brain, prompting it to pump out megadoses of the pleasure hormone dopamine. Dopamine, FYI, is the same hormone that your brain releases in response to highly addictive drugs like cocaine.[2] Yikes.

Of course, all good things have to end sooner or later. The problem with pounding back the junk food is that once you stop, the dopamine release shuts down. You're left wondering why the party ended—and craving more junk to get the good times going again. It might've taken a brain scientist to understand exactly how the process works, but it doesn't take one to figure out that that sort of habit could end up leaving you pretty moody—not to mention on a constant hunt for your next sugar fix.

Clean foods are free of the added sugars and refined carbs that send your dopamine levels into overdrive. But that doesn't mean that they can't make you happy, too! By delivering a steady source of energy and keeping you off the emotional roller coaster, clean foods work to keep your mood nice and even. Sure, the highs might not be as extreme as the highs that come from eating sugary, processed foods, but the lows won't be as low, either. What's more, research suggests that eating clean can actually lead to greater happiness overall. One Australian study of nearly 14,000 people found that those who ate nine or more daily servings (about 6 cups or more) of fruits and vegetables reported feeling more satisfied with their lives compared to those who consumed less.[3] People also report feeling calmer, happier, and more energetic on days when they eat fruits and vegetables, according to findings published in the *British Journal of Health Psychology*.[4] It all sounds pretty nice, right?

Notes from a Clean Eater

"Before I would get my period, I'd have bad PMS. I don't have that now. No mood swings, nothing. I'm going to keep eating clean. It's a no-brainer."—**Gigi D.**

Clean Eater

Gigi D.

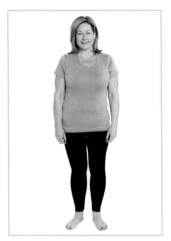

BEFORE

Want proof that eating clean can lead to amazing changes? Just look at **Gigi**. After Gigi had been eating clean for several weeks, a friend called her up at 6:30 in the morning to invite her on a 17-mile bike ride. Feeling energetic, Gigi decided to go. "Before that, the last time I [rode a bike], I was 10 years old! And it was *not* for 17 miles. So that was huge," she beams.

Huge, indeed. Gigi had been taking steps to eat better for about 9 months before fully committing to eating clean. She started getting serious about eating as much organic food as possible. She only had wine or sugar once in a while. She even made sure to bring clean food to social events like holidays and birthday parties so she always had something delicious to eat.

"I really was very careful with what I ate," she says. But for Gigi, going from pretty clean to squeaky clean was exactly what she needed. The sugar cravings that used to plague her at night disappeared. Her mind felt clearer. And her moods were consistently positive instead of up and down, as they had often been before.

What's more, she's sticking with her new habits. "If you want to be healthy, this is how you should be eating," she says. "It's really not a program, it's not a diet. It's a way of life."

Dr. Wendy Observes: Surprising things can happen when you start eating clean! Your mood shifts and you just might turn back the hands of time to tap some youthful energy you didn't realize you had. Small shifts paid off for Gigi in ways that she didn't expect. Sure, she lost weight and inches, which was great. But to engage life with a more positive, vibrant outlook? That's a reward worth seeking!

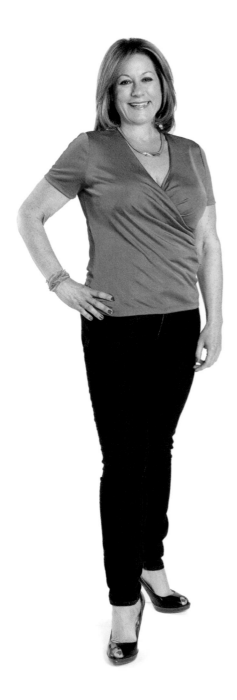

TOTAL POUNDS LOST

7.5 lbs

TOTAL INCHES LOST

6.5

MOST NOTABLE IMPROVEMENTS

Eating clean gave **Gigi** a major energy boost. Her moods were more even-keeled, too, even before her period, when she would usually deal with mood swings.

Big-Time Stress Busters

You know that tense, frazzled feeling that makes you want to run straight for something comforting, like a frosted doughnut or a gooey, melty bowl of mac and cheese? Of course you do. Scarfing down junk is a pretty normal response to feeling anxious or stressed—and at some point or another, we've all done it. But it won't help you relax for long, and it definitely won't help you lose weight!

Eating clean can actually help keep stress—and the snack-crazy urges that often come with it—at bay. When you eat foods that aren't packed with refined sugars and carbs, you avoid the extreme blood sugar spikes and dips that can leave you feeling moody, irritable, and ready to reach for the cookie jar. In fact, research shows that eating a diet based on whole, unprocessed foods is associated with lower risks for both anxiety and depression, while sticking to a Western-style diet of processed or fried foods, refined grains, and excess sugar is linked to higher risks for both conditions.[5]

That's important, because once you get tangled up in the vicious cycle of sugar and stress, it can be tough to find your way out. Say you're at the corner deli, planning to get a turkey-and-veggie sandwich on whole wheat with a side salad for lunch. As you're waiting in line, you get an e-mail from your boss asking if you can send over that report by the end of the day instead of by the end of the week. You immediately feel frenzied and start eyeing the pastrami sandwich and side of creamy coleslaw that the guy in front of you just ordered. Because stress makes it harder to exert self-control—even when you *want* to make healthy choices—you cave and copy his order. You'll get that more nutritious combo you had actually planned on tomorrow.

As you're inhaling your meal, your boss sends *another* e-mail asking you for a status update, ASAP. Now you're in full-on anxiety overload. Your body's levels of the stress hormone cortisol start surging, which sends your body right toward storing fat. If that's not bad enough,

Do This Now!

Why not start harnessing the feel-good powers of fruits and vegetables right now? Think about how you can ramp up the produce in each of your meals and snacks for the rest of the day—and reap the benefits of happier, more even moods. (Or do it tomorrow, if you're reading this before bed.) How about a banana instead of cookies with lunch? The carbohydrates will boost your brain's production of the feel-good hormone serotonin while the fiber promotes a steady, even mood. What about some nuts at snack time, or sprinkled on top of a salad? Almonds, cashews, and peanuts are top sources of magnesium, which promotes feelings of calm. Can you do a juicy orange or some crunchy broccoli florets with your dinner? Both are rich in folate, a vitamin that's linked to lower rates of depression.

If losing weight feels like one *more* thing to worry about, try shifting your perspective a little bit: While stress is inevitable, you have in your possession one simple tool that's proven to help you feel less frazzled—and that's eating clean. **Eating real, balanced meals on a regular schedule keeps your blood sugar steady so you stay focused and energized.** Plus, planning clean meals and snacks in advance saves you time—not to mention the anxiety of scrambling to figure out what's for dinner every night. So close your eyes and take a few deep breaths. (Really—try it now!) Don't you feel better already?

all of that unspent cortisol leaves you feeling ravenous and desperate for anything made with sugar and white flour. So you grab a giant chocolate chip cookie before running back to the office, thinking it will calm your nerves and help you plow through the crazy amount of work you now have to take care of.

At the end of what turns out to be an insanely long day, you finally hand in the finished report. Exhausted, you pick up a container of greasy stir-fry for dinner. Thanks to who-knows-how-much sugar in the stir-fry sauce and a mountain of white rice, your energy crashes half an hour after dinner and you fall asleep without even putting on your pj's. In the morning, you wake up totally frazzled, so you grab a sugary blueberry muffin at the coffee shop. So starts another day.

For many of us, these sorts of scenarios happen all the time. And of course, no one's saying that eating quinoa and salmon can stop stressful situations from happening. But picking clean foods over processed ones *can* help your moods stay more even. That way, when life throws you the inevitable curveball, you can remain (somewhat) calmer—instead of flying off the handle and reaching for the candy bowl.

Notes from a Clean Eater

"I think sugar was causing me to be short-tempered or easily frustrated. Little things would irritate me completely. Eating clean really changed that."—**Alan F.**

Sounder Sleep

Nearly half of all Americans say that they regularly struggle to get enough quality sleep.[6] If you're one of them, listen up: You might not realize it, but the way you eat has a major impact on how much—and how well—you snooze. And the better rested you are, the easier it is to reach or maintain a healthy weight. Want proof? When Harvard researchers followed some 60,000 women for nearly 2 decades, those who regularly slept for fewer

Stress-Fighting Snack Swaps

Feel a case of the crazies coming on? Resist the urge to nix those nerves with an empty-calorie snack, and try one of these clean, calming picks instead.

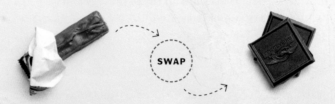

A CANDY BAR FOR I OUNCE OF DARK CHOCOLATE

Findings suggest that the flavonoids in dark chocolate could keep levels of the stress hormone cortisol from spiking during tense times,[7] while cocoa may help lower your blood pressure.[8] For the most phytonutrients and the least amount of added sugar, stick with dark chocolate that's at least 80 percent cacao.

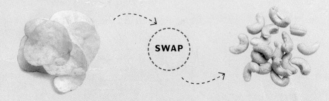

POTATO CHIPS FOR ¼ CUP OF ROASTED, SALTED CASHEWS

Both are rich, salty snacks. But cashews pack the mineral selenium and the amino acid tryptophan, both of which can elevate your mood. (As for potato chips, we don't need to remind you that they're practically devoid of nutrition, right?)

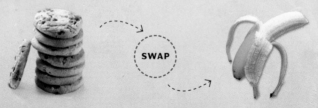

COOKIES FOR A MEDIUM BANANA

An all-carbohydrate snack ramps up your brain's production of the feel-good hormone serotonin within minutes of consumption, so you start to feel calmer—stat. And sure, cookies are loaded with carbs, but they don't offer much else. Eat a medium banana, instead, and you'll get the same chill-out benefits, plus fiber (to slow digestion and keep you happy longer) and loads of potassium.

than 5 hours per night were 32 percent more likely to gain 30 or more pounds compared to those who regularly slept for 7 or more hours.[9] Yup, when it comes to getting lean, sleep is *that* important.

Even so, the relationship between sleep and weight is complicated, and experts still have a lot to learn about how the two are connected. What does seem to be clear, though, is that a steady stream of highly processed, inferior food can make it harder to get the quality sleep you need. Research published in the *Journal of Clinical Sleep Medicine* found that people who eat diets high in sugar and refined carbs tend to take longer to fall asleep and wake up more frequently during the night.[10] Meanwhile, unhealthy fats could negatively affect the body's normal sleep–wake cycle, making it harder to doze off at night and wake up refreshed in the morning.

In part, that's because staying up later can seriously impact your ability to make choices that can help you get leaner. When you're zonked, you simply have less energy for things like shopping for fresh food, preparing clean meals, or even exercising. To make matters worse, running short on shut-eye actually makes it harder to resist junky snacks. In fact, one *SLEEP* study found that sleep deprivation actually cranks up the pleasurable effects of salty, sugary, and fatty foods by amplifying the body's endocannabinoid system—yes, the same one that responds to marijuana.[11] And to top it all off, when you don't get enough sleep, your body actually prompts you to eat *more* calories and burn *fewer* of them. If that's not an ugly recipe for spending countless unproductive hours zoned out on Netflix and sugary snacks, nothing is.

There's more to it, though. Eating clean doesn't just

(continued on page 32)

Dr. Wendy Says . . .

Ready to stop counting sheep? Pick an evening snack that actually helps you drift off to dreamland sooner, like one of these. Enjoy it 2 to 3 hours before going to sleep, since eating too close to bedtime can disrupt your sleep.

✤ **4 whole grain crackers topped with 1/4 cup of cottage cheese.** Cottage cheese is rich in protein, which your body needs to make the sleep-promoting amino acid tryptophan. And crackers have carbohydrates, which boost tryptophan's availability to your brain.

✤ **8 ounces of tart cherry juice.** Tart cherries are a top source of melatonin, the hormone responsible for regulating your sleep–wake cycle. Plus, research shows that tart Montmorency cherries can help people with insomnia sleep longer—and better.[12]

✤ **10 walnut halves.** Like tart cherries, walnuts contain melatonin—and eating them has been shown to increase levels of the hormone in your blood, according to a study in *Nutrition*.[13]

✤ **Half a slice of whole grain toast with 1 tablespoon of almond butter.** Both deliver magnesium, which can offer protection against sleep-disrupting leg cramps and insomnia.

✤ **8 ounces of low-fat milk.** Many of us struggle with getting enough calcium and vitamin D, but both can reduce the odds of having trouble falling asleep and staying asleep. Milk is one of the few foods that serves up *both*.

✤ **A cup of chamomile tea.** This naturally sweet herbal sipper has long been used to promote feelings of calm and relaxation. Plus, it's calorie-free, so no worries. It can help you doze off even if you've already reached your snack limit for the day.

Clean Eater

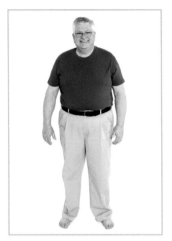

BEFORE

Sixty-four-year-old **Alan** had known for a while that he needed to lose weight. But getting motivated to do so wasn't easy. "My kids had been on me about it for a couple of years," he says. "Before this chance came along, I had decided that I was never going to change. I convinced myself that I was just going to be this way until I had a heart attack or something."

His decision to make a change couldn't have come at a better time. Three weeks into eating clean, Alan was diagnosed with prostate cancer. His doctors said his prognosis was good, but they also told him that losing weight could only help his health—and help him tolerate his treatments better. "I was glad that I had already started cleaning up what I was eating before I started the treatments," he remarks.

There were other benefits, too. Food had always been a way for Alan to deal with his feelings. As he started eating clean, he realized that the best way to avoid emotional eating was to simply be honest with himself. One time, driving home after treatment, he wanted to use a coupon to get a free coffee from a doughnut shop. In the past, he would've rewarded himself by buying a couple of doughnuts, as well. "But I didn't do that," he says. "I just figured, you're on this plan. And you're actually staying on this plan."

At the same time, Alan found that eating clean actually helped his moods stay steadier. At work, sugary snacks would give him a short-lived energy boost, only to leave him tired and irritated. "Being on the plan really changed that. I haven't felt the stress that I was feeling before," he gladly reports.

As he continues treatment, Alan's doctors say there's a great chance that he'll beat his cancer. In the meantime, he's working on losing another 26 pounds to reach his goal weight and is making continued progress.

Dr. Wendy Observes: By some estimates, we face nearly 200 food choices a day. Add life stresses into the mix, and it's absolutely no surprise that we fall into food traps guided by our emotions rather than our stomachs. That was what Alan did, until he started eating clean. That's when he realized that he was in charge of his choices—and that small decisions, like passing on the doughnut while still enjoying the coffee, add up to measurable progress. By taking those steps, Alan put himself well on his way, and now he's taking charge of his health instead of letting it happen to him. And his progress and prognosis are good!

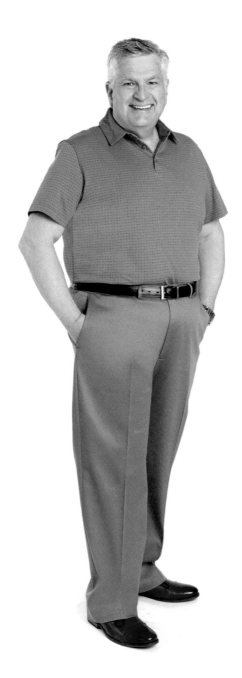

TOTAL POUNDS LOST

15 lbs

TOTAL INCHES LOST

7.75

MOST NOTABLE IMPROVEMENTS

Alan's cholesterol decreased by 57 points, moving from the high to the healthy range. His energy levels went up, and his stress levels went down.

Sleep Your Way Slim

Getting enough sleep doesn't just promote the kind of clearheaded thinking that helps you pick salmon over a bacon double cheeseburger or a handful of nuts instead of a handful of candy. Adequate sleep actually appears to play a role in keeping your metabolism humming along at a healthy rate, so you burn more calories. When University of Pennsylvania researchers tracked the metabolic rates of unlucky subjects who were limited to just 4 hours of sleep for 5 nights, they found that the subjects burned about 42 fewer calories per day than they did when they weren't sleep-deprived.[14] At that rate, a week of poor sleep could cause you to burn nearly 300 fewer calories—the equivalent of a breakfast of a creamy bowl of oatmeal with nuts and fruit. That's right! You can actually earn more calories just by making it a point to get more snooze time. Next time you're tempted to stay up and watch another hour of TV, remember your get-lean goal—and hit the hay.

pull you out of the cycle of eating junk food, sleeping poorly, and then eating more junk food because you're sleep-deprived. Clean foods actually deliver the nutrients your body needs to sleep *better*. Research shows that people with adequate levels of vitamin D—found in foods like eggs, mushrooms, fortified milk, and fatty fish—are 33 percent less likely to experience insomnia than those with insufficient levels of this nutrient.[15] And speaking of fatty fish, some findings suggest that the omega-3 fatty acids found in fish like tuna and salmon can actually contribute to a better night's rest.[16] (So far, the research has been conducted on kids, but it's likely that adults would reap similar benefits.)[17] Your body relies on potassium (found in foods like sweet potatoes and bananas) and magnesium (found in foods like avocados, nuts, and seeds) to help your muscles relax so you can drift off to dreamland sooner. And it needs the calcium in foods like plain yogurt and leafy greens in order to produce the hormone melatonin, which tells your body when it's time to feel sleepy. (A few foods, including tart cherries and walnuts, actually *contain* melatonin.) With all of that in mind, it might not come as much of a surprise to learn that people who eat diets high in fiber-rich foods, like many of those just mentioned, report getting deeper, more restful sleep than their processed-food-eating counterparts.[18]

Big Beauty Benefits

You know those days when you wake up in the morning and something just feels off? Maybe your skin is starting to break out, or your hair seems dull and lifeless. Or you feel weirdly bloated, and the jeans that always look good suddenly *don't*. Deep down, you know this kind of stuff is small and short-lived and that you shouldn't let it bother you. But often, it still does. So you head out the door feeling sort of down about yourself—and those negative feelings start to affect the decisions you make throughout the day. You're already feeling a little yucky, so why bother exercising or making healthy food choices?

When you make clean foods the mainstays of your diet, you're getting more of the important nutrients that can help you look your best—think clearer, more radiant skin; bouncier, shinier hair; and even a flatter, bloat-free belly. The sugar, refined carbs, and sodium abundant in processed foods can actually ramp up sebum production and promote breakouts, not to mention that it can cause water retention that can leave you feeling puffy. Overdoing it on the sweet stuff could be particularly bad because too much sugar can actually make your skin duller and more wrinkled. That's thanks to a process called glycation, where the sugar in your bloodstream attaches to proteins to form harmful new products called advanced glycation end products (or—appropriately—AGEs, for short). AGEs do damage to collagen and elastin, the protein fibers that keep skin firm and elastic. And the more sugar you eat, the more AGEs develop.

Eating clean can help fight *all* of this stuff. Fruits and vegetables pack powerful phytonutrients that actually keep sugar from attaching to proteins, helping your skin stay smooth and supple instead of turning tired or lifeless. Whole foods boost your beauty in other big ways, too. Fresh produce, whole grains, and nuts are all brimming with beta-carotene, iron, zinc, vitamin C, and B vitamins that can strengthen your hair follicles. Yogurt, raw sauerkraut, artichokes, and onions deliver probiotics and prebiotics that help promote good digestion and keep uncomfortable bloating at bay. And animal findings suggest that the good bacteria play a role in protecting skin against the sun's harmful UV rays[19]— and even stimulate the growth of healthier, shinier hair.[20]

In other words, clean foods are beautifying foods that can help jump-start a sort of feel-good feedback loop. When you're already happy with what you see when you look in the mirror, you're more likely to feel motivated to do *more* of the good-for-you things that can help you lose weight.

4.6 YEARS

Drinking 20 ounces of sugary soda a day can age cells by *this* much—or the same amount as being a regular smoker, according to findings from the *American Journal of Public Health.*[21]

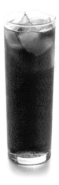

Flat-Belly Food Swaps

That yucky, puffy feeling that comes from overindulging? It can sometimes play weird mind games that can drive you to eat *more* junk. For a flatter belly that leaves you feeling good instead of bloated, swap bloat-causing snacks for these clean picks.

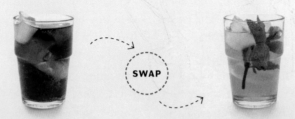

DIET SODA FOR UNSWEETENED ICED TEA WITH FRESH PEPPERMINT

The carbonation from the bubbles can get trapped in your belly and cause bloating. Iced tea is free of fizz (not to mention unhealthy artificial sweeteners), while peppermint leaves add fresh flavor and enhance your digestion.

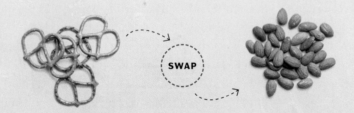

POTATO CHIPS OR PRETZELS FOR ¼ CUP OF UNSALTED ALMONDS OR WALNUTS

The sodium and refined carbs in salty snacks can cause water retention and puffiness. Unsalted nuts are free of both offending ingredients, but they still pack the same satisfying crunch.

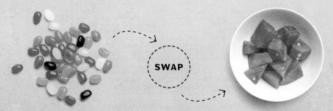

CANDY OR COOKIES FOR A BANANA OR 2 CUPS OF WATERMELON

The sky-high amounts of sugar in sweet snacks can be tough on your digestive system and can lead to gassiness. Bananas and watermelon still deliver a sweet flavor, but for way less sugar. They're also good sources of potassium, which can help fight water retention caused by eating too much sodium.

Yes, you can eat your way to lovelier skin! For a radiant, more healthful complexion, make an effort to work more of these into your meals and snacks.

For a radiant glow: Carrots, sweet potatoes, pumpkin, and butternut squash

Orange fruits and vegetables get their bright hue from the antioxidant beta-carotene. And when you eat them, findings show that they can quite literally give dull, sallow complexions a brighter, sun-kissed appearance—minus the UV-ray exposure.[22]

For younger-looking skin: Avocados, walnuts, flaxseeds, and chia seeds

The monounsaturated fats in avocado and omega-3 fatty acids in walnuts, flaxseeds, and chia seeds play an important role in helping your skin stay hydrated. As a result, skin looks smoother and more supple, and it shows fewer fine lines. Monounsaturated fats, too, are essential for the creation of healthy skin cells.

For extra sun protection: Coffee, green tea, grapes, tomatoes, and ginger

At first glance, these foods and drinks might not have much in common. But *all*

of them deliver dermis-friendly phytonutrients that can both help protect against future and fight existing damage and inflammation caused by the sun's UV rays. (They won't replace your sunscreen, though, so keep applying it daily!)

For healthy, nourished skin overall: Kiwifruit, strawberries, blueberries, and oranges

All of these are rich in vitamin C, an essential nutrient that speeds wound healing, prevents easy bruising, and staves off dryness. It also aids in the production of the protein collagen, which helps skin stay firm and elastic.

Putting It All Together

1 **Remember that food affects how you feel, so eat to feel good.** Clean meals and snacks boost your mood and energy levels, helping you stay revved to make more smart choices.

2 **Sleep well and stay calm to burn on.** Find ways to unwind and cope with stress, and prioritize getting 7 to 8 hours of shut-eye each night. Stress and sleep deprivation can wreak havoc on your metabolism and make you crave sugary, processed foods.

3 **Harness clean food's beauty-boosting effects.** From clearer skin to a flatter belly, the right foods can help you love the way you look *now*—which can motivate you to stay the clean-eating course.

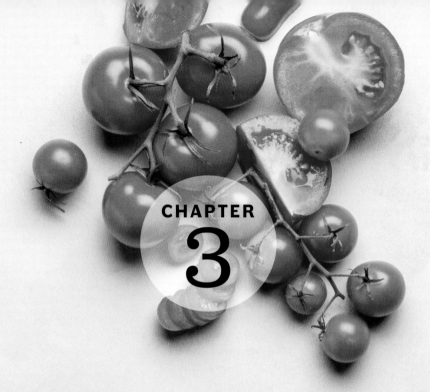

CHAPTER 3

Finding Clean Fare

Okay, *you get it!* If you really want to get serious about losing weight and keeping it off for good, living the clean-eating lifestyle is absolutely, positively, 1,000 percent the best way to go. So what exactly counts as a clean food, and what definitely doesn't? More importantly, how the heck can you find these foods—especially when there are so many sneaky imposters lining the supermarket shelves? If it all sounds like a lot to figure out, don't worry. By the end of this chapter, you'll be on your way to becoming a pro.

Clean Foods 101

Head into any local megamart, and you'll be bombarded by a dazzling array of foods that tout themselves as healthy, natural, or even capable of helping you lose weight. But what *actually* counts as clean food, and which ones will work the hardest to help you slim down? Thankfully, the answer is much more straightforward than you might think. Follow these principles, and you'll be eating a truly clean diet—and getting leaner—in no time.

Load Up on Fresh Produce

This likely isn't the first time you've been told that it's important to eat plenty of fruits and vegetables. But it's worth repeating, because fresh produce is the foundation of a clean diet. From apples to zucchini (and everything in between), fruits and vegetables are loaded with the vitamins, minerals, and phytonutrients that your body needs to function at full capacity and help you feel your best. And because produce tends to be low in calories and high in fiber, it plays an essential role in helping you lose weight while still feeling satisfied.

Opt for Organic

Organic produce, by definition, is grown without synthetic, industrial fertilizers or pesticides. That's a big deal, since billions of pounds of agricultural chemicals are sprayed on our crops each year. And believe it or not, most of these chemicals haven't gone through extensive testing to ensure that they're safe. Seems a little bizarre, right?

When you choose organic, you know that the fruits and vegetables you're getting are truly clean. That's because organic produce:

❊ Can only be grown on land that's been free of fertilizers and pesticides for at least 3 years.

❊ Can't be irradiated to kill bacteria.

❊ Can't be fertilized with sewage sludge (in other words, treated human waste).

❊ Can't be grown from genetically modified seeds.

Since many of the chemicals used to produce conventional food haven't been thoroughly vetted, it's tough to know for sure just *how* harmful they really are. But why take a chance? Research has already linked synthetic pesticides and fertilizers to annoying effects, such as headaches and nausea, as well as more serious issues, including cancer and reproductive problems. And some findings suggest that they could even be messing with the number you see on the scale.

But opting for organic isn't just about avoiding the

bad stuff—it's also about getting more of the good stuff. For a while, experts believed that organic produce packed the same nutritional punch as conventional. But more recently, a review of 343 studies published in the *British Journal of Nutrition* found that organically grown fruits and vegetables contain an average of 17 percent more polyphenolic antioxidants than their conventional counterparts.[1] Organic crops, experts think, probably get a boost from being grown in nutrient-rich soil that hasn't been sucked dry by years of exposure to chemical pesticides and fertilizers.

Basically, choosing organic can help you fuel your body with more of the nutrients it needs—which is key to losing weight and feeling your best. (We'll get to that in much more detail later.) Still, that doesn't necessarily mean that you need to go organic 100 percent of the time. Eating fruits and vegetables in abundance—even conventionally grown ones—delivers serious benefits for your health and your waistline. So go organic when you can, but when you can't, don't let that stop you from enjoying as much fresh produce as possible.

Where Organic Matters *Most*

Choosing organic meat, eggs, and dairy might be even more important than choosing organic fruits and vegetables. Of course, conventionally raised cows and chickens aren't getting sprayed with chemical-laden pesticides or fertilizers. But their food—which consists mostly of corn, soybeans, and grains—still is. So when you have a drum-

stick, a glass of milk, or a steak, *you* end up being subjected to the impact of that feed. Many conventional farmers also pump their cattle full of sex and growth hormones to increase meat and milk production, and some of these hormones are passed on to you. That's scary stuff, since the growth hormones rBHG and rBST are linked to

The 12 Best Fruits and Vegetables for Weight Loss

Eating more of practically *all* types of fruits and vegetables can help you slim down. But according to a recent *PLoS Medicine* study[2] that followed some 130,000 men and women for more than 2 decades, these picks seem to pack the biggest punch.

- Apples
- Berries
- Broccoli
- Brussels sprouts
- Cabbage
- Cauliflower
- Kale
- Mustard greens
- Pears
- Romaine lettuce
- Spinach
- Swiss chard

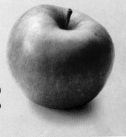

What makes these guys so great? According to researchers, they tend to be especially high in belly-filling fiber—so you stay fuller, longer. They also have a low glycemic load, which can help prevent blood sugar spikes that can cause cravings for sugary fare.

Who's Dirty, Who's Clean?

Different fruits and vegetables contain different levels of pesticide residues (even after being washed), so it makes sense to go organic when buying the worst offenders. The Environmental Working Group's "Dirty Dozen" list reveals which types of produce have the highest pesticide residues and are therefore the most important to buy organic when possible. Their "Clean Fifteen" list shows the produce with the lowest pesticide residues, which are therefore okay to buy conventional.

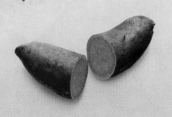

The Dirty Dozen Plus

1. Apples
2. Peaches
3. Nectarines
4. Strawberries
5. Grapes
6. Celery
7. Spinach
8. Sweet bell peppers
9. Cucumbers
10. Cherry tomatoes
11. Snap peas (imported)
12. Potatoes
13. Hot peppers
14. Kale/collard greens

The Clean Fifteen

1. Avocados
2. Sweet corn
3. Pineapple
4. Cabbage
5. Sweet peas (frozen)
6. Onions
7. Asparagus
8. Mangoes
9. Papaya
10. Kiwifruit
11. Eggplant
12. Grapefruit
13. Cantaloupe
14. Cauliflower
15. Sweet potatoes

an increased risk for breast and prostate cancers.

Evidence also suggests that all that added junk could affect your weight. One animal study from New York University found that mice who were given high doses of antibiotics had lower numbers of T-cells, which is associated with obesity.[3] And some experts suspect that the steroid hormones given to meat and dairy cattle could also be contributing to the obesity epidemic. While the FDA maintains that these hormones don't pose a threat to human health, it's worth thinking about: If steroids can make cows and steers get bigger, why wouldn't they have the same effect on the people who eat them?

Dr. Wendy Says . . .

Remember: A produce-rich diet is essential for losing weight and optimizing your health—whether that produce is organic or not. It's great to choose organic when you can. But when the organic option isn't possible, never let that stop you from eating an abundance of fruits and vegetables.

Pick Clean and Lean Proteins

When it comes to losing weight, protein is pretty darn important. First, it forces your body to work harder and burn more calories during digestion, since high-protein foods are tougher to digest than ones that are mostly carbohydrates or fat. These foods take more time to digest, too—which means that protein-packed meals can help you stay satisfied for longer. Most importantly, protein-rich fare supports healthy muscle tissue, which burns more calories than fat does. Add it all up, and it's easy to see why lean sources of protein—such as poultry, fish, eggs, dairy, beans, and moderate amounts of lean meats—are essential for getting lean.

Remember Plant Proteins

Protein doesn't only have to come from meat, dairy, and eggs. In fact, plant-based sources like beans and legumes, nuts and seeds, whole soy foods, and more deliver plenty of the muscle-builder, too—along with a side of belly-filling fiber and powerful antioxidants. Plus, people who eat a plant-heavy diet tend to weigh less than major meat eaters. Some important things to keep in mind:

- **Pick whole or minimally processed soy.** Edamame, tempeh (a fermented soybean cake), miso, and tofu are delicious, inexpensive sources of clean protein. Stuff like veggie "meats" or soy protein isolate are highly processed, so steer clear.
- **Don't worry about making "complete" proteins at a single meal.** You might have heard that you have to combine different plant foods to form a complete protein, such as beans and rice or whole grain bread and peanut butter. But as long as you're eating a variety of plant foods throughout the day, you don't need to worry about pairing different protein sources at the same meal. So much simpler, right?
- **Remember whole grains.** Yes, they're carbohydrates. But whole grains like spelt, kamut, teff, amaranth, sorghum, and quinoa also pack more than 8 grams of protein per cup.

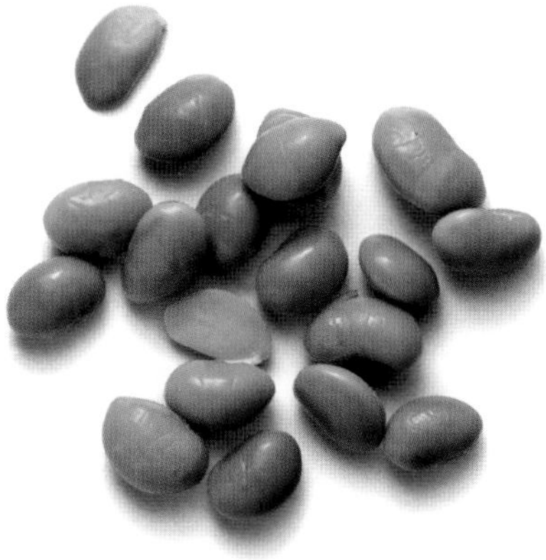

Protein Power!

Which plant foods pack the most fat-melting, muscle-building protein?
Glad you asked! Make these picks a regular part of your diet, and reap their get-lean benefits.

PLANT	PROTEIN PER COOKED SERVING (EXCEPT NUTS AND SEEDS)
Organic, non-GMO edamame	17 g per 1 cup
Organic, non-GMO tempeh	15 g per 3 ounces
Lentils	9 g per ½ cup
Organic, non-GMO tofu	8 g per 3 ounces
Black beans	8 g per ½ cup
Amaranth	8 g per 1 cup
Quinoa	8 g per 1 cup
Spelt	8 g per 1 cup
Kamut	8 g per 1 cup
Teff	8 g per 1 cup
Sorghum	8 g per 1 cup
Wild rice	7 g per 1 cup
Almonds or almond butter	7 g per ¼ cup almonds or 2 tablespoons almond butter
Peanuts or peanut butter	7 g per ¼ cup peanuts or 2 tablespoons peanut butter
Chickpeas	6 g per ½ cup
Lima beans	6 g per ½ cup
Pistachios	6 g per ½ cup
Walnuts	5 g per ½ cup
Chia seeds	5 g per 2 tablespoons

Catching Safer Seafood

Once upon a time, *all* of the seafood people ate was, of course, wild-caught. Over time, concerns about the harmful effects of heavy metals (such as mercury) and pollutants in our waters, combined with a higher demand for seafood, led to the rise of aquaculture, or farm-raised fish. But fish farms—especially those located outside the United States, which often lack strict regulations—are far from perfect: Like conventional livestock, the fish raised in these reservoirs are usually fed low-quality fish meal made from soy, wheat, and corn instead of the algae, krill, or smaller fish they'd normally eat in the wild. As a result, farmed fish can contain lower levels of beneficial omega-3 fatty acids than their wild counterparts. It's also common for farmed fish to be given a steady supply of antibiotics to help them avoid getting sick due to being crammed into small enclosures with too many other fish. Farmed fish can be exposed to harmful chemicals, too. For instance, farmed salmon grown on large-scale fish farms can contain up to 10 times more organic pollutants—including probable carcinogens like polychlorinated biphenyls (PCBs), pesticides like DDT, and even flame retardants—than their wild counterparts, according to tests conducted by the Environmental Working Group.[4]

Still, cutting farmed fish out of your diet completely can really limit your seafood options. Wild-caught seafood can be expensive—and it's getting tougher to track down. Roughly half of our seafood is currently farmed, and according to World Bank estimates, that number could climb to two-thirds by 2030. Fortunately, some types of seafood are being farmed in a cleaner, more responsible way. Many fish farms are growing their own algae to ensure that their fish eat a more natural diet, which helps them contain higher levels of omega-3s. And some high-end supermarkets have established standards for farmed seafood.

Something Fishy's Going On

Buyer beware! As demand for clean, wild seafood has skyrocketed, fish fraud has become a legitimate concern. Here are two things to watch for.

❋ **"Organic" seafood.** Though the USDA has yet to establish guidelines for organic seafood, you might come across imported farmed options that call themselves organic. These "organic" offerings aren't subject to regulation, and the producers who farm them may still add contaminants to their fish feed or employ chemicals to fight parasites in fish, according to experts at the Environmental Defense Fund.[5] Steer clear!

❋ **Mislabeled wild salmon.** A recent report[6] by the environmental nonprofit organization Oceana found that out of 82 samples of "wild" salmon sold at grocery stores and restaurants, nearly half were actually farmed. Often, retailers will purposely mislabel farmed salmon as wild—especially during winter, when wild salmon isn't actually in season.

Finding Cleaner Fish

Since organic standards don't apply to fish and seafood, finding clean options might not be as straightforward as just looking for the USDA organic seal. But with a little know-how, you can shop for wild or sustainably farmed seafood with confidence.

❋ **Look for specifics.** The more information that's available, the less chance that your wild seafood is a fake. For instance, salmon labeled Chinook or king is more likely to be the real deal than anything just labeled "salmon" or "wild salmon." But if the label doesn't specify . . .

❋ **Ask questions.** Specifically, "Where was this fish caught?" Your fishmonger or restaurant server should be able to tell you the country (domestic is better than imported) and name a specific body of water (like the Pacific Ocean). He should also be able to tell you whether farmed fish was raised in a clean environment and whether it was given antibiotics. If he can't tell you, or if it just doesn't seem to add up, pick something else. And if all else fails . . .

❋ **Consider the cost.** Wild-caught and sustainably farmed fish usually isn't cheap. If the price simply seems too good to be true, it probably is.

❋ **Or, just check with the pros.** The Monterey Bay Aquarium's Seafood Watch List is considered the top sustainable seafood shopping resource. Find their clean picks or download the app at seafoodwatch.org.

Get Friendly with Healthy Fat

Let's get one thing straight: That whole thing about fat making you fat? It couldn't be further from the truth. True, fat *does* have more calories than carbohydrates or protein, which means keeping your portions in check is important, especially if you're trying to lose weight. But a few slices of creamy avocado, a spoonful of nut butter, or a drizzle of fruity olive oil can leave you feeling fuller for longer and can even help your body burn more fat. Plus, let's be honest—fat makes food taste better.

The key is picking healthy types of fat, since not all fats are created equal. So how can you tell which is which? It's easiest to think about different types of fat like lights on a traffic light: Some are green lights (great anytime in moderate portions, of course), some are yellow (best once in a while, so be cautious), and some are red (stop and try to avoid these completely).

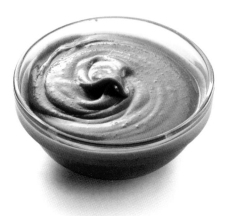

Green Light Fats

Unsaturated fats such as monounsaturated (MUFA), polyunsaturated (PUFA), and omega-3 fats can help lower your risk for heart disease. They also play an important role in keeping your blood sugar levels stable, which could help stave off cravings for sugary junk. You can find them in lots of whole, unprocessed foods.

❖ **MUFAs.** Olive oil, olives, avocados, nuts, and nut butters
❖ **PUFAs.** Safflower oil and sunflower seeds
❖ **Omega-3s.** Fatty fish, such as salmon, trout, mackerel, herring, and anchovies; walnuts; chia seeds, hemp seeds, flaxseeds; and flaxseed oil

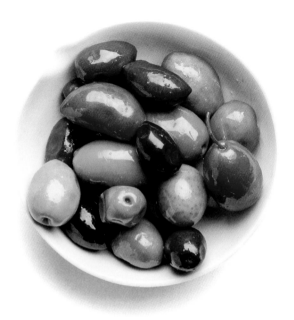

Yellow Light Fats

In large quantities, the saturated fats found in meat, full-fat dairy (whole milk, full-fat yogurt, butter, and cheese), eggs, and tropical oils (such as coconut oil) can raise your risk for heart disease. But in moderation, they can be perfectly fine. If you're having an egg or two (with yolks) for breakfast, some diced chicken in your salad, or a stir-fry with vegetables and lean beef, you probably don't have to worry.

But if you're eating more than that on a regular basis, it's worth trying to cut back for the sake of your heart. Just make sure you swap your saturated fat with a healthier pick. Slashing saturated fat won't reduce your risk of heart disease unless you replace that fat with healthier foods, such as unsaturated fats or whole grains, according to findings published in the *Journal of the American College of Cardiology.*[7]

Dr. Wendy Says . . .

Make the effort to seek out cleanly produced oils, like those labeled "cold-pressed" or "expeller-pressed." Cold-pressed oils are pressed at low temperatures, so they retain all the flavors, aromas, and nutrients that can get destroyed by heat. "Expeller-pressed" means that the oil was extracted mechanically (through good old-fashioned squeezing!) instead of with chemicals.

Can Coconut Oil Make Me Thin?

Coconut oil is often touted as a weight-loss wonder food, and there is some evidence to suggest that the medium-chain triglycerides (MCTs) in coconut oil could help you fit into your skinny jeans. One small study published in the journal *Lipids*[8] found that women who consumed roughly 2 tablespoons of coconut oil daily for 12 weeks lost more belly fat than women who downed the same amount of soybean oil. There's also some evidence suggesting that coconut oil's MCTs can rev your metabolism and boost satiety to help you eat less throughout the day.

So should you down it by the spoonful? All oils contain about 120 calories per tablespoon, so simply *adding* coconut oil to whatever you're already eating won't help with weight loss. But replacing other less nutritious things in your diet with coconut oil—using it instead of conventional canola oil in a stir-fry, for example—might help you lose weight faster. Just stick to less than 2 tablespoons of coconut oil per day as you're working to shed some pounds.

Red Light Fats

Trans fats are artificial fats that are made by adding hydrogen to liquid vegetable oils, which makes them solid. And they're straight-up bad for you: Aside from the fact that they have zero nutritional value, trans fats have also been shown to raise your "bad" LDL cholesterol, lower your "good" HDL cholesterol, and increase your risk for heart disease and diabetes. Trans fats tend to show up in packaged items like cookies, crackers, and margarine—and if you spot them on an ingredients list (usually under the name "partially hydrogenated oils"), it's a surefire sign that the food is *not* clean. Don't eat these fats!

Go with the (Whole) Grain

Repeat after us: You don't need to cut out carbs or gluten to lose weight. You just need to choose complex, fiber-rich carbohydrates instead of their refined counterparts. Quinoa, barley, millet, oats, and brown rice are tasty and filling. And they can have *big* benefits for your weight: In a *Nutrition Journal* study of more than 45,000 adults and children, those who ate the most whole grains had lower body mass indexes and smaller waist circumferences and were more likely to be at a healthy weight compared to those who ate the least.[9]

But you don't have to limit yourself to individual grains. Pasta made from whole wheat, quinoa, and non-GMO corn are all great choices, too. Clean eating can even include bread—as long as it's made from whole grains. Plenty of manufacturers add a touch of whole grain flour (or even just caramel coloring) to make their bread seem more wholesome than it is. But the only way to tell for sure whether a bread is whole grain is to check the ingredients list. First up should always be something with the word "whole" in the name, like "whole wheat" or "whole oats." If you don't see the word "whole," that's a sign that the grains in your bread are likely refined. (Head to page 165 for more on what to look for when buying a clean whole grain bread.)

Buy Clean Packaged Foods

Eating clean doesn't mean cooking every single thing from scratch and swearing off all foods that come in a box, can, or bag. (Though if you want to give it a try, we salute you!) Instead, it's about being conscious of choosing packaged items that help support your health and weight-loss goals—not leave you feeling like garbage. That means seeking out packaged foods that are made with real ingredients, that aren't overly processed, and that are free of artificial additives. Your body and waistline will benefit from a little label reading.

Common GMO Culprits

Good news! The majority of real, whole foods aren't genetically modified. So by eating clean, you'll automatically be avoiding most foods that contain GMOs. However, it's common for conventional packaged, processed foods to contain genetically modified ingredients such as soy, corn, rapeseed (used to make canola oil), and sugar beets (used to make white sugar). When buying packaged or processed foods, look for certified organic products since by law, organic foods cannot be grown using genetically engineered seeds. Another good option: Look for non-GMO labels from third-party certifiers, like the Non-GMO Project.

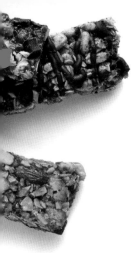

Check the Ingredients

Forget the marketing mumbo jumbo on the front of the package and bypass the nutrition facts chart for a minute. **Before you do anything else, read a packaged food's ingredient list.** Foods with fewer, more simple ingredients tend to be better for you than ones with lots of ingredients or ingredients that are unrecognizable. Think about, say, an energy bar. You might think that, in general, any energy bar is probably pretty good for you because it contains foods like oats, dried fruit, and nuts. But let's take a look at the ingredients lists for two different types of bars.

Energy Bar A: dates, almonds, unsweetened apples, walnuts, raisins, cinnamon

Energy Bar B: granola (whole grain rolled oats, brown sugar, crisp rice [rice flour, sugar, salt, malted barley extract], whole grain rolled wheat, soybean oil, dried coconut, whole wheat flour, sodium bicarbonate, soy lecithin, caramel color, nonfat dry milk), semisweet chocolate chips (sugar, chocolate liquor, cocoa butter, soy lecithin, vanilla extract), corn syrup, brown rice crisp (whole grain brown rice, sugar, malted barley flour, salt), invert sugar, sugar, corn syrup solids, glycerin, soybean oil. Contains 2 percent or less of sorbitol, calcium carbonate, salt, water, soy lecithin, molasses, natural and artificial flavor, BHT (preservative), citric acid.

Once you look at the ingredients list, it's easy to tell that energy bar A is the cleaner choice: There are only six ingredients, and none of them are processed. Energy bar B, on the other hand, is packed with processed ingredients (when was the last time you found freshly picked chocolate liquor at the farmers' market?), loads of sugar, and potentially carcinogenic colors and preservatives. Not exactly the stuff clean snacks are made of, right?

Watch for Hidden Sugars

The average American eats nearly 20 teaspoons of sugar every single day. Most of that comes from packaged foods—and not just desserts. Everything from jarred pasta sauce to microwave oatmeal packets to whole wheat bread can be loaded with added sugar. This is bad news if you're trying to eat clean, since loading up on sugar zaps your energy, ramps up your cravings, and sends your body toward fat storage—all of which make it nearly impossible to lose weight. But manufacturers are crafty. They know that sugary foods are addictive, so they add the sweet stuff to virtually all of their products, including many that might surprise you, such as bread,

The Different Names for Sugar

- Agave syrup
- Barley malt
- Beet sugar
- Brown rice syrup
- Brown sugar
- Buttered syrup
- Cane sugar
- Caramel
- Carob syrup
- Coconut sugar
- Corn syrup
- Date sugar
- Dextran
- Dextrose

- Evaporated cane juice
- Fructose
- Fruit juice
- Fruit juice concentrate
- Glucose
- Glucose solids
- Golden syrup
- Grape sugar
- High-fructose corn syrup
- Honey
- Invert sugar
- Lactose
- Malt syrup
- Maltodextrin

- Maltose
- Mannitol
- Maple syrup
- Molasses
- Raisin juice concentrate
- Raw sugar
- Refiner's syrup

- Rice/rice bran sugar
- Sorbitol
- Sorghum syrup
- Sucrose
- Sugar
- Turbinado sugar

tomato sauce, crackers, salad dressings, and frozen dinners. To make matters worse, you won't always spot "sugar" on the ingredients list. The sweet stuff goes by tons of different names, including some that sound pretty wholesome, such as agave syrup, honey, or maple syrup. But to your body, it's *all* sugar.

Beware of Weird Additives

Here's something that might blow your mind: Some of the additives in packaged foods haven't actually been tested by the FDA because they're considered by certain experts to be "generally recognized as safe" (GRAS). This makes sense for basic ingredients, like salt or pepper—do we really need to test those things to know that they're a-okay? But the GRAS program has effectively created a loophole for some potentially harmful ingredients to end up in our foods without adequate testing. Seems like a pretty terrible idea, right?

Unless you're growing and preparing all of your own food, it can be tough to avoid food additives completely.

But eating clean isn't about being perfect—it's about picking the best option that you can with the resources that you have at the time. For those instances when you have to pick up a packaged food, it's a good idea to try to avoid these potentially sketchy additives as much as possible.

❄ **Artificial sweeteners, including aspartame, sucralose, and acesulfame-K.** These fake sweeteners often pop up in "diet" or "sugar-free" items like diet soda, sugar-free gum or desserts, chewable vitamins, cough syrup, toothpaste, and cereal. And they might be messing with your weight. In part, that could be because the sweet flavor of aspartame and other artificial sweeteners appears to stimulate taste receptors in your taste buds and digestive tract in the same way that sugar does. That can trick your brain into thinking you're getting calories from real sugar when you're not, which can promote cravings for *more* sweet foods, as well as cause other ill effects. Even more serious? Some studies have shown that artificial sweeteners could also have a negative impact on the bacteria in your gut, which plays a role in metabolism. It's no wonder that groups like the Center for Science in the Public Interest recommend avoiding artificial sweeteners altogether—and we agree.[10] Bottom line: They're not natural and they're not clean.

❄ **High-fructose corn syrup (HFCS).** A highly processed version of fructose (the sugar that occurs naturally in fruit) that's added to bread, candy, yogurt, salad dressing, canned vegetables, cereal, and more. Too much HFCS can increase insulin resistance, which can raise your risk for diabetes and heart disease. If you spot it on a package, it's a dead giveaway that what you're looking at is not a clean food.

❄ **Monosodium glutamate (MSG).** A flavor enhancer found in potato chips and snacks, cookies, seasonings, canned soups, frozen meals, lunch meats, and some Chinese food. It's known to trigger migraines in some people, and it has a crazy addictive flavor that makes you want to eat and eat and eat.

❄ **Added trans fats.** This lab-produced fat is used to extend the shelf life and improve the flavor of

How to Find a Clean Packaged Food—*Fast*

We get it–there isn't always time to scrutinize every single detail on a product's label when you're rushing through the grocery store to get everything on your list and make it home in time to get dinner on the table. When you're racing the clock, find safe, healthy options with these simple guidelines.

1. Scan the ingredients. Do you recognize all (or most) of them? If you wanted to, could you buy these ingredients separately?

2. Opt for organic. This guarantees that the food was produced without synthetic pesticides, is free of artificial additives, *and* is made without genetically modified ingredients. Check, check, check!

3. Scrutinize the sugar. Stick to products with less than 15 grams of sugar per serving and with most of that sweetness coming from real foods, like fruit—not from added sugars.

4. Watch the salt. A snack should have less than 250 milligrams of sodium per serving; a meal should have less than 600 milligrams.

things like margarine, chips, crackers, baked goods, and fast foods. It's strongly linked to heart disease and diabetes, which is why the FDA ruled that added trans fats must be phased out of most packaged and restaurant foods by 2018. (Meat and dairy contain small amounts of naturally occurring trans fats, but if you're eating these foods in moderation, these trans fats aren't something to worry about.)

✽ **Food dyes: blue #1 and #2, red #3 and #40, yellow #5 (tartrazine) and #6.** Found in fruit cocktail, maraschino cherries, ice cream, candy, baked goods, American cheese, mac and cheese, and more, these colors might *look* pretty. But they're petroleum based, and several have been linked to hyperactivity in kids and cancer in lab animals. You don't *really* need pink yogurt, do you?

✽ **Caramel color.** This common food coloring shows up in soda, beer, brown bread, chocolate, cookies, doughnuts, ice cream, and even pickles. It can be processed with ammonia, which leads to the creation of the potentially carcinogenic compound 4-methylimidazole.

✽ **Sulfites.** These preservatives and flavor enhancers are found naturally in wine and beer, and they're added to soda, juice, dried fruit, condiments, and potato products. In some people, they can cause allergy-like symptoms ranging from hay fever to anaphylaxis.

✽ **Sodium nitrite and sodium nitrate.** A possible carcinogen, sodium nitrite is a synthetic preservative used in processed meats such as hot dogs, lunch meats, bacon, and smoked fish. Natural sodium nitrates, which are derived from celery, are often used in "uncured" meat products and may be safer, but even those aren't clean eats. Avoid sodium nitrites altogether, and limit your consumption of sodium nitrates as much as possible.

✽ **Butylated hydroxyanisole (BHA) and butylated hydroxytoluene (BHT).** These petroleum-based preservatives are found in potato chips, gum, cereal, frozen sausages, enriched rice, lard, shortening, and candy. BHA is a likely human carcinogen; BHT has been linked to cancer to a lesser degree.

✽ **Potassium bromate.** This flour-bulking agent is often used in breads and rolls, bagel chips, wraps, and bread crumbs to strengthen dough and shorten baking time. It could cause kidney or nervous system disorders and gastrointestinal discomfort.

Deciphering Food Claims

Whole foods are real, simple, and straightforward—usually! Sometimes, even things as basic as a carton of eggs, a jug of milk, or a package of chicken breasts can have an awful lot of *stuff* on the label. And while the terms can be a bit confusing, they're worth paying attention to if you're committed to eating clean. Here are a few biggies to get familiar with.

❋ **Organic.** For produce, this means that the plants weren't grown from genetically modified seeds; were not grown with pesticides, herbicides, or sewage sludge; and were not irradiated. For meats and poultry, this means that the animals were fed organic feed containing no animal by-products, were not given antibiotics or hormones, and had some (but not necessarily much) access to the outdoors. For a packaged food to be labeled organic, it must be made up of at least 95 percent organic ingredients; a label stating "made with organic ingredients" means the product must be made up of at least 70 percent organic ingredients.

❋ **Cage-free.** For eggs, "cage-free" means that the hens were not confined to cages—but they didn't necessarily have access to an outdoor space. Unless they're organic, cage-free hens can still be fed grains made from genetically modified crops that have been heavily treated with chemical pesticides, which can then be passed on to you. Since there's no mandatory third-party auditing for the term "cage-free," look for a third-party verification seal like "Certified Humane" or "Animal Welfare Approved."

❋ **Free-range.** Found on both poultry and egg packaging, free-range means that hens have some access to the outdoors. Like cage-free hens, free-range hens that aren't certified organic can still be given feed that contains antibiotics and pesticides. Since there's no mandatory third-party auditing for the term, look for a third-party verification seal like "Certified Humane" or "Animal Welfare Approved."

❋ **Pasture-raised.** This term can apply to meat, poultry, and eggs. Pasture-raised animals spend some time on grassland, where they're able to eat a more natural diet of grass and bugs. Because of this, their meat and milk often have a richer flavor and higher levels of nutrients, such as omega-3s. But since there's no mandatory third-party auditing, it can be tough to tell exactly how much time an animal actually spent on the pasture. For that reason, it's best to buy pastured meats and eggs with a third-party verification seal like "Certified Humane" or "Animal Welfare Approved." Or buy from a local producer who can offer details on how his animals are raised.

❋ **Grass-fed.** Due to recent changes to labeling standards, the USDA grass-fed label only means that beef, bison, lamb, goats, and dairy cattle were fed grass *at some point* in their lives. The label doesn't stop producers from feeding animals grain, giving them antibiotics or hormones, or keeping them in confined spaces. For true grass-fed products, look for those certified by the American Grassfed Association, or buy from a local producer who can offer details on how his animals are raised.

❋ **Natural.** "Natural" foods are those made without artificial flavors, colors, or other synthetic ingredients. But these foods can still contain high-fructose corn syrup, and many also contain genetically modified ingredients. In short, *natural* is a vague term, so don't rely on it exclusively when you're looking for clean products. Inspect the ingredient list, instead.

❋ **No hormones.** When you see this label on meat or dairy products, it means that hormones weren't given to the animals involved. The USDA already prohibits the use of hormones in poultry and pork, so you don't need to seek out this label for those products.

❋ **No antibiotics.** This term can be found on meat or dairy items, and it means that no antibiotics were given to the animals involved. That's a good thing, since antibiotic use in animals is linked to drug resistance, as well as obesity. But if you're going to pay more for antibiotic-free products, you might as well buy organic ones.

❋ **Certified humane.** This means that the animals had access to enough space to allow them freedom to move, which is good for your conscience. But it also means that the animals weren't treated with artificial growth hormones or antibiotics—which is good for your health.

(continued on page 56)

Everyday Essentials

Learning about all the weird stuff that goes into most conventional food might have you running to clean out your kitchen—stat. But once all the junk is out, what do you put back in? Don't worry about the goji berries and sprouted hemp seeds for now. The basic staples listed below are all you need in order to build a clean refrigerator, freezer, and pantry. Here's how to stock your kitchen so eating clean is easy, quick, and delicious.

Vegetables and Fruit

- Leafy greens, like kale, spinach, or romaine lettuce
- Cruciferous vegetables, like broccoli, cauliflower, or Brussels sprouts
- Other vegetables, like bell peppers, mushrooms, or sweet potatoes
- Fresh fruits, like apples, oranges, bananas, or peaches
- Citrus fruits, like lemons or limes
- Frozen fruits, like frozen berries or mangoes
- Frozen vegetables, like broccoli or spinach
- Avocados
- Olives
- Fresh herbs
- Dried fruits, like raisins or unsweetened dried cherries

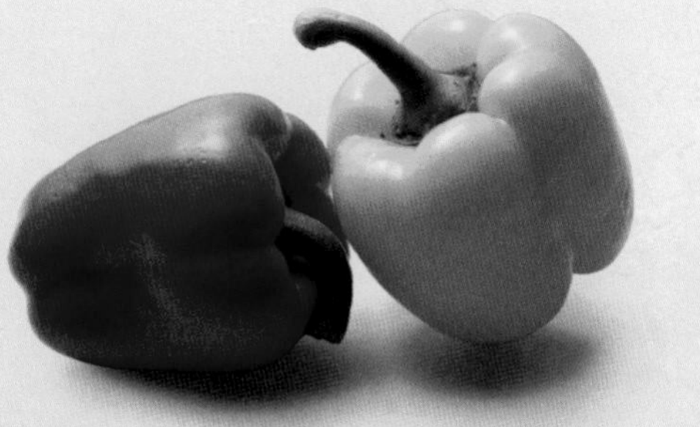

Clean Proteins

- Organic boneless, skinless chicken breasts
- Organic turkey breast cutlets
- Organic flank steak
- Organic ground chicken, ground turkey, or lean ground beef
- Organic pork tenderloin
- Wild-caught salmon fillets (fresh or frozen)
- Wild-caught shrimp (fresh or frozen)
- BPA-free canned tuna or wild-caught salmon

Dairy

- Plain organic yogurt (Greek or regular)
- Organic dairy milk or organic unsweetened nondairy milk, like almond, soy, coconut, or hemp
- Organic unsalted butter
- Parmesan cheese and a few of your other favorite cheeses, like ricotta, feta, or mozzarella

Grains and Beans

- Whole grain or sprouted breads, tortillas, or pitas
- Whole grain or gluten-free pasta
- Whole grains, like quinoa and brown rice
- Whole wheat flour
- Rolled oats
- Dried lentils
- BPA-free canned no-salt-added or low-sodium beans, and/or dried beans
- Organic, non-GMO edamame

Nuts, Seeds, and Nut Butters

- Raw nuts, like almonds or walnuts
- Raw seeds, like pumpkin seeds or flaxseeds
- Natural nut butters, like peanut butter or almond butter

Cooking Staples and Flavor Enhancers

- Anchovies
- Boxed low-sodium chicken or vegetable stock
- BPA-free canned light coconut milk
- BPA-free canned or jarred crushed tomatoes
- Capers
- Dijon mustard
- Dried herbs and spices and clean spice blends
- Low-sodium tamari
- Oils, like olive oil, organic non-GMO canola oil, or coconut oil
- Tomato paste
- Unsweetened cocoa powder
- Vinegars, like balsamic vinegar or apple cider vinegar
- White miso paste

Clean Eater

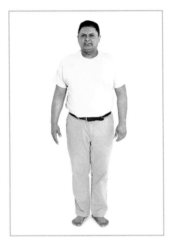

BEFORE

Vimal P.

A single guy with a stressful job who was heading toward his 50th birthday, **Vimal** never spent much time thinking about what he ate. He didn't bother reading labels to learn about what was going into his food. He couldn't tell what counted as a proper serving size, versus what was way too big. And he didn't cook.

But things began to change when he started eating clean. He started making an effort to buy higher-quality foods made without chemicals and preservatives, and he began shopping for fresh fruits and vegetables at his local farmers' market. And most importantly, he began paying attention to his portion sizes. "I didn't really know when to say enough was enough. Especially if I was watching TV or a movie," he admits.

Cutting out his nightly beer or Scotch helped Vimal become more aware of how much he was eating, too. In the past, he'd come home and have a predinner drink or two, which would lower his inhibitions and make him more prone to piling too much on his plate. But when he removed the alcohol, he found that he naturally wanted to eat less at dinner because he wasn't as hungry as he used to be. What's more, he was no longer drinking hundreds of empty calories from the drinks themselves.

He still hasn't turned into much of a cook, but he has learned that you don't need to make elaborate meals in order to eat clean. By homing in on just a few things—eating cleaner proteins and more fruits and vegetables, and watching his salt use and the sodium content in packaged foods—Vimal focused on building simple meals, such as grilled chicken or fish and salad, or Greek yogurt with fruit.

And his hard work paid off. "I didn't think I'd see results," he says. "But if I can do it, I think anybody can."

Dr. Wendy Observes: Work pressure, peer pressure for daily lunches out and cocktails after work, a successful single guy's lifestyle, and disinterest in cooking make for a perfect weight-gain storm. Or, as Vimal learned, an ideal opportunity for a smart man to tackle each of these challenges head-on by keeping his health goals firmly in focus. He kept it simple and learned how to make eating clean work for him—two strategies that helped him succeed now and will help him in the long-term, as well.

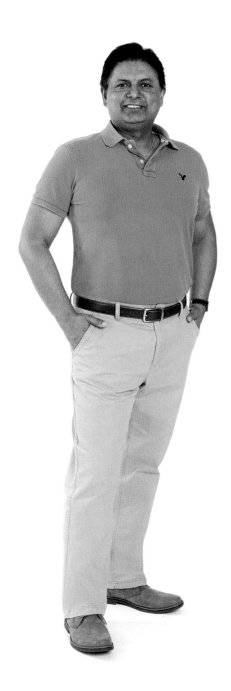

TOTAL POUNDS LOST

11 lbs

TOTAL INCHES LOST

8.25

MOST NOTABLE IMPROVEMENTS

Vimal increased his HDL ("good") cholesterol by 9 points, and his systolic blood pressure (the top number) dropped by 18 points.

✤ **Heart healthy.** The American Heart Association's Heart-Check program's standard certification requires that a product have less than 6.5 grams of total fat, 1 gram or less of saturated fat (or less than 15 percent of total calories), less than 0.5 gram of trans fats, and 20 milligrams or less of cholesterol per serving. It also requires that a food contain less than a certain amount of sodium, depending on the food category. The food must contain 10 percent or more of the daily value of one of six beneficial nutrients (vitamin A, vitamin C, iron, calcium, protein, or dietary fiber). While nuts are higher in fat than many foods (such as fruits and vegetables), they can also get the Heart-Check mark, thanks to the enormous amount of evidence backing their benefits for heart health. Still, because of the label's emphasis on certifying lower-fat foods—even as mounting research shows that quality fats are good for you—take the label with a grain of salt and read the ingredients list and nutrition panel before you make a decision.

✤ **High-fiber.** High-fiber foods must contain at least 5 grams of fiber per serving, according to the Whole Grains Council. Whole grains typically contain between 0.5 and 3 grams of fiber per serving, so you'll usually see the "high-fiber" label on processed foods that contain added fiber in the form of resistant starch, inulin, or cellulose. If you're already eating a whole foods diet that contains plenty of vegetables and grains, you don't need to bother looking for this label.

✤ **Raw.** This label typically shows up on juices, fermented drinks and vegetables, dairy, and some snack foods—and it means that the product was not cooked or heated to a temperature that destroys certain beneficial nutrients and enzymes. In the case of things like kombucha, sauerkraut, and kimchi, it means that the product has retained its good bacteria and still offers probiotic benefits. The jury's still out for juices, since pasteurized juice still retains many vitamins and minerals. When it comes to raw milk, many experts believe the benefits may not outweigh the risks of food-borne illnesses. For packaged snack foods, such as kale chips, look for more specific quality indicators in addition to raw, such as organic or non-GMO.

✤ **Non-GMO or GMO-free.** Both terms imply that a food is free of genetically modified organisms—but neither one is regulated. To be most certain that the food you're buying is free of GMOs, look for foods that are certified organic and have a "Non-GMO Project Verified" seal.

Savvy Shopping for Clean Eaters

It's true that distinguishing clean foods from their not-so-healthy counterparts can sometimes be tricky. (Though it's nothing you can't handle and it gets easier with practice.) The good news is that more and more people are waking up to the fact that clean foods are key to losing weight and feeling great. This means that

Package Deal?

Stroll through the supermarket, and it'll only take about 30 seconds for you to notice that packaged foods—from cereals to energy bars to frozen dinners—flaunt a whole lot of health claims on their labels. And while some of them might sound impressive (antioxidant-fortified waffles and probiotic chocolate bars, anyone?), most of these claims aren't as great as they seem. For instance, foods that tout themselves as being loaded with protein are often pumped up with soy protein isolate—a highly processed form of soy made from genetically modified soybeans and processed with the chemical hexane. As for foods that boast that they pack an extra antioxidant, omega-3, or probiotic punch, no one can say for certain whether those items actually deliver any real benefits. Part of what makes whole foods so good for you is that they contain an entire suite of nutrients—and experts suspect that many of these nutrients may be their most potent when they work in harmony. It's a lot like an orchestra: One violin on its own might sound nice, but when all of the instruments play together, you get a symphony. The bottom line? Try to avoid getting seduced by tempting claims on package labels, and get your nutrients from real foods as much as possible.

whole, unprocessed fare is more widely available than ever. Gone are the days when you had to drive 50 miles to reach a store that carried quinoa—only to find that it cost $20 a bag. We're living in a golden age for clean shopping, and there are more places than ever that offer fresh, clean foods at prices that won't break the bank. So grab your reusable bags and let's go!

Clean Food Lives Here

Where exactly can you find clean food? The question should really be, where *can't* you find it? All of these spots are stocked with the staples you need.

❇ **Supermarkets.** These days, even most megamart chains offer at least some organic produce, meat, dairy, and eggs. They also have a smattering of truly clean packaged goods. Just be sure to check those ingredients lists!

❇ **Natural food stores.** Whether it's a Whole Foods Market or a small indie shop, these stores tend to offer a bigger selection of clean produce, animal products, and more. Even better, they usually have huge selections of bulk items—everything from whole grains to dried beans to nuts and seeds. And since you're avoiding all of the extra packaging, these bulk foods tend to be more affordable.

❈ **Farmers' markets.** More and more farmers' markets are popping up all across the country, which is good news for clean eaters. In addition to selling fresh, seasonal produce, most markets also offer locally produced eggs, dairy products, meats, and breads. The best part? You can talk to the farmers and producers to find out *exactly* what goes into growing or making their food.

❈ **CSAs.** CSA stands for community supported agriculture. Buying a share of a CSA means that you're investing in a local farm and receiving a weekly box of produce in exchange. (Some CSAs also offer eggs, dairy, and meats.) Like shopping at the farmers' market, this gives you the opportunity to learn more about how your food is produced and to get to know what's truly local and seasonal in your area.

Smart Ways to Save

At some point, you might've walked into a high-end grocery store and balked at a $6 bunch of broccoli or an $8 carton of eggs. It's easy to drop big bucks on clean fare, but fueling your body with the good stuff doesn't have to be expensive. In fact, when you start trading processed, packaged items for their whole-food counterparts, you might end up spending less! Consider these tips to save big.

❈ **Make a list—and stick to it.** It sounds obvious, but it's essential for sticking to your budget and avoiding the little impulse buys (fancy organic chocolate bar, anyone?) that can lead to sticker shock at the checkout counter. Make it a point to plan your meals and snacks ahead of time, and make a shopping list of all the ingredients that you'll need. (This will be a huge help with making clean choices and losing weight, too—but more on that later!) If you didn't write it down, it doesn't go in your cart.

❈ **Buy in season.** Produce grown out of season isn't just lacking in flavor. It's usually flown in from far, far away—so it's also really expensive. Stick to in-season fruits and vegetables that were grown nearby, and stock up on extras to freeze or even can so you can enjoy them all year long. Or look for produce that's available year-round, like apples and broccoli.

❈ **Go veggie more often.** Plant-based proteins are considerably less expensive than their animal counterparts. Commit to eating vegetarian or vegan meals more often, or eat meat, poultry, or fish in small quantities instead of as the main event. Bonus: A largely plant-powered diet has been shown to help with losing weight—and keeping it off.

Where's *My* Farmers' Market?

Looking to buy local but aren't quite sure where to go? Head to localharvest.org to find farmers' markets, CSAs, farm stands, and even pick-your-own farms in your area.

Shop the Perimeter

Distracted by the endless rows of chip bags and soda bottles at your supermarket? It's a grocery store's job to tempt you into filling your cart at every turn, but you don't have to cave to the pressure: Focus on the outer perimeter of the store, which is where whole foods like fresh produce, meat, poultry, seafood, and dairy are generally kept. As for the center aisles, that's where most of the processed stuff lives. Be on high alert when you walk through that zone, and check the ingredients list on any box or bag you pick up so you can find your best clean options.

✳ **Join a co-op.** Co-ops are member-owned grocery stores that focus on whole foods, including organic produce, dairy products, and meats. Usually you pay a small membership fee up front to own a share of the co-op and then you reap the rewards in the form of significantly discounted fare.

✳ **Grow your own.** Whether it's a raised bed in your yard that's brimming with vegetables or a pot of fresh herbs on the windowsill of your kitchen apartment, every bit of food you grow is food that you don't have to pay for out of your wallet. Plus, it's as fresh as you can get!

Putting It All Together

1 **Make whole foods the mainstays of your diet.** Fresh fruits and vegetables, lean proteins (including plant proteins like beans and nuts), whole grains, and healthy fats are the building blocks of clean eating.

2 **Scrutinize packaged foods.** Packaged foods can have a place in your diet. But read those labels carefully to make sure that boxed and bagged goods are truly clean!

3 **Buy organic when you can.** Prioritize meat and dairy first, then produce. But remember, if you can't buy organic, it's not the end of the world—you can still eat clean and succeed.

4 **Spread out from the supermarket.** You'll find plenty of clean options at most grocery stores. But when you can, try branching out! Hit the farmers' market, join the local co-op, or even try your hand at gardening.

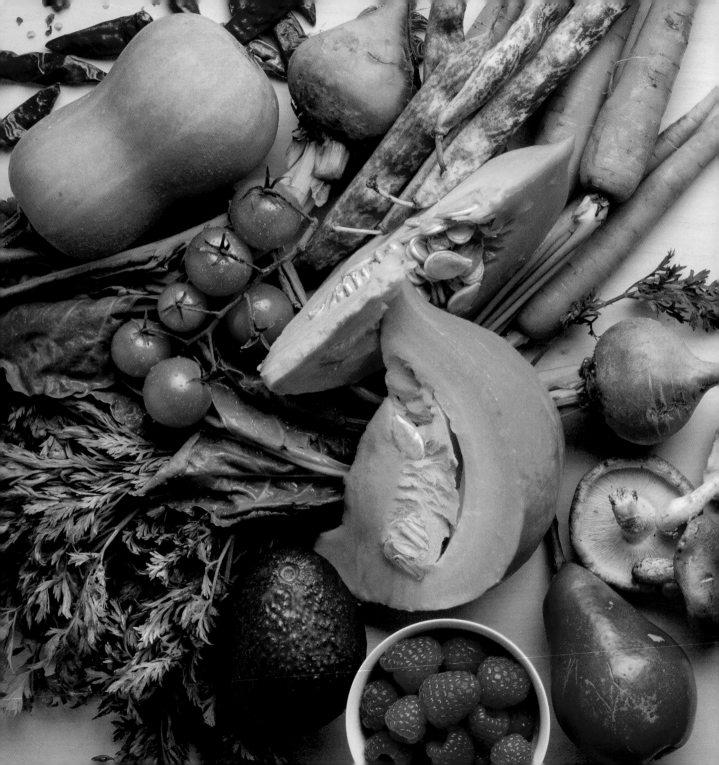

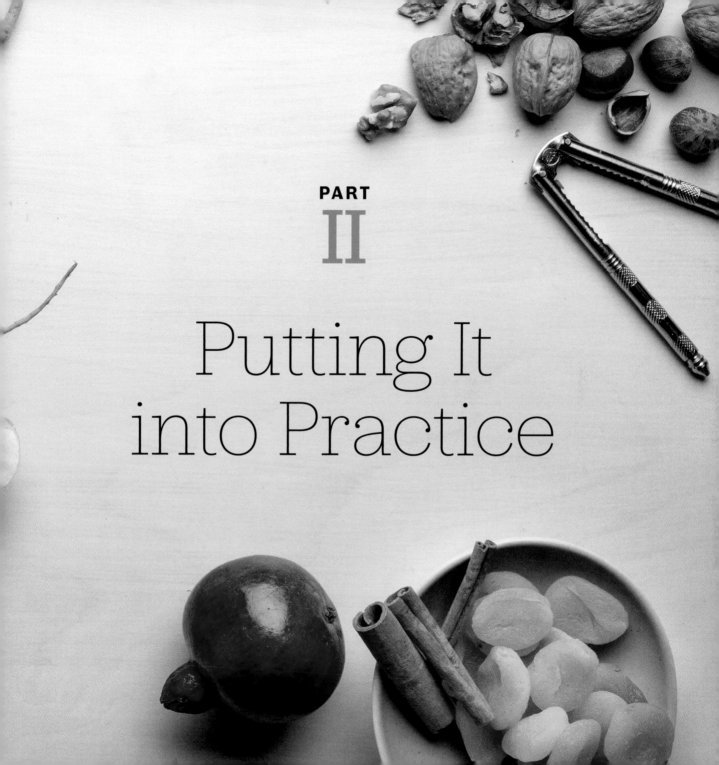

PART

II

Putting It
into Practice

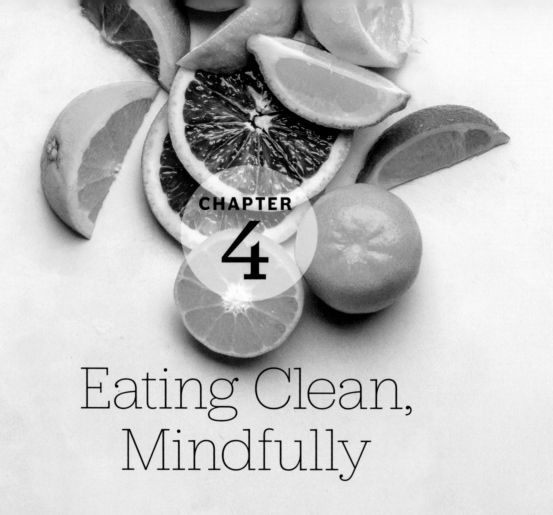

Eating Clean, Mindfully

Eating clean is all about giving your body the nourishment it needs to thrive and shed excess weight. And in order for your body to work optimally, you have to listen closely to what it's telling you. That's where mindfulness comes in. By tuning in to your hunger, your emotional state, and even your cravings, you can learn how to make clean choices that are right for you. And that can play an important role in helping you get the maximum enjoyment from your food, feel great about what you eat, lose weight, and keep that weight off—for life. Ready to learn how to give it a try? C'mon, let's go.

What Is Mindful Eating?

Mindfulness is a bit of a buzzword these days, so this might not be the first time you've heard it. But what exactly does it mean? In short, being mindful means paying attention. You can walk mindfully by focusing on your surroundings—like the birds chirping or the people around you—instead of staring at your phone. You can have a mindful conversation by listening closely to what the other person is saying instead of only thinking about what you'll say next. You can even fold the laundry mindfully by homing in on the fresh scent and soft feel of your freshly dried towels. (Which is actually pretty relaxing. Try it!)

In short, you can perform practically any activity with mindfulness—including eating. When you eat mindfully, you pay closer attention to your food. How does it look on your plate? How does it taste and smell? How does it feel in your mouth? More importantly, you zero in on how your food makes you *feel*. Are you phys-ically hungry, or do you just feel like eating because you're bored or stressed? Are you eating until you feel satisfied, or are you polishing off everything on your plate just because it's there? Do you feel content and energized after you eat, or do you feel sluggish or guilty?

Mindful eating is the part of losing weight—and keeping it off—that takes *you* into account. At this point, you're likely convinced that following the princi-ples of clean eating is the best way to lose weight. But mindfulness is the awareness that helps you figure out *how* to make those things work for you. Do you stay fuller after eating a breakfast of cornflakes and fruit or after a vegetable omelet? Do you really need a handful of almonds to satisfy your hunger in the afternoon, or do you just reach for them out of habit? Does splurging on two cookies leave you feeling crabby and stuffed, and if so, can you enjoy that same treat more fully by only having one cookie? When you're mindful of the way you

Dr. Wendy Says . . .

What is it about mindfulness that seems to help the pounds melt off? Let us count the ways!

1. **It helps you take in fewer calo-ries.** When you start paying closer attention to your hunger and full-ness signals, you'll probably start to eat less. Plus, when you begin noticing how different foods make you feel, you'll start to naturally gravitate toward cleaner, leaner options rather than their processed counterparts.

2. **It improves your relationship with food.** By becoming aware of the non-hunger feelings that trigger you to eat, you can take steps to change how you respond to those situations. And that can make eating a less emotionally charged event.

3. **It makes you feel good about your food choices.** When you eat accord-ing to your true hunger and stop when you're full, you'll probably feel less deprived and learn how to enjoy the foods you love without feeling bad about it. By taking the guilt and anxiety out of eating, you'll be able to satisfy your hunger, enjoy your meal, and move on.

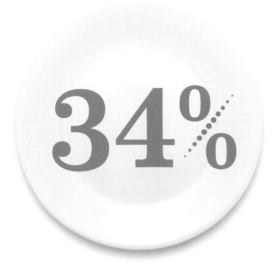

34%

People who don't practice mindful eating behaviors are this much more likely to be obese compared to those who are more conscious of what they're eating, according to a study published in the *International Journal of Behavioral Medicine.*[1]

eat, you uncover the answers to these questions. In turn, you get the maximum amount of enjoyment out of your food—and you learn how to approach it in a more balanced way. That can add up to more pounds lost—and kept off for the long term.

Eating Clean, Sustainably

Taking time to continually check in with yourself might sound like a lot of work—especially when you want to lose weight quickly. After all, isn't it easier to just follow a bunch of rules that tell you exactly what to do and what to avoid? In the short term, yes. And following an expert plan like the one in this book will absolutely jump-start your weight loss, as well as give you the tools you need to eat cleaner and work toward achieving your goals in a mindful way.

But most other weight-loss plans aren't designed to be followed forever. And even if they were, the truth is, you'd have a tough time sticking with them for the long haul. Eventually, you'd get bored of eating the same dinners and lunches over and over again. Or after saying no to your favorite dessert for 2 months straight, your worn-out self-control muscles would finally give up. Or your circumstances would change, and following a detailed plan just wouldn't work for your lifestyle anymore. Mindfulness tunes you in to what your body truly needs and how to feed it accordingly. And staying in touch with yourself as you stick with the clean-eating lifestyle you're learning here—instead of trying to keep up with a rigid set of prescribed diet rules—is how you stay lean for life.

How Mindful Are You?

As you work to make more conscious food choices, it can be helpful to know where you're starting from. To find out, read each one of these statements and check off how many of them apply to you. (Sure, it might feel a bit hard, since it calls for some brutal honesty and self-reflection. But knowledge is power, right?) After completing the Eat Clean, Stay Lean plan, you can revisit this list to see just how much progress you've made.

☐ When I'm stressed-out or overwhelmed, I basically eat whatever I want.

☐ Once I start eating junk, I keep eating because I've "already blown it."

☐ I tend to give up on healthy eating goals when I'm busy or have a lot going on in my life, waiting until sometime I think will feel right to start.

☐ Sometimes I have a plan in place to eat well, but other times, I have no strategy at all.

☐ What people might think or say about me sways my food choices.

☐ I keep myself busy with food when I'm bored.

☐ Sometimes I eat when I'm putting off doing something else.

☐ Eating helps distract me from how I'm feeling. It calms me and comforts me when I'm stressed, sad, or anxious.

☐ When I celebrate something, I usually eat larger amounts and more indulgently.

☐ I make better food choices in the morning and worse choices at night.

☐ I spend a decent amount of time worrying about my weight, appearance, and eating habits.

☐ I often eat when I'm checking e-mail, watching TV, or doing work.

☐ I typically finish everything on my plate.

☐ I often have intense cravings for unhealthy foods, to the point where I think about those foods continuously.

☐ I often eat most of my food for the day in one sitting or over the course of a few hours.

☐ I couldn't tell you what I ate for breakfast 2 days ago.

☐ I regularly binge eat, or consume too much food in one sitting, to the point where I feel uncomfortable or ill.

Clean Eater

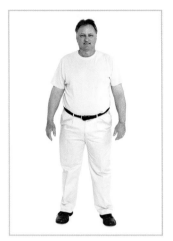

BEFORE

George S.

George had always been a self-described food addict who loved sugary treats and letting loose at happy hour on Friday night. But as he got older, he realized that his free-for-all eating style could be putting his health at risk. (Not to mention that many of his clothes no longer fit.) Having lived with type I diabetes for 40 years, the 58-year-old knew that he needed to start building better habits if he wanted to be around for his children as they began starting families of their own. "I'm in pretty good shape. But as I get older, I have to work harder and harder to stay there," he acknowledges.

Transitioning to cleaner meals and snacks wasn't always easy. A business owner, George had a tendency to get lost in his work and skip meals. When he finally remembered it was time to eat, he'd usually just order something from the deli for lunch or dinner. So he started packing clean lunches, dinners, and snacks to take to work, and he made an effort to eat every couple of hours to avoid getting too hungry. "I told myself, you have to focus on good meals. So I'm stopping [my old habits] and this is what I'm doing," he resolves.

Eating smaller portions came with a learning curve, too. George had long been used to eating or drinking what—and as much as—he wanted, whenever he wanted. But soon after starting on the plan, he realized that he didn't need as much food as he had thought. George also confessed that sometimes he'd eat out of habit, not because he was actually hungry. "I realized I actually don't need to eat as much as my 24-year-old son," he says. "I'd be watching golf on TV and think that I should be having chips. Then I'd think, no, I don't really need that. I'm good."

Dr. Wendy Observes: Sometimes it's hard to break out of certain eating habits when you're successful and productive in other areas of your life, such as work. But George realized that something had to change. And once he gave clean eating with smaller portions and regular timing a real try, he discovered that he could have success in work and weight loss, too.

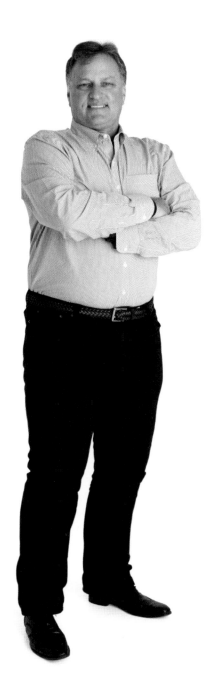

TOTAL POUNDS LOST

11.5<small>lbs</small>

TOTAL INCHES LOST

4

MOST NOTABLE IMPROVEMENTS
George's cholesterol fell by 15 points and went from too high to healthy. His high triglycerides dropped to a healthy level, too.

Getting Rid of Good and Bad

Many of us tend to think of food in black-and-white terms. If you eat a salad or a bowl of oatmeal, you're being good. If you eat a slice of pepperoni pizza or a cinnamon roll, you're being bad. And though you might think that that kind of mind-set would help you make better choices, it can often do the exact opposite. When you eat something that you think is "bad," you likely end up feeling shameful and guilty. As a result, you throw in the towel and start making rationalizations. Since you already blew your diet, you figure that you might as well keep on pigging out for the rest of the day. Or, just as unproductive, that you need to make up for it tomorrow by being extra good—which is often code for eating the foods that are lowest in calories, not necessarily the ones that are the most nutritious. It's this cycle of guilt that tends to be the downfall of most diets.

When you practice mindfulness, though, you learn how to enjoy your food without feeling guilty, so you're less susceptible to the cravings and binges that can throw you off the clean-eating wagon. **Foods are no longer good or bad, and they aren't grounds for reward or punishment.** Instead, *all* foods sit on a spectrum of more nutritious to less nutritious, and more clean to less clean to highly processed—and there's no judgment over what's on your plate. Sure, you can still have a slice of pie for dessert sometimes. But since it's on the less healthful side of the spectrum, it's better to have

Dr. Wendy Says . . .

Three o'clock cookie fix? After-work glass of wine? Pizza for dinner because, well, that's what you always have on busy nights? We eat for many reasons—and one of those reasons is habit. Habits can be tricky to change, especially when they're easy, comforting, and delicious. Still, even though it sometimes *seems* like the cookie jar is in charge, that's just not so. Using mindfulness-based strategies, *you* have the power to override those old habits while still acknowledging your feelings and forming healthier new practices.

Make a sometimes, not always, plan. Decide that you'll have your habitual food twice a week instead of every day. (And pick the days and amounts in advance, to minimize on-a-whim eating.) Twice a week is far from deprivation, but it's not often enough for your brain to actually form a habit. Especially if you . . .

Change up the timing. This takes practice, but it's a surefire way to unwire old associations, like wine when you get home from work or a candy bar during your afternoon break. If 3:00 p.m. is when you always treat yourself, try doing it at a completely different time, instead.

Try a new behavior in a new place. If you're used to snacking on sweets while sitting at your desk at a certain time of day, enjoy a clean snack while sitting in the break room, instead. Always walk in the door and head straight to the kitchen after work? Put on your sneakers and take a 15-minute walk, or take 15 minutes to lie on your bed and flip through a magazine.

Be positive and open-minded. Eating clean matters, and *you* matter. You can do this!

something more nutritious, like fruit, *most of the time*. And when you *do* have your pie, you take the time to really enjoy the way it tastes and smells, and even how it feels in your mouth. And you walk away from the table feeling content instead of guilty, and satisfied instead of stuffed.

What You Want versus *Whatever* You Want

When you decide to eat mindfully, you're making choices about what and how to eat based on what your body wants. At first, this might make mindfulness just sound like a woo-woo name for chowing down on chips and ice cream whenever the mood strikes. But eating what you want and eating *whatever* you want, *whenever* you want it, are not the same thing. And as you start to make mindfulness the name of your clean-eating game, you'll learn to tell the two apart.

Practicing mindfulness is about learning to tune in to your feelings—both physical and emotional—to figure out what it is that you really need and how to meet that need in a way that will help you feel your best. Sometimes, that might mean treating yourself. But most of the time, it means eating the clean, wholesome foods that help fuel you. And when you pay attention, you'll come to find that knowing the difference between the two is easier than you think.

> **Eating what you want and eating *whatever* you want, *whenever* you want it, are not the same things. As you start to make mindfulness the name of your clean-eating game, you'll learn to tell the two apart.**

When brain fog sets in at 3:00 p.m. on a Tuesday afternoon and you get a hankering for a candy bar, being mindful means that before you hit the vending machine you pause to ask yourself, *Am I actually hungry for chocolate and caramel right now, or am I really just running low on energy?* Chances are, the real answer is that you're just in the middle of an afternoon slump—and that you can get the boost you need from drinking some water or taking a quick stretch break. Or maybe you just found out that you're getting a promotion, and you want to treat yourself to a cupcake. Being mindful might mean remembering that you're still full from lunch or that you actually packed a wonderful snack that you're looking forward to eating in a couple of hours. This mindful, momentary pause might also help you realize that maybe it's better to celebrate by getting a manicure or pedicure after work than by serving up a short-lived infusion of sugar. See? It's pretty simple.

Making Mindfulness Work for You

How can you tell whether you're truly hungry or just in the mood to eat for a completely different reason? How can you enjoy your food fully so you finish eating feeling satisfied instead of wanting more? And how the heck can you feel good about splurging on a treat instead of feeling completely guilty? Eating mindfully might sound sort of difficult at first. But the longer you do it, the easier it gets.

Remember, this isn't about being perfect. In fact, when you choose to eat mindfully, you're pretty much throwing the idea of perfection out the window. Diets that fail you have excessive rules, so if you follow them 100 percent, you'll be successful for a while. But there are no hard-and-fast rules to mindfulness other than listening—*and responding* appropriately—to what your body needs.

Okay, but how exactly are you supposed to figure *that* out, and how can you tell the difference between what you really need and when you just want that muffin because it's sitting in front of you on the conference room table? Learning to read your hunger and cravings sounds complicated, but once you get the hang of it, it really will start to feel like second nature. Ready to give it a try?

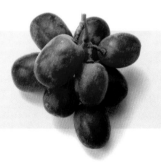

Gut Check

Is it genuine hunger—or something else? **Ask yourself if fruit or veggies would be satisfying.** If the answer is yes, have some. If your mind says no and insists that it's a cookie or bust, you're probably not actually hungry.

Ask, Am I *Really* Hungry?

Do you sometimes find yourself eating out of stress, boredom, or loneliness? Or, on the flip side, because you're happy or downright giddy? Don't worry, you're definitely not the only one. At some point, most people have been driven to eat for emotional reasons that have absolutely nothing to do with how empty—or full—their stomachs were. But learning to listen to your appetite—and in particular learning (or *re*learning) your true hunger cues—is the cornerstone of eating mindfully. And it can go a long way toward helping you lose weight.

Hunger is your body's way of saying that you're running low on energy and need to start thinking about fueling up. Unlike the other feelings that can drive you to eat, hunger comes with some distinct physical sensations that make it pretty tough to miss. When you're hungry, your stomach feels empty and hollow. The hungrier you get, the stronger that feeling becomes. And when you get *really* hungry, you might also start to feel light-headed or shaky, or you might have trouble concentrating.

Your goal is to eat when you're hungry, not starving. Not only does getting *too* hungry feel terrible, but it also increases the risk that you'll scarf down whatever's around instead of taking the time to pick something healthy and balanced. So when's the right time to eat? The next time you think about wanting to have a certain food, ask yourself if you'd also be up for eating fruit or veggies, such as an apple or some celery sticks. If the answer is yes, you're genuinely hungry, and you should eat. If the answer is no, you probably aren't physically hungry, and you should hold off on eating. Instead, reach for a cup of hot tea, which can quell your urge to nibble on something.

Notes from a Clean Eater

"As we age, our bodies don't need all the food we've been programmed to eat. When I get the urge to eat [for reasons other than hunger], I remind myself that it's not necessary. This program is rewiring my thoughts about food."—**George S.**

Focus on Your Food

You know how food always seems to taste more delicious when you're hungry? Well, it's true: Eating after you've worked up an appetite will go a long way toward helping you get the maximum amount of pleasure out of your food—whether it's your regular lunchtime Israeli Couscous Salad with Salmon (page 245) or a decadent slice of devil's food cake. But paying more attention to what you're eating also goes a long way toward helping you feel more satisfied, so it takes less food to fill you up and you're less tempted to scrounge around for more after getting up from the table.

Of course, paying attention to your food doesn't

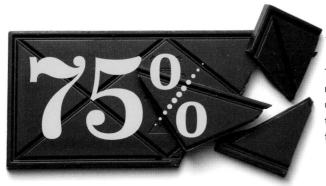

That's the percentage of study participants who ate for reasons other than hunger when they were offered an unexpected treat immediately after eating as much as they wanted of another chocolate snack, according to findings published in the journal *Eating Behaviors.*[2]

mean doing something crazy like talking to your chicken breast. It just means making your meal or snack the main focus—and taking the time to *really* enjoy it. Here are three simple ways to do just that.

To maximize your satisfaction with your meal, devote at least 20 minutes to eating.

- **Eat sitting down.** You might tell yourself that the calories in that bite of pasta or handful of crackers don't count if you're standing up, but they do. Plopping yourself at the kitchen table, the counter of your local sandwich shop, or even on a bench in the park can help you acknowledge that you're eating an actual meal or snack. And that in and of itself can make you less inclined to start noshing again in an hour or two.

- **Ditch the distractions.** TVs, phones, computers, and books (even this one!) all count as distractions. Make eating the main event instead of eating while

Dr. Wendy Says . . .

Mindful eating can seem sort of wishy-washy until you experience it for yourself. So give it a try with this simple experiment that engages all of your senses. All you need is a ripe strawberry (or another piece of fruit) and a few spare minutes.

1. **Look and touch.** Place the strawberry on a small dish, and place the dish on the table in front of you. Pick up the strawberry to feel its weight, and gently squeeze it to feel its ripeness. Now take a look at the berry: Is it bright red all over, or are some parts white or pink? Are the berry's seeds evenly distributed, or are they mostly concentrated in one area? Is the berry's texture smooth, or is it bumpy?
2. **Smell.** Bring the strawberry to your nose and inhale. Does it smell sweet? Tart? Can you smell the grassiness of the leafy green top? Slice the berry in half, and smell it again. Is the aroma stronger? Can you almost taste it? Do you sense the saliva building up in your mouth?
3. **Taste and listen.** Take a small bite of the strawberry and let it sit in your mouth. Close your eyes and count to five. Don't chew yet. What do you notice? Does the strawberry get sweeter? Do your salivary glands kick in? Does your body keep telling you to chew? Now chew three times and wait 5 more seconds. Does the flavor get more intense, or does it start to become muted? While you are chewing, listen closely. The sound may be subtle, but you should be able to hear the slight movement of your teeth as they break down the berry.
4. **Swallow the bite.** Stay present and feel your throat tighten momentarily as your tongue pushes the strawberry toward the back of your mouth and down your throat. Close your eyes for a few seconds, and see if you can feel the bite travel down toward your stomach. Visualize it happening even if you can't actually feel it.
5. **Repeat.** Perform steps 1 through 4 with the second half of the strawberry. There! You did it—a moment of mindful eating. Now think about how you might apply this to your meals and snacks.

What's *Your* Trigger?

Keeping a food journal is one of the most effective ways to become more aware of your triggers. If you're consistent, journaling can help you pinpoint the emotions that trigger you to eat and the specific foods that you like to reach for. That can help you figure out what tends to prompt you to eat mindlessly—and to avoid those triggers in the future.

Every night or after every meal, write down what you ate along with at least three adjectives to describe how you felt at the time. Try to be as descriptive as possible. For instance, instead of just writing *angry,* maybe you write *frustrated, sad,* or *overwhelmed.* Digging deeper helps you learn more about how you're feeling—

and expose the triggers that cause you to overeat so you can start figuring out other ways of dealing with them.

Of course, remember to write about the good stuff, too! Jotting down the small victories or what you're doing well can encourage you to keep doing it.

---

you do something else—and home in on the flavor, texture, aroma, and appearance of your food. Chances are, you'll feel satisfied sooner than if you ate with your eyes glued to a screen or a page.

✳ **Slow down.** This isn't a race! Eating at a more relaxed pace gives your body time to pump out fullness-signaling hormones that tell you when

you've had enough, and those hormones are key to weight loss. Research shows that when people at a healthy weight eat their meals slowly, they take in fewer calories and feel fuller for longer, compared to when they eat their meals quickly.[3] Sure, it's tough to always make eating a leisurely event—but try to devote *at least* 20 minutes to meals as often as you can.

Zero In on Your Triggers

A lot of us have foods that we can't stop eating once we start. For most of us, these foods tend to be high in sugar, fat, or salt—or, very often, a combination of all three. Throughout most of human history, these kinds of calorie-dense foods were tough to come by, and we evolved to binge on them when we found them in order to avoid starvation. Unfortunately, our brains haven't caught up with the fact that we now live in an environ-

ment where binge-worthy fare is available 24/7. So it's no surprise that once you start munching on chips or cookies, it can be really hard to stop.

Of course, that doesn't mean we're completely powerless against the lure of sugary, fatty, high-calorie treats. Often, the compulsion to eat junky stuff is triggered by something completely unrelated to food, such as stress at work, a fight with your spouse, the loneliness of

Dr. Wendy Says . . .

Have you heard people joke that they're on the *see-food* diet? You know, where they see food—and then they eat it? Turns out, there's some truth behind this funny play on words. Findings show that when food is in our visual path, we actually *are* more likely to eat it. Of course, that can spell bad news when you're trying to lose weight. (If the first thing you see when you open your pantry is a box of cookies, you'll be pretty tempted to eat it.)

The good news? The whole see-food thing can work to your advantage to help you make *cleaner* choices, too. All it takes is know-how in the kitchen. Here are five simple steps that can have a significant impact on what you do—and don't!—decide to eat.

I. **Declutter those counters.** On your countertop, swap sugary or processed snacks for a bowl or basket of fresh fruit. Women who keep things like potato chips, cereal, or soda on their counters tend to weigh more than women who don't, according to one study. And those who keep fruit on their counters tend to weigh *less*.[4] Opt for fruits like apples, oranges, bananas, pears, apricots, and peaches, which ripen best at room temperature. (They're also pretty, so they practically serve as a decoration for your kitchen.)

2. **Reconfigure your fridge and pantry.** Make fruits and vegetables more visible by moving them up to the shelves instead of storing them in the crisper, and store less-healthy items on the bottom shelves or toward the back of the fridge. In your pantry, put the healthy grains, dried fruits, and other clean staples front and center, and push sweets and treats toward the back. Better yet, if you have the space, store special-occasion treats in a less-visible space altogether, like another drawer or cabinet that you don't open often. When food is out of sight, it's more likely to be out of mind.

3. **Designate a clean-eating snack drawer.** Just like you have your own closet and drawer space for your clothes, it's perfectly reasonable to designate a drawer or two for yourself in the kitchen. Having your own space means that you'll only see *your* snacks when you open the drawer, not any of the more tempting stuff that might be stocked in the pantry for other members of your family.

4. **Rethink your serving dishes.** Consider rearranging your cupboards to put smaller dishes, bowls, and cups right up front; that way,

you'll get into the habit of reaching for them when it's time to eat. We serve ourselves more when we use bigger cups, plates, and utensils, and research shows that we eat 92 percent of what we serve ourselves—regardless of how hungry we are.[5]

5. **Keep the kitchen for cooking and eating.** Cook and prep in your kitchen, and eat sitting down at the kitchen table. (No spoonfuls over the sink or loitering in front of the fridge. Small bites add up!) Chat, play, or work in another part of your home. If your family tends to congregate at the kitchen table even when it isn't mealtime, consider setting up another gathering spot. A desk or a small table in your family room is a good spot to be together while going through the mail, doing homework, or flipping through magazines.

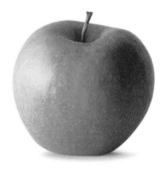

coming home to an empty house, boredom, or sheer exhaustion. Or it could just be a habit: Maybe you're just used to eating a bowl of pretzels while you watch your favorite show. Or maybe you used to eat chocolate ice cream for dessert growing up, so you get an urge to treat yourself to a scoop whenever you visit your parents.

The point is, we each have our own triggers—and it doesn't really matter what your specific ones are. If they happen regularly and prompt you to eat for reasons other than hunger, they can lead to mindless overeating and weight gain. But simply becoming more aware of your triggers and the effect that they have on you can actually help you deal with them in a healthier way.

Find Nonfood Rewards

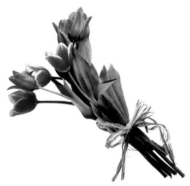

Remember how foods that are high in sugar, salt, and fat activate the reward center in your brain? Negative trigger emotions cause you to seek out those highly processed foods—often without even thinking about it!—because they make you feel good. But eating a brownie won't actually solve whatever problem you're dealing with, and the happy feeling it gives you disappears as soon as you've polished off the last bite. And to make matters worse, it's usually replaced with guilt over eating something junky.

When you become aware of your triggers and the foods that they drive you to eat, you can find ways to reward yourself without food. Think about the feeling you need to achieve to get past your trigger, then brainstorm ways to get it without eating. Say you start to notice that unexpected situations at work stress you out and drive you to eat junk. Now, if your boss has the tendency to pile on projects at the last minute, you might not be able to get him to change. But you *can* change how you react to it. Instead of snacking on candy the next time he throws an unexpected assignment your way, start a new habit of taking a 5-minute walk. Not only will the walk boost your levels of feel-good hormones, it will also give you time to get some air, gather your thoughts, and come up with a game plan for how you'll get the work done. Or maybe you realize that you feel lonely when you come home to an empty house, and maybe that loneliness drives you to eat something comforting. Instead of soothing your feelings with some cheesy pasta or a pint of ice cream, you can fill your desire for companionship by calling a friend.

Of course, you can harness the power of nonfood rewards for smaller situations, too. If you're just feeling tired, do some jumping jacks in your office to increase blood flow to your brain instead of popping a piece of chocolate. When you want a quick mood boost, watch a viral video of a kitten doing something silly. Need a temporary escape when you just can't deal? Keep a novel in your bag and read a couple of pages.

Cope with Cravings

If you've ever experienced the sudden, intense desire to devour a hot slice of pepperoni pizza or indulge in a fudgy brownie, you know that cravings can be pretty tough to resist. You should absolutely feel good about enjoying treats once in a while. But when you're plagued by overpowering urges to eat those kinds of foods every day, it can get in the way of your weight loss.

Clean foods can help keep cravings in check because they're free of the refined carbs and added sugars that send your blood sugar on a roller-coaster ride and drive you to eat more junk. Still, even the cleanest eater isn't immune entirely. So often, we're surrounded by delicious, easy-to-access food—everything from the doughnuts in your office break room to the free chip-and-dip samples at the grocery store to the well-meaning neighbor who thanks you for mowing her lawn by bringing over a plate of freshly baked cookies. Sooner or later, temptation is bound to happen. And when it does, mindfulness can help you keep a clear head: Reminding yourself of the fact that you're in the throes of a craving—and aren't actually *hungry*—can often be enough to snap you back to reality.

And when it's not? Don't worry, you still have plenty of other tools to help you curb that craving. Try some of these.

✳ **Take a walk.** A quick bout of exercise can help slash stress, reducing your urge to eat. And it doesn't take much: Walking for just 15 minutes can curb cravings for sugary snacks, according to one Austrian study.[6] Take a brief stroll in your neighborhood and see how you feel.

✳ **Get distracted.** Text your friend. Check your e-mail. Take a couple of minutes to play a game on your phone. Grab a magazine or book. Your brain can only juggle so much stuff at once before it forgets about that cupcake, so take advantage.

✳ **Use your nose.** Keep a vanilla or green apple candle around and give it a sniff when a craving strikes. Smells that are sweet but that don't remind you of specific junky foods are thought to help curb appetite.

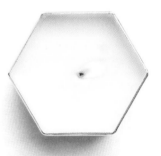

✳ **Imagine yourself indulging—a lot.** Thinking repeatedly about eating the thing that you're craving might be enough to make you want it less, according to research published in the journal *Science*.[7] Enjoy the experience through the visual exercise, and then move on.

✳ **Just have a small taste.** You might find that it's all you really wanted, anyway. Eating less than half an ounce of chocolate or potato chips satisfied subjects' cravings just as well as eating a portion as much as ten times bigger, according to one Cornell University study.[8] (Just be careful if you know that the food in question is a trigger for you. In that case, it's probably better to save the snack for a time that you planned ahead for, rather than eating it on impulse.)

✳ **Have a zero-calorie beverage.** Sip some water, sparkling water, or green tea. (Add a squeeze of fresh lemon or lime, for extra flavor.) Drinking can satisfy the urge to have something in your mouth, plus you might find that your hunger was really just thirst in disguise.

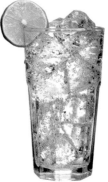

Notes from a Clean Eater

"When I have this urge to eat, I'll go out and walk. It takes the urge away, and it takes me out of that space of wondering, *What can I put in my mouth?*"—**Melissa R.**

Is It Hunger or a Craving?

Cravings are intense desires for *specific* foods and usually aren't signs that you're actually hungry. Remember: If your stomach is truly rumbling, something simple and

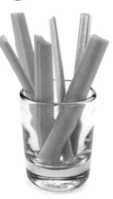

nutritious, such as an apple or celery sticks, will probably be appealing. But if only a double-fudge brownie or a pile of cheesy nachos will do? *That's* a craving.

Clean Eater

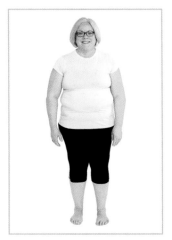

BEFORE

Mary Pat S.

As a self-described emotional eater, **Mary Pat** was quite literally used to eating whenever the mood struck her. Eating clean not only helped her learn to tell the difference between her hunger and her cravings, it also helped her find a daily rhythm for her meals and snacks that kept her from ever getting overly hungry.

"I felt like I had a lot of knowledge in my head about nutrition and what's healthy for you. But I wasn't able to sync it up with my actions," she says. Since she woke up to see her teenage daughter off to school, Mary Pat was used to eating breakfast early. She'd usually start to feel hungry by midmorning, but she'd try to hold off on eating. As a result, she'd be ravenous by lunchtime and would often end up overeating. "When I started following a schedule and having my morning snack, I noticed that what I ate for lunch satisfied me," she says.

Mary Pat reinforced the regular eating schedule by taking time to pause and fully enjoy her snacks. "I'd have a pumpkin ball (page 229) or some walnuts and tart cherries with a cup of herbal tea, and it was very satisfying," she says. Often, she'd even picture the hot water from the tea causing the nuts, seeds, or whole grains to expand in her stomach, which helped her feel fuller.

And when the urge to nosh off-schedule did strike? She'd try to respond with her head instead of her heart. "In the evening, when I'd be most likely to want to snack, I'd tell myself, *You know you just ate dinner. Those growls from your stomach are just digestion, not hunger,*" she observes. "It worked like a stop-pause for me."

Dr. Wendy Observes: Learning to differentiate between hunger and cravings can seem overwhelming, especially when you're prone to energy ups and downs that come from eating on an irregular schedule. I like to remind clients like Mary Pat to use their intellect as well as their emotions (*both* matter) and consider that often, we really do confuse healthy digestive sounds and rumblings for hunger. It's important to simply pause to consider that possibility before choosing to eat. Learning about balanced timing and snacks helped Mary Pat have foods ready to go and stable energy to make smart decisions about eating.

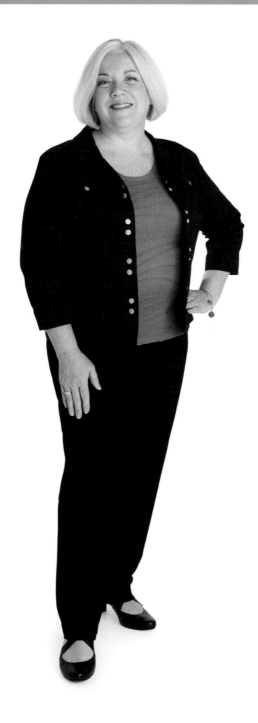

TOTAL POUNDS LOST

9 lbs

TOTAL INCHES LOST

7.5

MOST NOTABLE IMPROVEMENTS
Mary Pat lowered her fasting blood sugar by 38 points and increased her HDL ("good") cholesterol by 5 points. Plus, her systolic blood pressure (the top number) dropped by 21 points, which took it out of the risk zone.

Your Cravings Rx

Got chocolate and curly fries on the brain? That could be a sign that you're among the 90 percent of Americans missing out on at least one important vitamin or mineral. While a blood test is the only sure way to diagnose a nutrient deficiency, cravings can sometimes be a red flag. Here's a list of six common nutrients that are tough to get enough of and some tips on how to eat to beat cravings.

CALCIUM AND MAGNESIUM

Craving: Sweet or salty
Food fix: Make it a point to get more calcium from plain Greek yogurt, low-fat milk, or leafy greens. Get more magnesium from almonds, spinach, edamame, or avocados.

B VITAMINS

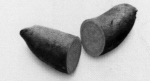

Craving: Sweet or salty
Food fix: B vitamins are found in many foods, but in varying quantities and combinations. Eating the following would give you a good mix: animal protein (such as poultry, lean beef, or salmon), yogurt, green veggies, beans, lentils, sweet potatoes, winter squash, sunflower seeds, avocados, and bananas.

ZINC

Craving: Sweet or salty
Food fix: Only certain proteins, such as oysters, crab, liver, and dark chicken meat, are high in this mineral. It's found to a lesser extent in eggs, black beans, cashews, and oatmeal.

IRON

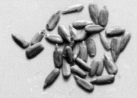

Craving: Fatty meat
Food fix: Beef, poultry, and fish have the most absorbable iron, but you can also increase your levels by eating dried fruits, cashews, pumpkin seeds, legumes (such as white beans and others), leafy greens, and iron-enriched pastas and grains. Boost the absorption of plant-based iron sources by eating them with vitamin C-rich foods such as citrus fruits, kiwifruit, berries, broccoli, or bell peppers.

OMEGA-3S

Craving: Cheese
Food fix: Focus on fatty fish, such as salmon, sardines, and canned tuna, as well as plant sources, such as walnuts, flaxseeds, and chia seeds.

Adapted from S. Eckelcamp, "Take Control of Your Eating & Never Diet Again," Prevention, January 2016, 119-21.

Putting It All Together

1 **Harness the power of mindful eating.** Focusing on your food can help you make choices you feel good about and can help you eat less overall.

2 **Remember that _what_ you want doesn't mean _whatever_ you want.** Occasional treats in reasonable portions can help you eat cleaner most of the time. Just don't overdo it.

3 **Listen to your stomach.** Check in to make sure you're hungry before you eat. And eat slowly to make sure that you stop when you're satisfied, not stuffed.

4 **Take the time to learn your triggers.** Keep a food journal to learn more about the feelings and situations that drive you to eat when you aren't hungry, and find other ways to cope.

5 **Know that cravings happen—but you can fight back.** Everyone gets struck with an urge to eat an ice cream cone or a bag of chips once in a while. But there are lots of tactics that can help you avoid giving in. Use them, and you'll have success!

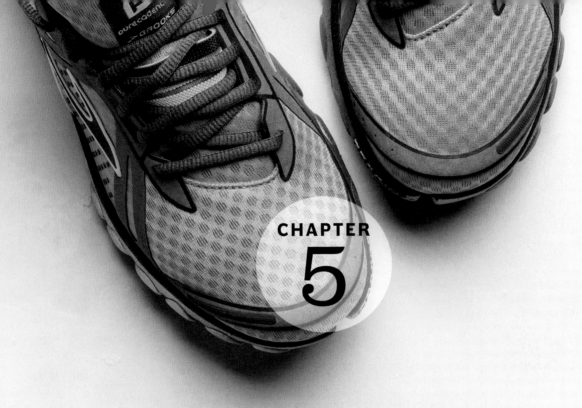

Moving Clean

Wait, isn't this supposed to be a book about eating clean? Well, yes. But eating clean and being active go hand in hand—and if you want to get serious about getting lean and feeling great, you've got to commit to both. Don't worry, that doesn't mean you need to turn into a gym rat or a triathlete! You just need to commit to building movement into your day—every day. Which, sure, might sound daunting now. But once you start reaping the feel-good (and get-lean) benefits of regular physical activity, you'll start to wonder how you ever got along without it. C'mon—let's take that first step!

Get Moving!

Maybe you try to exercise a few days a week when you have the time or if you're feeling up to it. Or maybe the last time you exercised voluntarily was during high school gym class. Either way, you're hardly alone: Two-thirds of American adults don't get the recommended 150 minutes of moderate physical activity per week. And more than one-quarter of us aren't active at all.[1]

Of course, there are a million reasons *not* to exercise. (I don't have the time! I can't afford a membership to that swanky gym! Working out is boring! I hate getting sweaty!) But here's the truth: **If you want to lose weight and keep it off, movement has to be a regular part of your life.** You don't have to devote hours to training for a marathon. You don't have to spend tons of your hard-earned cash on a deluxe gym membership, fancy sneakers, or designer workout clothes. You don't have to participate in an activity that you think is boring, uncomfortable, or just plain awful. You don't even have to get all that sweaty.

But you *do* have to move. Sure, you probably *could* lose weight through diet alone. But it wouldn't be much fun. Without burning those extra calories through exercise, you'd have to watch what you ate really, really carefully. Your portions would have to be smaller, so you'd be more likely to feel hungry between meals. And you wouldn't have much room for an afternoon snack, much less the occasional treat like a glass of wine or your favorite ice cream. Not so great, right?

There's more. Active folks tend to have more lean muscle mass than couch potatoes do, and muscle plays an important role in keeping your metabolism fired up. But most importantly, being active supports a clean lifestyle as a whole. When you exercise, your body pumps out feel-good endorphins that boost your energy and mood and lower your stress levels. Expending all that extra energy throughout the day also means that you'll likely sleep better at night. In short, exercise helps you feel better overall. And the better you feel, the more likely you are to want to eat clean and make other choices that promote your overall health and well-being.

Dr. Wendy Says . . .

Remember, being active can—and should!—be *fun*. The key is finding forms of exercise that you can enjoy doing instead of ones that feel like work. Often, that means aligning your workout with another pleasurable activity, which can make it more tolerable even at a time when you're not feeling particularly enthusiastic. Think bicycling while you listen to your favorite music or podcast, taking an aerobics class with your friends, or walking—and bonding—with your dog. And you know what else? Every bit of movement counts. Give yourself an extra boost by taking steps to build more movement into your everyday activities. Whether you're taking another lap around the mall before heading home or carrying in those heavy grocery bags yourself instead of asking your kid to do it, those short bouts of exercise can add up to a seriously healthier—and leaner—body.

Moving Your Way

If eating clean is all about making better choices without actually having to follow a traditional, rule-crazy diet, moving clean is all about living an active lifestyle without having to follow a rigid workout plan. Yup, that's right! There's no law saying you have to slog it out on the treadmill or elliptical; navigate those clunky, confusing weight machines; or even step foot inside a gym. The only thing you have to do is make sure you build physical activity into your day—every day. Don't worry; even if you're brand new to exercise or totally strapped for time, it's easier than you think.

Eat Clean, Stay Lean Exercise Essentials

What counts as a workout versus a leisurely stroll? And how long do you need to be active each day in order to support your weight-loss efforts? Here's exactly what you need to know in order to exercise effectively.

❊ **Move daily.** Aim to be active at least 6 days a week for a minimum of 30 minutes each day. If you can squeeze in 45 minutes or an hour, that's even better! The more you move, the more benefits you'll reap with regards to your weight—and your health.

❊ **Find something fun.** When it comes to exercise, consistency is key. So pick an activity that's worth looking forward to! Whether it's walking briskly through the park, taking a dance class, or playing tennis with your pals, it won't feel like work if you're having a good time. Just plain don't enjoy being active? Okay—find something that you can at least *tolerate*.

❊ **Make a rock-solid plan.** Each week, look at your schedule and figure out how you'll meet your movement quota. Will you walk before work? Meet your friend for kickboxing class in the evening? Whatever you decide, put it on your calendar. When you treat exercise like an appointment, you're less likely to skip out.

❊ **Amp up the intensity.** Your workout doesn't have to leave you panting or sweating buckets. (Though if you want to do something intense, get your doctor's okay and go for it!) But it does need to be vigorous enough to get your heart rate up. To find your sweet spot, just use the talk test: You should be able to carry on a light conversation but be a little too winded to be able to sing a song. At that level of intensity, your body will start to feel a bit warmer, and your breathing rate will begin to increase.

✳ **Break things up.** Can't fit in a full workout in one fell swoop? No problem. A few chunks of activity can be just as effective as one long sweat session, so feel free to spread your exercise out over the course of your day. Just try to work in at least 20 minutes at a time. Aiming for this amount will help you burn more calories and—just as important—will lead to better blood sugar control. After about 20 minutes of movement, your cells start working more efficiently to pull extra sugar from your blood to transform it into usable energy instead of letting it turn into fat. Amazingly, this effect can last for up to 24 hours.

The World's Easiest Exercise

We're talking about walking! A quarter of people who lose weight and keep it off rely on this simple activity for their daily exercise. And if you're new to being active or you just want to keep things simple, walking is a fantastic tool for achieving your weight-loss goals and improving your overall health.

Of course, easy doesn't mean that you don't have to put in any effort. (You do. Remember the talk test?) Instead, it means that it's easy to *do*. No matter what your current fitness level, you can start walking—even if you've never exercised before in your life. And you don't need any fancy equipment or a gym membership to get started. All you have to do is put on some comfortable clothes and sneakers, swing open the front door, and put one foot in front of the other. That's all there is to it. As long as you're keeping a brisk pace for at least 20 minutes, you're doing walking right.

You can walk when it's warm or cold, when it's sunny or rainy (just bring an umbrella!), and when it's morning, afternoon, or evening. An a.m. walk is a great way to ramp up your energy for the day ahead, while an after-lunch walk can combat the dreaded midday slump. As for walking after dinner? When it comes to decompressing after a long day, it beats watching TV on the couch by a landslide. Try it—you'll see. And remember, if you'd rather walk indoors, you can do that, too. Stock up on a few different walking workout DVDs, or take laps around the mall. If it gets you walking, it *works*.

Notes from a Clean Eater

"I try to walk outside no matter what the weather is like. I'll take a big umbrella sometimes. But if I get wet, it's not a big deal."—**Kathy C.**

Rise and Shine!

The best time to exercise is whatever time works for you. But for a lot of us, that time might be first thing in the morning. Research shows that a.m. exercisers tend to be more consistent than p.m. exercisers—in part because they run into fewer workout-derailing scheduling conflicts. What's more, you'll start your day on an energized, productive foot because exercise floods your system with feel-good endorphins. So set that alarm and give it a try. When 5:30 p.m. comes and the inevitable late-day meeting or unexpected dinner invitation comes through, you'll be so glad you did.

Stepping It Up

Maybe you already have a habit of walking regularly, and you want to take things up a notch in order to accelerate your weight loss. That's great! Ramping up the intensity of your workout is a smart move, and it doesn't have to get complicated. Here are two ways you can start feeling the burn.

1. Add in some intervals. Injecting brief periods of intense effort into your regular walks (or runs, swims, bike rides, or other types of cardio) kicks your metabolism up to a slightly higher rate—and the boost can last for hours. As a result, you keep on burning more calories even *after* your exercise session is over. Talk about more bang for your buck!

Not sure how to introduce intervals into your routine? If you're a walker and you typically exercise for 30 minutes, sprinkle in a 30-second burst of jogging every 5 minutes. As you become more fit, you can

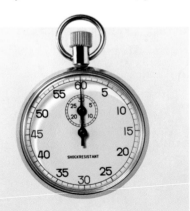

Walk This Way

For some people, the beauty of walking is that it doesn't feel like a formal workout. But what if you want to add a little more structure to your strolls? Bring along a wristwatch or stopwatch, and try alternating walking with other get-fit moves, like:

✳ **Walking lunges**
✳ **Pushups or modified pushups**
✳ **Jumping jacks**

For more ideas, look up our favorite walking workouts at bazilians.com/ECSLdiet/extras.

2,800

This is the number of calories burned per week by individuals who successfully lose weight and keep it off. Sounds like a lot, right? But the number is actually much more manageable than it seems. When you break it down, 2,800 calories a week equals . . .

❋ 400 to 500 calories per day
❋ *or* 4 to 5 miles per day
❋ *or* 10,000 steps per day

increase the length of your intervals to a full minute and decrease the walking segments to 4 minutes. For the biggest metabolism boost, the interval portion needs to be challenging, so go all out! If you're breathing very hard by the end, you're doing it right.

2. Start strength training. While your heart and other organs demand fuel around the clock, there's little you can do to increase their metabolic needs. However, your muscles—which also require constant feeding—are changeable. Make them bigger, and they will demand more calories day and night. (Not to mention that they'll give you a leaner, more sculpted shape.)

Happily, you don't need tons of time or a gym membership to strength train effectively. With the right moves and a basic set of dumbbells, you can work all of your major muscle groups in the time it takes for you to watch your favorite sitcom. Perform strength-training exercises two or three times a week, and your muscles will soon turn into furnaces that burn up extra calories before your body can convert them into fat. Find our effective, easy-to-follow 30-minute routine at bazilians.com/ECSLdiet/extras.)

Tips for Trackers

Pedometers and other wearables count the number of steps you take throughout the day to estimate how much distance you've covered. Some also come with a stopwatch to literally clock the amount of time you spend exercising. You don't *need* these devices to exercise, but they can make it easier to figure out whether you're meeting your daily movement goals. Plus, a tracker can deliver a major motivational boost: You'll likely find yourself trying to beat yesterday's step count or sneak in another half mile. If you opt to use one, here are a few tips for making the most of it.

✳ **Pick a step goal.** For general health, aim to work up to 10,000 steps per day. In order to lose weight or maintain your weight loss, you may need to bump it up to 12,000 to 15,000 steps per day.

✳ **Work your way up.** If you're new to exercising, taking 10,000 steps per day might seem daunting. That's okay! Can you manage 3,000 or 5,000 steps? Once that feels good, try adding in another 1,000 steps. Every time you increase your step goal, you're getting a little bit more fit.

✳ **Track daily.** For the most accurate picture of your overall movement, wear your pedometer or tracker every day. Put it in a prominent spot that makes putting it on first thing in the morning easy to remember—next to your alarm clock or near your toothbrush are both good choices. Don't think you'll remember to don your device? Use a step counting app on your smartphone, instead. Findings show that they're just as accurate as other trackers,[2] and chances are, you always have yours with you.

Everyday Activity

Moving clean is about more than just exercising for 30 or 60 minutes a day. In order to live a truly active lifestyle, it's important to find ways to weave more movement into all aspects of your day. For instance, taking the steps instead of the elevator. Or visiting your coworker's office to talk about a project instead of sending an e-mail or instant message. Or walking into the coffee shop instead of cruising through the drive-thru. See how many opportunities there are to sneak in some extra steps?

We get it. You might be thinking, *I already* did *my workout. Why do I need to worry about getting even more activity?* For starters, because every little bit of movement counts. Parking at the far end of the lot on one grocery shopping trip or skipping the escalator at the mall might not burn many calories on its own. But over the course of a day, a week, a month, or even more, all of that extra effort adds up—and it can help support your efforts to get leaner. On the other hand, spending hours and hours sitting can send your body into Fat Storage Land. It can zap your energy, too—which only encourages you to spend *more* time in your chair or on the couch.

The Scary Side of Sitting

Most of us sit while we work. We sit while we drive to work or to the store. And we sit at home while we eat, watch TV, and scroll through our phones. Problem is, all of that sitting can be pretty harmful to your health—even if you're a regular exerciser.

Just how bad is keeping your keister in a chair all day? In terms of your heart and lung health, 2 hours of sedentary behavior (sitting, driving, or working on your computer) is as bad for you as 20 minutes of exercise is good for you, according to *Mayo Clinic Proceedings* research.[3] Too much time on your tuckus is also associated with a higher risk for obesity, type 2 diabetes, metabolic syndrome, and even cancer.[4]

What is it about sitting that's so bad for you? One line of thought is that when you're sitting all day long, your muscles produce fewer fat-burning enzymes, which can raise your blood sugar. Another theory is that your body becomes so accustomed to sitting that your muscles don't work as well when you try to do other activities, which hurts your posture and your ability to exercise. Are you jumping out of your seat yet?

Do This Now!

Take a look at the clock. How long have you been sitting here reading? If it's been more than 30 minutes, put down your book, stand up, and take a movement break. Stretch your arms and legs, walk to the kitchen for a glass of water, or head outside to grab the mail. We'll still be here when you get back!

Moving More, All Day Long

Okay, so you'll make a mental note to take the stairs more often instead of the elevator or escalator. And you'll try to park as far away from the supermarket or the drugstore as you can. (Fine—as long as it's not raining.) But aside from those oft-repeated tips, what else can you realistically do? Moving more throughout the day might seem tough if your job has you chained to a desk or if you live in a neighborhood that's within walking distance of, well, nothing. But you can do it—and chances are, making the extra effort to move will leave you feeling great. Here are some ideas to get you started.

WHEN YOU'RE AT HOME . . .

✽ **Be an inefficient cleaner.** Sure, putting things away in one big haul is the *fastest* way to tidy up, but making several smaller trips nets you way more steps. (And you won't end up dropping stuff all over the floor!)

✽ **Axe the TV ads.** When you're watching the tube, get off the couch and take a lap around the house every time there's a commercial break. They're boring anyway, so why sit there watching them?

❋ **Go *find* your family members.** Do you usually make a habit of yelling for your spouse or kids from the other side of the house? Swap the shouting for walking over to talk to them, instead. Bonus: You may never again have to hear anyone bellow, "Whaaaaat?!"

❋ **Adopt an audiobook habit.** If reading is your favorite type of downtime, trade your hard copy for an audiobook. Download it to your smartphone and listen while you walk the dog, tend the garden, or cook dinner.

❋ **Pretend your cell phone is a landline.** Leave it in a central location, like the kitchen, and turn the ringer way up. Whenever you hear a ping, you'll have to *get up* to grab the phone. What a throwback, right?

WHEN YOU'RE AT WORK . . .

❋ **Walk and talk.** When you're on the phone, pace around instead of sitting at your desk. Rather than drafting a lengthy e-mail to your coworker, head over to her office and talk in person. Got a meeting? Suggest that the gang go for a walk instead of gathering around the conference room table.

❋ **Set an alarm.** It's easy to go hours without getting up when you're buried in projects or e-mails, so set an alarm on your phone or computer to go off every half hour. When it goes off, walk or stretch for a full 2 minutes before sitting back down.

❋ **Be the picker upper.** When your gang places an order for coffee or lunch, give the intern or delivery guy a break and offer to go fetch the stuff yourself.

❋ **Hack a standing workstation.** March in place while you file paperwork, sit on an exercise ball instead of an office chair, or do squats while you brainstorm or dictate notes. Have the resources to make some bigger changes? Consider investing in a treadmill and securing a tray to the front where you can put your laptop and phone while you work. (Just walk slowly—think 1.0 to 2.0 mph, max—so you are active, productive, *and* safe at the same time!)

❋ **Trash your wastebasket.** When you have to throw something out, get up and toss it in a common area trash can.

WHEN YOU'RE ON THE GO . . .

❋ **Stroll the supermarket.** Take a lap around the perimeter of the store before you start filling your cart.

❋ **Do a power pickup.** Walk to pick your kids up from school instead of driving, if you can. If you have to drive, get out and greet them with a big hug instead of waiting for them in the car.

❋ **Walk off your wait times.** Have time to kill before the doctor, dentist, or hairstylist is ready for you? Head outside for a walk instead of waiting in the reception area, and ask for a call or text when it's time to come in.

❋ **Get off at another stop.** If you travel by bus or train, hop off a couple of stops early and walk the rest of the way to your destination.

✻ **Give yourself permission to window shop.** Go ahead—take a detour to check out what's new at your favorite store. If you find something you love, decide that you'll reward yourself after you lose *X* number of pounds.

Eating and Exercise

The idea of exercising might conjure up notions of energy bars and protein shakes. After all, don't you need extra energy to fuel all of that movement?

It may surprise you to learn that for most people, the answer is no. Sure, athletes who train for hours on end certainly need more food to supply their muscles with adequate energy and to avoid zonking out on the field. But for the average person, 30 minutes or even an hour of moderate exercise probably isn't enough to justify an extra snack before or after a workout. Especially when you're trying to lose weight. Even though your 30-minute jog or hour of brisk walking *felt* like tons of hard work, it only takes an extra fruit-and-yogurt smoothie or whole wheat bagel with peanut butter to undo all of that effort. That's not to say that your everyday workout isn't good

enough—it *is*, and you should be proud of the fact that you put in the effort. But most of the time, it likely isn't enough to justify eating extra food. (If you regularly do longer or more intense workouts, consider consulting with a sports nutritionist. Together, you can fine-tune your meals and snacks to fuel your performance and reach your weight-loss goals.)

Still, it can be tough to forget the pre- or postworkout snack advice that most of us have heard over and over. And depending on what time you exercise, you might feel legitimately hungry when it comes time to start moving. But with a little extra planning, you can be active at any time of day without feeling too hungry.

It's All in Your Head

Think of your workout as pleasure instead of business, and your urge to snack just might subside. In one study from Cornell University, people who saw their walk as formal exercise took more than twice as much candy postworkout compared to those who saw their walk as a leisurely, scenic stroll. In a second study, those who perceived their walk as exercise instead of fun opted for a dessert of chocolate pudding and soda instead of applesauce—and took in 42 percent more calories.[6] The next time you're tempted to grab a bite as you slip on your sneakers, try looking at your daily activity in a different light. A simple shift in mind-set could make a major difference. Have fun!

❊ **If you exercise in the morning . . .** If you tend to be hungry when working out first thing in the a.m., split breakfast into two mini-meals. You can literally eat half of your breakfast before exercising and have the rest after your shower, or you can eat two snack-size breakfasts. Half a slice of toast with peanut butter and sliced banana or half of a fruit-and-protein smoothie are both good options. Not interested in food when you wake up? No problem. Just exercise first and eat breakfast afterwards. You don't *need* any extra fuel.

❊ **If you exercise after work . . .** Save your afternoon snack, and eat it an hour or so before your workout. You'll get the energy you need to make it through your exercise (and showering and getting dinner on the table), but since you're having a planned snack that you would have eaten anyway,

Dr. Wendy Says . . .

Whether you're walking around your neighborhood for 30 minutes or going all-out during an hour-long spin class, hydration is an essential part of healthy exercise. You need to get the right amount of water to replace the water you lose from sweat while you're active in order to feel energized and perform your best. Skip your regular sips, and you're more likely to feel fatigued, get muscle cramps, and even feel dizzy. (And there's no need for sports drinks. They're high in calories and sugar that you don't need. Plus, plain old water is nature's perfect source of hydration!)

So how much water do you need? A good rule of thumb is to drink water throughout the day, sip 6 to 12 ounces about 15 minutes before you start working out, and rehydrate with another 2 to 3 cups of water after you're done.

you're not actually taking in any extra calories that you don't need.

One more thing: Remember to always home in on your true hunger level. For many of us, it's common for exercise to act as a trigger for snacking—whether our stomachs are rumbling or not. So try to forget about what you *think* you should be doing or what you feel like you might deserve as a reward for exercising, and just think about how you actually feel. If you're eating three clean meals and two or three clean snacks per day, you should be pretty satisfied!

Putting It All Together

1 **Move more, period!** Being active helps you burn more calories, have more energy, and make healthier choices overall—which helps you lose more weight.

2 **Make it a habit.** Consistency is key, so find ways to be active every day—even if you don't have time for a full workout.

3 **Have fun!** You're more likely to stick with an activity that you enjoy than you are one that feels like drudgery. As long as it gets your heart rate up and you do it for at least 20 minutes, it counts!

4 **Add more activity into the rest of your day.** Being sedentary is bad for your health—even if you exercise. Plus, being more active throughout your day can help you burn extra calories and boost your energy.

5 **Skip the extra snacks.** Pre- and postworkout snacks aren't usually necessary, and they can slow your weight loss.

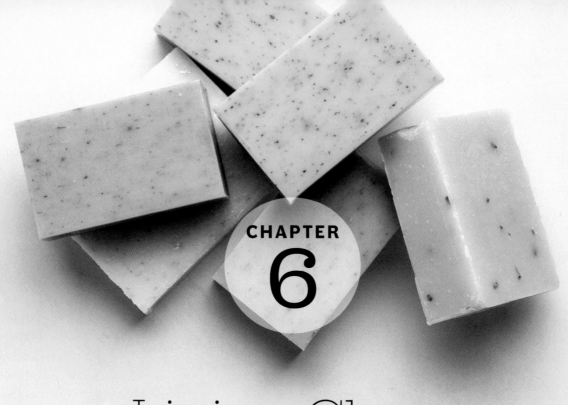

Living Clean

You've already made the important decision to choose clean, wholesome foods over their processed and artificial counterparts. It's a big step that empowers you to take charge of your health and lose weight—and you should feel good about it! Now it's time to take a closer look at the *other* stuff you use on a daily basis that could be exposing you to chemicals that may have a negative impact on your weight. After all, if you're already making the effort to nourish your body with the right food, why derail those efforts with other dirty products? Eating clean is an important first step, but you can go further. The pages ahead will show you how.

Taking the Next Clean Step

Learning about the weird ingredients in processed foods—and how they affect your moods, energy levels, and weight—can feel like a major wake-up call. And for many people, making the shift to a cleaner diet is the first step toward living a cleaner life overall. Because, unfortunately, dirty ingredients don't just lurk in foods. They can also hide in the cleaner you use to wipe your countertop after cooking, the soap you use in the shower, and even the makeup you apply when you're getting ready for a night out.

We know. You're probably thinking, *I already get that the chemicals in heavy-duty products like drain cleaner can mess with the environment or that breathing in fumes from, say, oven cleaner might leave me woozy (or worse). But can a tube of moisturizer or a bottle of window cleaner really be hurting my health—and be the thing that's keeping me from getting lean?* At first glance, we know it might seem a little far-fetched. So just hear us out.

On its own, it seems unlikely that the ingredients in one measly product could have a significant impact on your overall health *or* your weight. (Though for the time being, there haven't been any studies to prove *otherwise*.) But here's the thing: You don't use just one product. No one does. We use gels and soaps and lotions and lipsticks and deodorants to make our bodies look and smell nice, along with sprays and wipes and detergents to do the same thing for our homes and workplaces. **So even if you're eating a squeaky-clean diet made entirely from unprocessed foods, it's likely that you're *still* being exposed to hundreds of different chemicals every day. And a heavy chemical load could have unintended consequences for your body—including making it harder for the pounds to come off.**

Dr. Wendy Says . . .

Trying to steer clear of every potentially harmful chemical out there would be overwhelming—not to mention almost impossible! After all, you can't control what type of cleaner the custodian at your bank uses to wipe down the counter where you make your deposits, or the type of hand soap that your neighbor keeps in her guest bathroom.

What you *can* do? Make a conscious decision to seek out safer products for yourself and your home when you can. Remember, it's not about being perfect!

By surrounding yourself with cleaner goods most of the time, you'll reduce your exposure to toxic chemicals in a major way. And that could spell the difference between a scale that won't budge and one that starts trending downward.

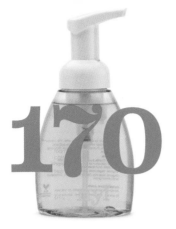

170

That's how many chemicals the average woman is exposed to from the 12 personal-care products she uses each day. And guys don't fare much better: The average man uses 6 products per day, exposing him to close to 90 different chemicals.[1] Think about the good you'll do just by swapping out one or two conventional products for cleaner ones.

Indecent Exposure

You don't eat shampoo or soap or the spray that you use to wipe down your kitchen counter. So how exactly are you being exposed to the unsavory ingredients found in your personal-care or cleaning products? Believe it or not, you don't actually have to put any of this stuff in your mouth in order for it to have a potentially harmful effect.

Consider your skin. You might think of it as being like a brick wall, with nothing going in or coming out unless you have a cut or wound. But in reality, your skin is a lot more like a sponge. It's porous, and most of what you put on it—from lotions to hair gel to makeup—gets absorbed right into your bloodstream. (Still skeptical? Think about topical medications like nicotine patches or fungal creams. If they can't get inside your body, how do you think they work?) The same goes for stuff that *isn't* designed to go on your skin, such as cleaning products. Most cleaners contain wetting agents called surfactants, which allow a product to carry away oils. Because they're designed to help cleaners penetrate surfaces, surfactants are also really good at allowing cleaners—and their toxic ingredients—to penetrate your skin. In fact,

Watch Your Mouth!

If you ever use lipstick, lip gloss, or lip balm, you could be eating some of these not-so-savory ingredients after all. A recent FDA test of more than 400 products showed that, on average, lipsticks contain 1.11 parts per million of lead.[2] According to the FDA, these numbers are considered safe because people don't actually ingest lipstick. Still, think about it: If you've ever finished a meal and found that all of your meticulously applied lip color disappeared along with your food, that lead-containing lipstick had to go *somewhere,* right? Swap your conventional lipstick, gloss, or balm for a cleaner alternative, and you just might save yourself a side dish of heavy metals.

one study published in the *American Journal of Public Health* found that the skin absorbs, on average, 64 percent of the chemicals that it's exposed to.[3] And when it comes to fragrance ingredients like phthalates (more on those later), researchers theorize that the skin's absorption rate could be as high as 100 percent.[4] Yikes.

That's not all. You know how the fumes from things like glass cleaner, hairspray, and even nail polish or polish remover tend to make you cough or even feel a little dizzy if you get too close to them or use them in a poorly ventilated space? These products (and many others) contain volatile organic compounds (VOCs), chemicals that are emitted into the air as a vapor or gas. The health effects of some VOCs remain unknown, but exposure to others is linked to a range of problems—including headaches and dizziness, as well as kidney, liver, and central nervous system damage, according to researchers at the US National Library of Medicine.[5]

Tipping the Scales

Okay, so you get that most of us are exposed to a ton of questionable chemicals through our personal-care and cleaning products. But how exactly do these chemicals affect your weight loss? Back in Chapter 1, we talked about the endocrine-disrupting effects of the BPA and BPS found in plastic containers and canned food linings. But these chemicals show up in personal-care and cleaning products, too. And because endocrine disruptors are capable of mimicking or blocking hormones like estrogen, androgen, and thyroid hormones, they can play some weird tricks on your body—like prompting your cells to store more fat.

Indeed, a growing number of studies are now linking exposure to endocrine-disrupting chemicals with weight gain.[6] In fact, experts writing in the *Journal of Clinical Endocrinology and Metabolism* estimate that endocrine-disrupting chemicals could be responsible for nearly 54,000 cases of obesity and more than 20,000 cases of diabetes in older women living in the European Union,[7] where use of these chemicals is *more* tightly regulated than it is in the United States. Who would've thought that a little tube of hand cream or a bottle of window cleaner could possibly have such a significant impact on your body?

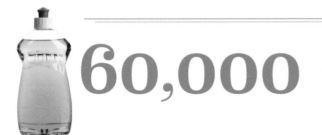

60,000

The number of ingredients regularly used in consumer goods and cleaning products that have not been adequately tested for safety, according to estimates from the Environmental Working Group.[8]

But that's not all. While endocrine disruptors appear to have a more direct impact on your weight, there are plenty of other chemicals that could have an indirect influence by affecting your health in other ways. For instance, chemicals that are derived from the preservative formaldehyde are linked to issues like asthma, headaches, dizziness, and fatigue. Others, like triclosan, have been shown to have a negative impact on your immune system.[9] And when you just feel lousy, it's a lot harder to muster up the energy to eat right or be active.

Of course, those are just the weighty effects of some of the chemicals that we *do* know about. Like many of the chemicals found in processed or conventional foods, we're still in the dark about much of what goes into our personal-care products and cleaners. Similar to packaged food additives, many of the ingredients used in cosmetics haven't actually been tested by the FDA because they're considered to be "generally recognized as safe." (For more about GRAS ingredients, see page 48 in Chapter 3.) Things get even sketchier when it comes to cleaning products. The federal government doesn't require them to disclose their ingredients, *period*, so you'll be hard-pressed to figure out what, exactly, goes into making

Scent Heavy

Laundry detergent that smells like you let your towels air-dry in the sun. Air fresheners that turn your house into a pine-scented forest. Perfume that instantly transports you to a gorgeous rose garden. The fragrances in many of our personal-care and household products smell surprisingly realistic. But you can be almost certain that they're completely artificial.

The truth is, the vast majority of natural-smelling scents are developed in test tube–filled labs. The International Fragrance Association readily admits that manufacturers use nearly 3,000 chemical ingredients to create the scents that are added to most consumer products.[10] And some, including phthalates, are known endocrine disruptors with ties to obesity.

Considering the fact that scented products are pretty much everywhere, it comes as no surprise that most of us are exposed to chemicals like phthalates on a daily basis: According to nationally representative data from the National Health and Nutrition Examination Survey, more than 75 percent of participants had detectable levels of phthalates in their urine.[11] And if you regularly spritz on perfume, your exposure could be considerably higher. Compared to women who hadn't recently worn a scent, those who had used perfume within the previous 24 hours had nearly three times more phthalates in their urine, one University of Rochester study found.[12]

Fortunately, there *are* ways to reduce your exposure. Start by steering clear of products that contain ingredients like "fragrance" or "parfum," as both are often code for phthalates. If you love using perfumes or other scented products, consider seeking out chemical-free alternatives that are certified organic and made with plant-derived ingredients such as essential oils.

that bright blue bottle of glass cleaner or dish gel.

Added together, the effects that all of these chemicals have on the scale might be more significant than you think. On average, people are around 10 percent heavier today than they were in the 1970s.[13] But all of the extra weight we're carrying around these days isn't *just* the result of eating more and moving less, as we're often told. Exposure to environmental chemicals and pollutants, including those found in many personal-care products and other goods, may also play a role, say experts writing in *Obesity Research & Clinical Practice*.[14]

Cleaning Up Your Personal Care

Ready to get the gunk out of your gels, lotions, cosmetics, and creams? Cleaner personal care has come a long way from the crunchy natural products once confined to dusty health food stores. Today, there are more options than ever made from easy-to-recognize, plant-based ingredients that help you scrub, primp, and preen just as well—if not better!—than their conventional counterparts. Here's how to track them down and work more of them into your routine.

Build Your Ingredient Blacklist

Personal-care product labels are often a jumble of sciencey words that might as well be a foreign language. Rather than trying to learn them all, focus on this manageable list of dirty ingredients. By skipping products that contain them, you'll scrub the most offensive chemicals and additives out of your hygiene routine.

1. Phthalates. A group of endocrine-disrupting chemicals, phthalates show up regularly in lipstick, lotions, makeup, nail polish, perfumes, and other products that contain artificial scents. Phthalates have been linked to weight gain and diabetes, and one study even tied certain phthalates to potentially increasing

Dr. Wendy Says . . .

Replacing all of the products in your medicine cabinet or makeup bag in one fell swoop can be a big, expensive job. **Instead, take the one-out, one-in approach: When you run out of an existing product, just replace it with a cleaner alternative.** Each time, you'll reduce your chemical exposure by around 15 unique ingredients, according to data from the Environmental Working Group.[15] And within a few months, you'll have cleaned up your entire personal-care routine.

the risk for breast cancer.[16] Choose organic or phthalate-free products, instead.

Other names: You'll never actually see the word "phthalates" on a list of ingredients. Instead, look for "fragrance" or "parfum."

2. Parabens. These preservatives are used to keep bacteria, yeast, and mold from growing in your deodorant, shampoo, conditioner, aftershave, moisturizer, and makeup—which sounds like a good thing. But they also mimic estrogen in the body, which research suggests could increase the risk for breast cancer.[17] Look for organic products or those that are paraben-free.

Other names : Ethylparaben, butylparaben, methylparaben, propylparaben, isobutylparaben, isopropylparaben, other ingredients ending in -paraben.

3. Formaldehyde-releasing preservatives. Like parabens, these chemicals are designed to keep bacteria at bay in products like shampoos, conditioners, moisturizers, cleansers, lotions, hair gels, and shaving creams. But they expose you to formaldehyde—a probable human carcinogen—whenever you suds up. Choose organic products or those that are free of preservatives.

Other names : Diazolidinyl urea, DMDM hydantoin, quaternium-15, and sodium hydroxymethylglycinate

4. Sulfates. Found in shampoos, facial cleansers, and body washes, sulfates are responsible for creating suds and bubbles. But they're harsh detergents, and they often contain a potentially cancerous chemical called 1,4-dioxane that—frighteningly enough—isn't required to be listed on product labels. Look for organic or sulfate-free products.

Other names: Sodium lauryl sulfate, sodium laureth sulfate, ammonium lauryl sulfate, sodium lauryl sulfoacetate

5. Toluene. Wanna know what gives nail polish and hair dye that glossy, eye-popping shine? It's toluene, a petroleum-based chemical used in paint thinner that can cause dizziness, nausea, and fatigue. Some research also suggests that toluene could be an endocrine disruptor, and the chemical may also be linked to immune system toxicity.[18] And since toluene is a volatile organic compound (VOC), you can be exposed to the stuff just by breathing it in. Choose organic or toluene-free products, instead.

Other names: Butylated hydroxytoluene, benzoic acid, benzyl

6. Other petroleum-based chemicals. Used in deodorant, aftershave, hair gel, and shampoo, these chemicals are often contaminated with formaldehyde or 1,4-dioxane. Many are also classified as skin irritants. (And remember what we said about skin? It's like a sponge.)

Other names: Propylene glycol, polyethylene glycol (PEG)

7. Butylated hydroxyanisole (BHA). An endocrine disruptor and possible carcinogen, this preservative typically shows up in makeup—including concealer, mascara, blush, eyeliner, and lip gloss.

Other names: Antioxyne B, Antrancine I2, EEC No. E320, Embanox, Nipantiox I-F, Protex, Sustane I-F, Tenox BHA

Find Trustworthy Replacements

Poring over ingredients lists is one way to make sure the products you buy are free of potentially harmful chemicals. But if you're not quite sure of your label-reading prowess, you can get some extra assurance from a third party.

❊ **Go for organic.** Like with food, the term "natural" is unregulated—and it doesn't necessarily mean that the ingredients in your lipstick, shampoo, or shaving cream came from nature. To know that you're truly steering clear of synthetics and additives, look for personal-care products that bear the USDA certified organic seal, which ensures that a product is made with at least 95 percent organic ingredients. And if you spot an "organic" product without the seal, do some homework before you buy it. The *word* "organic" isn't actually regulated—only the USDA certified organic seal is—and some manufacturers do use the term even when their products actually aren't organic. (Crazy, right?)

❊ **Check up on your brands.** If you can't seem to find a certified organic version of the item you're looking for? Head to a trusted cosmetics database like the Environmental Working Group's Skin Deep (ewg.org/skindeep). It rates the safety of more than 60,000 personal-care products, making it easy to find the cleanest alternatives out there.

❊ **Find your favorites and stick with them.** Sure, tracking down trustworthy products takes a little bit of time up front. But remember, that little bit of research is a long-term investment in your health. Plus, once you find your new go-tos, there's nothing left to do but toss a fresh bottle in your cart when the old one goes empty.

❊ **Don't discount DIY.** You don't have to worry about funky ingredients when you use personal-care products made from items found in your refrigerator or pantry. And many are easier to whip up than you might think. (See "Clean Enough to Eat" on page 102.)

Clean, Green Goods

Overwhelmed by all the options? These easy-to-find clean brands are ideal places to start.

❊ **Shampoo and conditioner:** Whole Foods Market 365 Everyday Value, Avalon Organics
❊ **Facial care:** Weleda, Origins
❊ **Body wash:** The Honest Company, Yes To
❊ **Lotions and moisturizers:** NOW Solutions, J. R. Watkins
❊ **Cosmetics:** Jane Iredale, Tarte

❊ **Nail polish:** Butter London, Zoya
❊ **Toothpaste and mouthwash:** Tom's of Maine, Nature's Gate
❊ **Shaving cream and aftershave:** Dr. Bronner's, Aveda

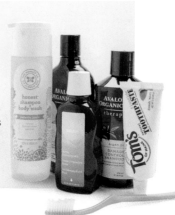

Clean Enough to Eat

When it comes to natural beauty, whole foods are some of the most powerful ingredients around. Whip up these DIY masks, scrubs, and moisturizers for more youthful skin, healthier hair, and a head-to-toe glow.

FOR YOUR FACE

FOR BRIGHTER SKIN

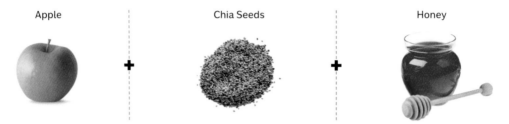

Apple   +   Chia Seeds   +   Honey

In a blender or food processor, combine ½ cup of chopped raw green apple, 2 tablespoons of chia seeds, and 2 tablespoons of honey. Blend or process until smooth, adding a few drops of water if necessary. Massage the mixture into dry skin and rinse well.

Why it works: The antioxidants and alpha hydroxy acids in green apples help brighten, soothe, and plump skin, while the chia seeds and honey exfoliate and deep clean.

FOR DEWIER, MORE YOUTHFUL SKIN

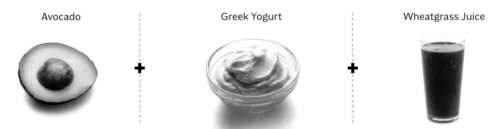

Avocado   +   Greek Yogurt   +   Wheatgrass Juice

In a blender or food processor, combine ½ avocado, 2 tablespoons of plain Greek yogurt, and I tablespoon of wheatgrass juice. Blend or process until smooth. (You can find wheatgrass juice frozen at natural food stores, or get it fresh at juice bars.) Apply the mixture to your face, let it sit for 20 minutes, and rinse with warm water.

Why it works: Avocado's healthy fats deliver moisture, while its vitamin E helps improve skin's texture. The lactic acid in yogurt gently loosens dead skin cells, and the wheatgrass adds a punch of vitamins A and E—antiaging powerhouses.

FOR YOUR FACE *(cont.)*

FOR CALMER SKIN AND LESS REDNESS

Blueberries	Almonds	Oats	Honey + Milk

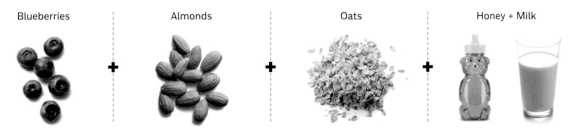

In a blender or food processor, combine ¼ cup of blueberries, ¼ cup of raw almonds, 2 tablespoons of rolled oats, I tablespoon of honey, and I tablespoon of milk. Blend or process until smooth. Apply the mixture to moistened skin and let it sit for 20 minutes, or until dry. Massage the mixture in a slow, circular motion until it crumbles away. Rinse with warm water.

Why it works: Oats have anti-inflammatory properties that help reduce redness, while milk and honey help cleanse and brighten skin. Blueberries and raw almonds deliver phytochemicals and skin-soothing vitamin E.

FOR YOUR HAIR

FOR HEALTHIER, SHINIER HAIR

Avocado	Honey	Olive Oil

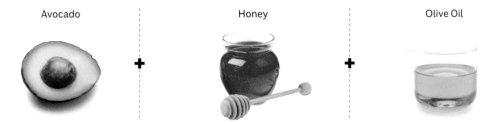

In a small bowl, mash I ripe avocado with I to 2 tablespoons of honey and 3 to 5 tablespoons of olive oil. Apply to your hair from the roots to the ends, and let it sit for 30 to 60 minutes. Rinse well.

Why it works: Avocado and olive oil's monounsaturated fats soften dry, brittle hair, while honey coats and conditions your strands, giving them extra shine.

FOR YOUR HAIR *(cont.)*

FOR MORE VOLUME

Beer

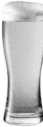

Open a bottle of hoppy beer, like an IPA, and let it sit for 30 minutes to let the bubbles settle. Shampoo your hair, rinse, and then pour on the beer, roots to ends, and massage briefly. Let the beer sit for 15 to 20 minutes before rinsing and styling.

Why it works: The yeast and hops in the brew help swell your hair cuticle, making strands thicker.

FOR LESS GREASE

Chamomile Tea   Mouthwash

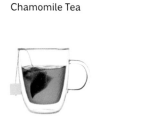   +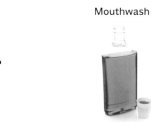

Brew chamomile tea and let it cool, then combine the tea with an equal amount of clean mouthwash. (Any kind will do.) Shampoo, condition, and towel-dry your hair. Then sprinkle the tea mixture over your scalp, rub it in lightly with your fingertips, and style as usual.

Why it works: Because both ingredients are mildly astringent, they absorb excess oil.

FOR YOUR BODY

FOR AN EXFOLIATING SCRUB

Milk

Brown Sugar

Vanilla

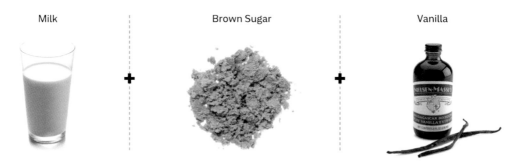

In a bowl, combine ½ cup of milk, ¼ cup of brown sugar, and a few drops of pure vanilla extract. In the shower or bath, gently scrub your skin using small circular motions. Rinse as usual.

Why it works: Brown sugar acts as a gentle exfoliator, while milk softens your skin. And the vanilla? It smells amazing!

FOR DRY, TIGHT SKIN

Cilantro

Buttermilk

Honey

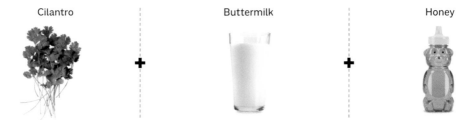

In a blender or food processor, combine I cup of fresh cilantro, 2 cups of buttermilk, and I tablespoon of honey. Blend or process until smooth, and strain. Pour the mixture into a warm bath and soak for at least 30 minutes.

Why it works: Cilantro has a cooling, soothing effect on skin. The natural lactic acids in dairy products like buttermilk help loosen dead cells, making skin soft and supple. Honey acts as a potent moisturizer and offers up antibacterial properties, too.

FOR YOUR BODY *(cont.)*
FOR ALLOVER MOISTURE

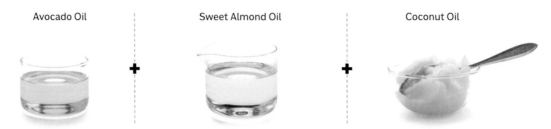

Avocado Oil	Sweet Almond Oil	Coconut Oil

In a jar with a tight-fitting lid, combine ¼ cup *each* of avocado oil, sweet almond oil, and melted coconut oil. Shake well and apply from your shoulders to your toes daily.

Why it works: The fatty acids in the oils penetrate your skin to deliver deep hydration.

Cleaning *Cleaner*

It might not come as much of a surprise that many of the same toxic chemicals that are used in personal-care products tend to pop up in common household cleaners. What you might *not* realize? Cleaning product manufacturers aren't actually required to list their ingredients on their labels—but they *are* allowed to use words like *natural, green, eco-friendly,* or even *organic* to create the impression that their products are safe and natural. Put these two mind-boggling facts together, and it can be tough to figure out exactly what's inside of those bottles sitting underneath your sink—and how they might be impacting your health and your weight.

Thankfully, change could be coming. Congress is currently considering legislation that would require cleaning product manufacturers to disclose their ingredients on their product labels.[19] Manufacturers may also be forced to share more health and safety data on the chemicals they use—and to prove that those chemicals are safe.[20] But until that happens, it's up to consumers to do the legwork to seek out safer products.

And you *can* do it. Sure, wading through the sea of colorful containers to find truly clean alternatives might seem like a task best left to a chemist. But with a little know-how, it actually becomes pretty easy to spot healthy cleaning products—as well as harmful imposters.

Beware of Greenwashing

As with practically anything that comes in a box or bag these days, cleaning products are often tricked out with wholesome-sounding names and nature-inspired designs to make them appear trustworthy and safe. But most of the terms on cleaning product labels are unregulated—and if you're not a savvy shopper, it's pretty easy to get duped. Keep an eye out for these wishy-washy terms.

- **Biodegradable.** Biodegradable products are supposed to break down when they enter wastewater treatment plants, landfills, or rivers and streams. But because the term is unregulated, there's no way of knowing whether a cleaner is *truly* biodegradable or not.

- **Natural.** Like with packaged foods, you can't take "natural" at face value. In the world of cleaning products, the word is entirely unregulated.

- **Nontoxic.** This term suggests that a cleaning product is safe for your health. But there's no official definition of what nontoxic actually means, so slapping it on a label doesn't guarantee that a product is healthy or safe.

- **Plant-based.** Products will often use this term if some of their ingredients come from plants or minerals. The catch? They don't have to say how much—or how little—of those ingredients are *actually* present in the product.

- **Organic.** Manufacturers use this term to imply that their products are made from plants grown

Germ Theory

Those disposable wipes are a godsend when you need to clean off the kitchen counter fast. And you're convinced that the little bottle of hand sanitizer in your bag helped you avoid a run-in with the flu last winter. But these products could come with some downsides.

Antibacterial products like wipes, soaps, and sanitizers get their germ-fighting power from triclosan, a chemical that, weirdly enough, could actually be hurting your health. By now, it's widely thought that triclosan-containing products could be increasing our resistance to antibiotics and depressing our immune systems. But they may be affecting the number you see on the scale, too. A recent review published in the journal *PLoS One* found that people with greater levels of triclosan in their urine had higher BMIs than those whose urine contained less triclosan.[21] In part, that could be because the chemical boasts endocrine-disrupting abilities that could mess with metabolism by affecting thyroid hormones. Triclosan's germ-killing powers could lead to negative changes in gut bacteria that might impact weight gain, too.

Don't worry, there's also some good news: Experts say that triclosan isn't actually any more effective at killing germs than plain old soap and water are.[22] That means you can trade in your antibacterial products *without* having to worry that scary germs are going to take over your life. To find triclosan-free goods, start by checking a product's label. Triclosan will be listed as an ingredient in things like soap, since it's considered a personal-care product. As for cleaning products like sprays or wipes, triclosan might not be listed because manufacturers aren't required to list ingredients. So check the front label, instead. If it says "germ-killing" or "antibacterial," there's a good chance the product contains triclosan.

without synthetic fertilizers or pesticides. But unless the label bears the USDA Organic Seal, you can't trust that an "organic" cleaning product is the real deal.

✳ **Phosphate-free.** Sounds nice, but it's not very meaningful. Phosphates—which can be harmful to aquatic life—were banned in many states decades ago. So these days, almost *all* cleaners are phosphate-free.

Seek Safety Certifications

When faced with marketing mumbo jumbo that can mean almost anything and no ingredients list to scan, how exactly are you supposed to find cleaning products that are truly clean? The simplest—and most effective—way is to look for items that have been vetted by third-party certifiers, like Green Seal or ECOLOGO. In order to be verified by either, a product is required to disclose all of its ingredients and sources, and the ingredients must be shown to have a minimal effect on health. What's more, the product has to undergo testing to prove that it actually *works*. If a cleaner is Green Seal or ECOLOGO certified, you'll spot the seal right on the product's label.

Another option is to buy from retailers or cleaning product manufacturers that offer up trustworthy standards of their own. Whole Foods Market's Eco-Scale rating system evaluates each product that it sells for safety and prohibits more than 40 toxic ingredients found in conventional cleaners, so you can feel assured that you're getting a truly clean product. Or search for a product in the Environmental Working Group's Guide to Healthy Cleaning at ewg.org/guides/cleaners. With safety ratings for over 2,000 products, it's easy to find a spray, soap, gel, or detergent that meets your standards.

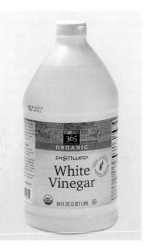

Vim and Vinegar

It might already be a staple for your salad dressing, but a simple bottle of vinegar can be your go-to for tackling to-dos around the house, too. (Opt for white or apple cider vinegars, which won't cause staining or discoloration like red wine or balsamic vinegar would.) Three genius ways to use it:

✳ **Brighten your whites.** White vinegar is a tried-and-true stain remover for clothing, towels, and sheets. Add a cup to the rinse cycle to keep your whites bright (*and* to get rid of soap scum inside your washing machine) without using harsh bleach.

✳ **Nix nasty odors.** Got a funk lingering in your car, closet, or bathroom? Leave a bowl of vinegar in the area overnight to absorb the stench.

✳ **Clean your toilet bowl.** Pour 16 ounces of white vinegar into the toilet bowl and let it sit overnight to dislodge dirt and eat up odors. Come morning, you just need to give it a quick scrub.

Squeaky-Clean Solutions

All it takes to fight dirt and grime around your home without toxic chemicals are a few simple ingredients—and most of them are likely already in your cabinets. Whip up your own all-purpose spray, tile cleaner, furniture polish, and more with these easy (and insanely inexpensive) recipes. Start your spray bottles!

ALL-PURPOSE CLEANER

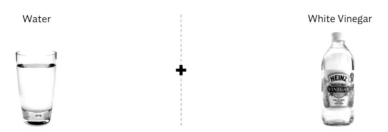

Water   +   White Vinegar

In a spray bottle, combine 9 parts water with I part white vinegar. Clean away on most nonporous, stone, tile, and porcelain surfaces. (Avoid using on porous wood surfaces or soft metals.)

Why it works: Vinegar boasts natural antibacterial properties. (It won't kill *all* germs, though. For really dirty messes, wipe down the area with a clean liquid soap and water, then follow with a squirt of straight vinegar and a separate squirt of hydrogen peroxide.)

TILE CLEANER

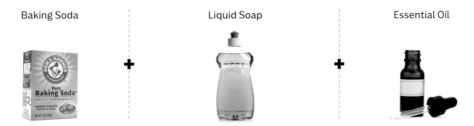

Baking Soda   +   Liquid Soap   +   Essential Oil

Place ½ cup of baking soda in a bowl and slowly pour in liquid soap, stirring until it is the consistency of frosting. (Skip the harsh detergents and antibacterial agents. Instead, opt for castile soap, such as Dr. Bronner's, which is vegetable oil-based.) Add 5 to I0 drops of your favorite essential oil, such as lavender or rosemary. Scoop onto a sponge, scrub, and rinse.

Why it works: The soap deep cleans, while the baking soda acts as a mild scouring agent.

Squeaky-Clean Solutions *(cont.)*

WINDOW CLEANER

Vinegar	Liquid Soap	Water

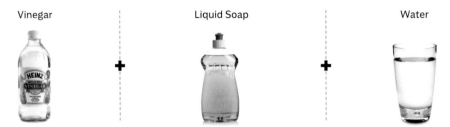

In a spray bottle, combine ¼ cup of vinegar, ½ teaspoon of liquid soap, and 2 cups of water. Shake to blend. Spray on a window, scrub with a kitchen sponge, and squeegee off. You can also scrub with crumpled newspaper.

Why it works: Vinegar and liquid soap cut grime and waxy buildup, and wiping with newspaper prevents streaking.

FURNITURE POLISH

Lemon Oil	Lemon Juice	Olive Oil

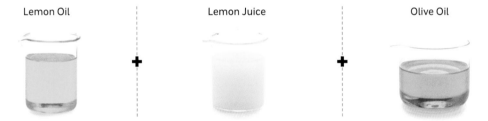

In a small spray bottle, combine 10 drops of pure lemon oil, 2 tablespoons of lemon juice, and several drops of olive oil. Shake to combine. Spritz on wood furniture and wipe dusty surfaces with a cotton flannel cloth.

Why it works: The acid in the lemon juice cuts through grease, while the olive oil protects and shines the wood. And the lemon oil smells fresh.

Squeaky-Clean Solutions *(cont.)*

FABRIC SOFTENER

Baking Soda or White Vinegar

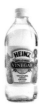

Pour I cup of baking soda into the rinse cycle for clothes or ½ cup of white vinegar for towels.

Why it works: Both baking soda and white vinegar eliminate soap and mineral buildup that can cause fabric to feel stiff.

OVEN CLEANER

Hot Water   Liquid Soap   Borax

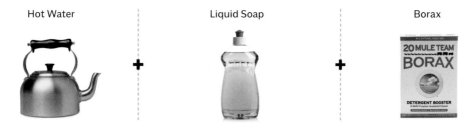

In a spray bottle, combine 2 cups of hot water, I tablespoon of soap, and I teaspoon of borax. Spray on the spill, let sit for 20 minutes, and wipe off with a clean cloth. For extra-greasy messes, wipe off as much goop as possible with crumpled newspaper first, then use the spray.

Why it works: Hot water and liquid soap cut grease. Borax, a naturally occurring mineral, has a texture similar to baking soda and dislodges stuck-on grime.

Squeaky-Clean Solutions *(cont.)*

DRAIN CLEANER

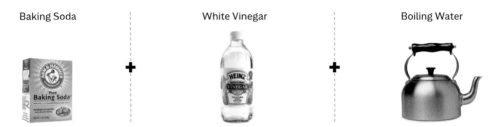

| Baking Soda | White Vinegar | Boiling Water |

In a heatproof glass measuring cup, combine equal parts baking soda, white vinegar, and boiling water. Stir carefully and slowly pour the mixture down the drain. Let it sit for a half hour, then rinse with hot water.

Why it works: The baking soda and vinegar fizz will eat through clogs.

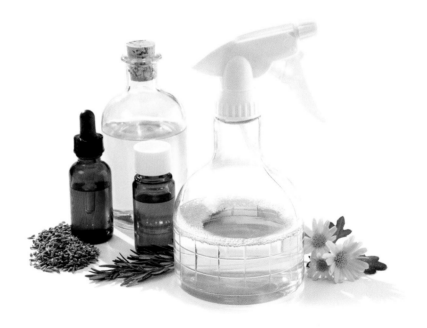

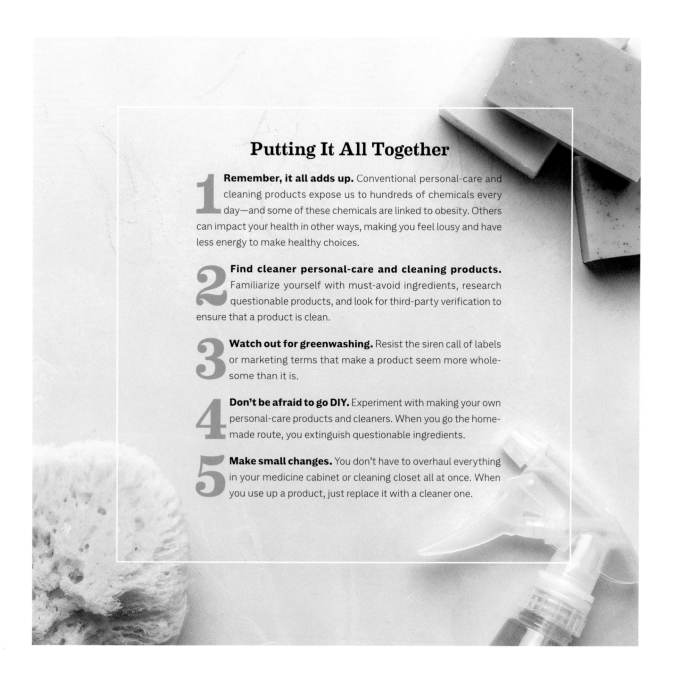

Putting It All Together

1 Remember, it all adds up. Conventional personal-care and cleaning products expose us to hundreds of chemicals every day—and some of these chemicals are linked to obesity. Others can impact your health in other ways, making you feel lousy and have less energy to make healthy choices.

2 Find cleaner personal-care and cleaning products. Familiarize yourself with must-avoid ingredients, research questionable products, and look for third-party verification to ensure that a product is clean.

3 Watch out for greenwashing. Resist the siren call of labels or marketing terms that make a product seem more wholesome than it is.

4 Don't be afraid to go DIY. Experiment with making your own personal-care products and cleaners. When you go the home-made route, you extinguish questionable ingredients.

5 Make small changes. You don't have to overhaul everything in your medicine cabinet or cleaning closet all at once. When you use up a product, just replace it with a cleaner one.

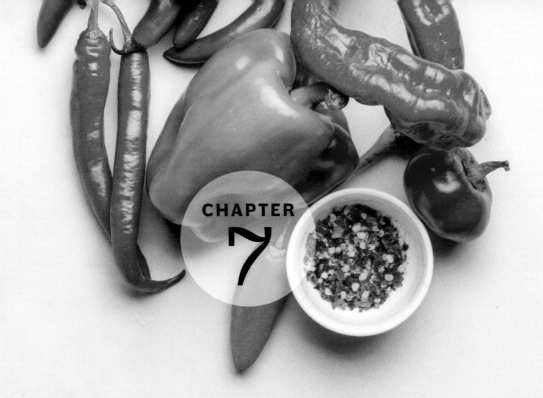

Keeping Clean
in the Real World

If you've ever tried to lose weight before, you know what usually happens: Things go along great for a little while, and you even lose a couple of pounds. But then, something comes up. Maybe work gets crazy and you find yourself relying on takeout more often than usual. Perhaps you take a well-deserved vacation and your eating habits get nudged off track. Or you finally give in to the friend who always insists that you get a giant bucket of popcorn at the movies.

Whatever that something is, it leaves you thinking that you've messed up big-time. As a result, you feel like you've blown it completely—so you throw in the towel and let loose for the rest of the day, or the rest of the week. Before you know it, you're back to your old way of eating, and the pounds have piled right back on.

It's an all-too-typical story, sure. But it doesn't have to be this way! From restaurant meals to relentless naggers, let's look at the strategies that can help you continue to eat clean when the going gets tough. Plus, we'll talk about how you can deal with slip-ups in a healthier way so your weight loss doesn't get derailed.

Getting Real

In a perfect world, the clean choice would be the easiest one every time. You'd have an extra free hour to put toward prepping all of your meals and snacks from scratch. Clean, delicious options would be the default whenever you went to a restaurant or traveled. You'd never have to worry about how you'd find something relatively healthy at your neighbor's annual holiday party. And instead of bringing home a gallon of double fudge ice cream ("It was on sale!") or inviting you to dinner at the new buffet down the street ("*Everyone* is raving about it!"), your family members and friends would do what they could to support your clean choices.

It all sounds pretty wonderful. But of course, we don't live in a perfect world. We live in the *real* world—and with it comes challenges to eating clean and getting leaner. After all, hardly anyone would struggle with her weight if making the best food choices was always easy! Packing a healthy snack or making time to cook after a long day can be tough. Finding clean options at restaurants, on the road, or at social events often feels like a hunt for buried treasure. And dealing with the strange ways that other people sometimes react to your decision to eat clean can be emotionally exhausting.

But guess what? *You can do this*. The road to achieving any goal is almost guaranteed to have a few speed bumps along the way—and losing weight is no exception. The key to overcoming obstacles when they do crop up is to anticipate them ahead of time—and have strategies for success already in place. Let's take a look at some of the most common stumbling blocks that strike when you're trying to eat clean and lose weight and discuss how to keep them from getting in your way.

Obstacle #1: I Don't Have Enough Time!

It's true—eating clean takes more time than picking up a burger and fries at the drive-thru does. But that doesn't mean that you need to spend hours following elaborate recipes or that you can't rely on healthy convenience foods when you pull together balanced meals and snacks. **By finding food-prep tactics that work with** your schedule and lifestyle, you're more likely to stick with clean eating for the long haul—even when things get hairy. These simple tips can help.

Plan ahead. A little bit of advance planning can go a long way toward helping you get clean food on the table, fast. Take time on the weekend to map out your meals and shop for groceries. Then, prep components that can be made ahead of time, such as marinara sauce or long-cooking whole grains. Similarly, you can put together easy options that make breakfast and snacks a breeze so you don't end up having to rely on a muffin from the café or a sugary granola bar from the vending machine. For instance, if you like eggs in the morning but never have time to cook them, make Mini Spinach Mushroom Quiche (see page 224). Pack the quiches in individual containers that you can grab and take before heading out the door. Love snacking on hummus or homemade trail mix? Make bigger batches and divvy them up into snack-size portions so you have

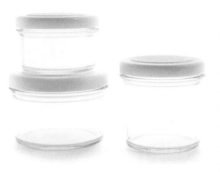

servings for the entire week.

Learn to love leftovers. They literally make your meals work double duty. Instead of cooking a new meal every night, cook double batches so you've got dinner for two nights in a row, or freeze half for later on, when you know things will be hectic. And remember: There's no reason to pack an entirely new lunch every morning before you run out the door. Have leftovers, like Maple Mustard Glazed Pork Tenderloin with Roasted Vegetables and Apples (page 256) for lunch, instead. Or repurpose your leftovers into an entirely new meal: Stuff Tuna and Cannellini Salad (page 233) into a small whole wheat pita pocket. Shred roast chicken and throw it into a salad, or toss last night's Roasted Broccoli with Chile and Lemon (page 277) with some quinoa and black beans. It's convenient and clean, and it saves you the time you'd spend trying to find a decent option at the sandwich shop next door to your office.

Notes from a Clean Eater

"I can't cook during the week because my kids are all involved in sports. So instead, I cook on Sunday for the week."—**Kelley S.**

Find fast-cooking favorites. Having a few meals in your repertoire that you can make at lightning speed means that you're less likely to order takeout when you're crazy busy and don't already have something prepped in the fridge. Chicken-and-vegetable stir-fries come together in minutes, as do veggie scrambles, omelets, and whole wheat pasta with sautéed greens and canned beans. For a full list of quick-

Three Frozen Meal Hacks

Keeping a few clean frozen entrées on hand can help you avoid greasy takeout on nights when cooking just isn't going to happen. Still, even the best boxed meals aren't usually quite as nutritious as something you'd make yourself. So when you pull one out of the freezer, try one of these easy tricks.

1. Start with a salad. It doesn't have to be fancy! Romaine lettuce or baby spin-ach, some chopped carrots or slices of tomato, and a drizzle of olive oil and vine-gar are all you need.

2. Have a steamed vegetable on the side. How about some broccoli or spin-ach? Asparagus or green beans? Pick whatever you like best.

3. Add a flavor booster. If your meal is on the lower-calorie side, try topping it with some diced avocado, chopped nuts or seeds, or even some Greek yogurt. (Just measure out the proper portions, since the calories from these extras can add up—and slow your weight loss—fast.) And don't forget those herbs and spices! Sprinkle freshly chopped basil over an Italian-style entrée, or dust chili powder over a burrito bowl for an extra kick. You'll amp up the flavor *and* add an extra dose of nutrition.

cooking Eat Clean, Stay Lean recipes, see page 220.

Think outside the (meal) box. There's no rule that says you have to stick to traditional breakfast, lunch, and dinner foods. As long as the foods you pick are clean, nutritious, and leave you feeling satisfied, it doesn't matter whether they fit the idea of a "normal" meal. Don't have time to cook your usual oatmeal for breakfast? Smear some almond butter on a slice of whole grain toast, grab a piece of fruit, and you're all set. Get home late and don't feel like making dinner? Put down the take-out menu and make a clean snack plate with some hummus, roasted red peppers, olives, and whole grain pita bread, instead.

Smoothies are another option. No, we're not talking about the sugary, milkshakelike concoctions that can be found at so many smoothie shops and cafés these days. (They're often made with powdered mixes, sugary juice, and even sorbet or ice cream, and they tend to contain little or no actual fruit.) We're talking about *real* smoothies that contain fresh or frozen fruits and vegetables, healthy fats (such as nut butters or seeds), and clean proteins (such as Greek yogurt or even some protein powders). When made with whole foods, you might be surprised by how satisfying a blended drink can be! For tips on how to build your own Clean and Simple Smoothie, see page 172.

Count on clean convenience foods. Remember, you don't have to cook every single thing from scratch in order to eat clean. Whether it's a box of clean, whole grain cereal for breakfast or a jar of salsa to liven up your chicken fajitas, there's *no* shame in using packaged foods selectively if they help you make healthier choices overall. The key, of course, is to use products that are minimally processed, low in added sugar, and made without unrecognizable ingredients or additives. If you need to brush up on the basics of choosing clean pack-aged items, just flip back to Chapter 3.

Clean Eater

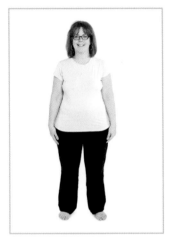

BEFORE

As a mom of three athletes, much of 50-year-old **Kelley's** free time is filled with cheering on her kids at games and shuttling them to tournaments. Her hectic schedule doesn't leave much time for cooking clean meals during the week, which meant that she had to get creative with prepping food for herself and her family.

"If I preplanned, I was successful. But if I didn't preplan, I wasn't successful," she says. Kelley got into the habit of shopping for groceries and cooking meals for the week on Sundays. But when one weekend got particularly busy, she didn't have time to do her usual prep work—and that threw her off. "So I felt like a failure. I was having cereal for dinner. I didn't go off the plan, I just didn't have great meals," she says.

That setback almost made her lose her resolve altogether. But then, someone noticed that she looked leaner. "When you work so hard and somebody notices, it's huge," Kelley says. Around the same time, *she* started picking up on the positive effects of eating clean, too. "The last 2 weeks, I could feel the weight loss," she remarks.

That's when she knew that she'd be able to stick with eating clean for the long haul. At the same time, she realized that always trying to aim for perfection might end up doing her more harm than good. For instance, when the teacher appreciation luncheon was held at the school where she works, she knew that she wanted to indulge without feeling guilty. "Once a week, I might want to have a treat that isn't part of the plan," she admits. But even so, "I think that I'll be eating in more moderation than I would have normally."

Dr. Wendy Observes: It's easy to get sidelined when you hit a speed bump. But when Kelley ran into the all-too-common challenge of navigating a time-crunched schedule, she adapted instead of giving up. Sure, some of her meals during that challenging week may not have been as tasty or pretty, but they were still clean—and that's a success. It's about progress, not perfection.

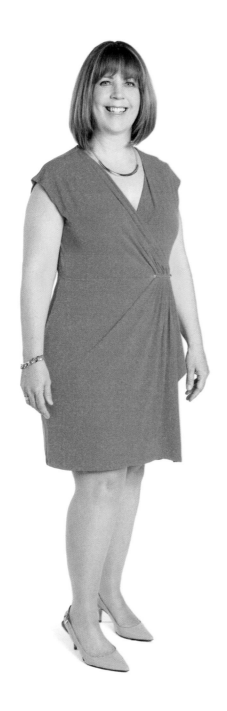

TOTAL POUNDS LOST

11 lbs

TOTAL INCHES LOST

13.25

MOST NOTABLE IMPROVEMENTS

Kelley's cholesterol was high before she started eating clean. But afterwards, it dropped into the healthy range.

Obstacle #2: The Restaurant Trap

Is it possible to eat out *and* eat clean at the same time? Findings show that people who usually cook at home tend to eat fewer calories, less sugar, *and* higher-quality foods than those who dine out often.[1] Why? Most restaurant meals pack way more salt, sugar, fat, and refined carbs into their dishes than you'd probably have at home. Not to mention the fact that the portions are enormous! If you were to eat breakfast, lunch, and dinner at a restaurant today, you'd take in nearly 1,600 more calories than if you'd eaten the same meals at most restaurants 20 years ago, according to estimates from the National Institutes of Health.[2]

With numbers like that, it's no surprise that **sticking to mostly home-cooked fare can make it easier to lose weight.** But that doesn't mean that once you've committed to eating clean, you can never step foot inside a restaurant again. (Though it's a good idea to stick to eating at home while following the Eat Clean, Stay Lean plan for the first 3 weeks or more. We'll talk more about why in Chapter 8.) Dining out is fun and delicious, and enjoying the occasional restaurant meal is a treat that's worth looking forward to. These simple principles can help you enjoy eating out without wrecking your weight-loss progress.

Arrive hungry, not starving. Eating less during the day (or not eating at all) means you can eat more at the restaurant, right? Well, not exactly. "Saving up" for your meal throughout the day might seem like a smart weight-loss strategy. But in reality, it means that you'll probably get to the restaurant starving—which is a sure-fire recipe for overeating. So stick with your normal meal and snack schedule, instead, and enjoy a moderate

Dr. Wendy Says . . .

Birthday cakes. Specialty cocktails. Multicourse tasting menus with optional wine pairings. Celebratory meals and treats to commemorate anniversaries, promotions, or big wins. Any of these treats might feel like splurges worth savoring—and they can be! But because there are *so many* food-centric occasions these days, it's essential to ask yourself: **Is this particular occasion important enough for me to bend my healthy habits?**

Of course, there's no right or wrong answer. You know what works for your weight-loss goals and what doesn't, and no one's judging you but you. So if it's a special occasion that you've been planning for a long time, or you finally got that reservation at the hottest restaurant in town, enjoy it to the fullest and savor every bite. What if you're celebrating another wonderful life moment, like a birthday, a holiday, or a winning game? There's no reason you can't enjoy those

events, too. But you might decide that, frankly, a clean and healthy meal and a bite of the cake is just as good or meaningful as having the entire piece and feeling lousy (or worse, guilty) later on. **Remember, there are lots of ways to make a special occasion feel special.** Pay attention to those opportunities, and you'll probably find yourself making great decisions around your food without unraveling your progress. You've got this!

portion of something delicious when you eat out. You'll feel better and more energized during the day, and you won't leave the restaurant feeling stuffed.

Be the first to order. Putting your order in before anyone else does means you'll be less tempted to copy your dining companion's decadent order. ("She's treating herself to the fried chicken platter, so maybe I should, too!") In fact, you might even influence others at the table to pick cleaner meals.

Pick a balanced plate. Just like at home, you want your meal to be a mix of lean protein, complex carbohydrates, and healthy fats. So steer clear of entrées that are total carbfests (like a heaping plate of spaghetti) or pure protein (like a giant steak) in favor of dinners that deliver a little bit of everything. Think a piece of fish with olive oil, roasted potatoes, and steamed green beans, or black bean soup with brown rice and diced avocado served with a side salad.

Look for clean menu descriptions. Not sure what to order? Zero in on dishes that are baked, steamed, grilled, broiled, or poached. They're lighter than those that are fried, crusted, or stuffed, for sure. But they're also cleaner, since many restaurants use unhealthy fats, such as hydrogenated vegetable oils or margarine—both of which contain trans fats.

Sideline your sauces. A little bit of stir-fry sauce, pesto, or salad dressing adds flavor to your meal. But most restaurants tend to pour on way more than you actually need. The solution? Ask for sauces on the side, and dip into them with your fork. You'll still get the taste, but without turning your meal into a calorie bomb.

Be a portion pro. When it comes to losing weight, the *size* of your meal matters almost as much as the ingredients. The thing is, it can be tough to stop yourself from devouring an entire plate of food once it's sitting in front of you—even if it's really, really big! So find simpler ways to keep your portions in check, such as by ordering an appetizer instead of an entrée. Split a full-size entrée with one of your dining companions, or ask your server to bag up half of your entrée before it comes to the table.

Remember the rule of one. Part of the fun of going out to eat is splurging on extras like wine, fresh bread,

Smart Substitutions

Tweaking or customizing your order can do a lot to make it cleaner. (And you shouldn't feel bad about doing it. Restaurants *want* to make you happy!) Some simple swaps to try:

- **Instead of:** White rice or pasta
- **Ask for:** Brown rice or whole wheat pasta

- **Instead of:** Mashed potatoes
- **Ask for:** Roasted potatoes or sweet potatoes, or a baked potato

- **Instead of:** Cheese, mayonnaise, or sour cream
- **Ask for:** Sliced avocado, guacamole, hummus, or mustard

- **Instead of:** French fries or potato chips
- **Ask for:** A side salad

- **Instead of:** Croutons, crunchy noodles, or fried tortilla strips (on a salad)
- **Ask for:** Beans, such as chickpeas or black beans

Clean-Eating Picks on Any Menu

Dining out? No matter what the cuisine, there's a clean pick to be found.

Asian: Shrimp stir-fry with brown rice and vegetables

Make it even cleaner: Get the sauce on the side so you can control how much you actually eat. Eat four good forkfuls of your rice, and pack up the rest.

Diner: Three egg-white (or two-egg) vegetable omelet

Make it even cleaner: Skip the home fries and have a fruit cup or a side of sliced tomatoes, instead.

Indian: Chicken tikka

Make it even cleaner: Order chapati—a whole wheat flatbread—instead of the typical naan, which is usually made with white flour and topped with melted butter.

Italian: Whole wheat pasta primavera (with red sauce, not white)

Make it even cleaner: Order it with extra vegetables. And since pasta portions are usually way too big, ask for half of your meal to be bagged up before your server brings your plate to the table.

Middle Eastern: Chicken shish kebab

Make it even cleaner: Skip the white pita bread in favor of an order of grilled vegetables or a side salad.

Seafood: Any fish, grilled, with lemon

Make it even cleaner: Eat only a checkbook-size portion of the fish and polish off all of your vegetables.

Southwestern: Vegetable fajitas

Make it even cleaner: Ask for corn or whole wheat tortillas instead of white flour tortillas, and get a side of plain black beans instead of refried ones. Top your fajitas with a spoonful of guacamole instead of sour cream and cheese.

Steak house: Flank steak

Make it even cleaner: For your side, order a plain baked potato (eat only half) or spinach sautéed with garlic (instead of the calorie-laden creamed version).

Notes from a Clean Eater

"Now I'm very conscientious of what I eat when I go out. At happy hour, I'll have oysters and thinly sliced salmon with some salad, instead of fried calamari and fries."—**George S.**

and delicious desserts. Always saying no to all three might help you lose weight faster, but it's also likely to leave you feeling deprived. So strike a compromise: Instead of having a glass of wine, a piece of bread, *and* a dessert, pick just one—and enjoy it.

Obstacle #3: Packing Your Bags

Whether you're on the go for work or headed out for vacation, being away from home can make eating clean more challenging. Though healthy options are more widely available than they used to be, most airports and roadside pit stops still aren't exactly known for being beacons of clean fare. And once you actually arrive at your destination? Temptation lurks around every corner—whether it's free soft serve by the pool, a round (or two) of cocktails before dinner, or the surf-and-turf special that everyone is raving about. Fortunately, a little bit of know-how can help you navigate the tempting terrain.

Notes from a Clean Eater

"While on vacation in Italy, we'd order one pasta or meat dish and one veggie or salad dish, and we'd share both. We also ordered soups that were loaded with beans and vegetables."

—Richard and Suzanne M.

On the Road

Is there any way to avoid the fate of stale gas station hot dogs and giant airport cinnamon buns? Absolutely. Whether you're driving or flying, packing clean fare at home can help you avoid being stuck with a not-so-appealing option—as well as minimize temptations—when the pickings are slim. Portable, protein-rich snacks like trail mix or roasted chickpeas are always an easy choice. But don't stop there! If you'll be traveling for hours and need to have a meal on the way, pack up something that's easy to eat on the run, like a turkey and avo-cado sandwich with a piece of fruit or a peanut butter and banana sandwich on whole wheat bread. Sure, it's nothing fancy—but it's clean and satisfying, so it gets the job done.

What should you do when there's just no time to pack food? When it comes to snacks, your best bets are also the simplest: nuts and seeds. Even the tiniest gas stations usually have a couple of packages on the shelf (think walnuts, almonds, peanuts, or sunflower seeds), and they save you the hassle of having to scrutinize ingredients lists when you're in a hurry. Pick raw, roasted, or salted over any flavored options (which could be higher in sugar), and watch your portions. A snack portion of nuts is $\frac{1}{4}$ cup, which is roughly a handful, but most packages offer two or three times that much.

Dr. Wendy Says . . .

Plan clean pit stops! At first, it might seem smart to save calories by avoiding eating *anything* until you get where you're going. But going too long without eating means that you'll likely be starving when you reach your destination—which can set the stage for plowing straight into a plate of gooey nachos or greasy wings. Instead, aim to keep up with your schedule of eating a snack or meal every 3 to 4 hours while en route to wherever you're going. It will take some planning, but staying on track will leave you feeling better about your food choices, as well as more energized. Have a big bottle of water, too, to help you stay hydrated and mentally sharp.

At Your Destination

Whether you're at the world's most boring work convention or a luxury resort, merely being away from home can make you want to forget about your weight-loss goals and throw caution to the wind. And while it might not be realistic to expect to follow your usual clean-eating routine to a tee, you don't want to let every meal turn into a free-for-all, either. Having a special meal or a cocktail can be fine. But go all out for your entire trip, and the number on the scale will probably read a few pounds higher once you get back home. Plus, a lot of indulging could make it harder to get back to normal, eating-wise. After all, it only takes a few nights in a row of splurging on key lime pie or double chocolate cake to get you into the habit of wanting something sweet after dinner every night.

How do you strike a balance? Eating clean while you travel is a lot like eating clean when you go out to a restaurant—you just have to do it for a longer period of time. Most of the time, try to stick to the same clean-ordering principles. When you feel like treating yourself, go for it—but indulge mindfully on the things that you *really* want and think about *how much* is really the perfect amount to satisfy you. As for the stuff that's just okay, simply skip it. For instance, if you're truly looking forward to having wine with dinner, pass on the so-so complimentary croissants at breakfast. Being choosy means that you can enjoy what you eat on vacation without feeling guilty—or completely derailing your weight-loss goals.

Once You Get Home

Hopefully, you feel pretty good about the choices you made while you were away. But what if you overdid it a bit? You might feel guilty, bloated, and even sluggish, which can set the stage for continuing to eat larger portions and less nutritious foods once you get home. In that case, your goal is to stop that negative cycle before it starts. Instead of dwelling on the unhealthy stuff you ate during your trip, start planning the clean foods you'll eat now that you're home. The sooner you get back on track, the sooner you'll start feeling good again—both physically and mentally. After a day or two, you'll start to crave the energizing effects of your favorite clean foods once again.

Obstacle #4: Sticky Social Situations

Whether it's a cocktail party with friends, a dinner event for work, or a holiday celebration with your family, all of these events have something in common: At them, you're likely to be surrounded by lots of foods that aren't particularly clean—and lots of people who are encouraging you to eat them. Sure, you might be perfectly content cruising along with your kale, white bean, and quinoa salad or Greek yogurt and berries when you're on your own. But when a well-meaning friend flags you down with a plate of deviled eggs or bacon-wrapped shrimp, it can be extra tough to say no. After all, you don't want to seem like a party pooper—or worse, hurt the feelings of someone you care about!

Of course, steering clear of all social events isn't exactly an option. (At least it's not a very fun one.) So how can you hang out with the crowd and still avoid succumbing to peer pressure to abandon your clean-eating principles? Stick with these rules of thumb.

Go in with a plan. Before the event, think about how you want to eat. Are you going to a dinner party where the host always serves an outrageously delicious homemade

(continued on page 128)

When Should I Weigh In?

Eager to hop on the scale as soon as you get back home? Try holding off for a day or two. The combination of salty restaurant food and travel-related dehydration means that your body is likely holding on to more water than usual, which could translate to an unexpectedly high number on the scale. Don't worry—just focus on getting back to eating clean right away, and you'll lose any water weight after just a couple of days!

Clean Eaters

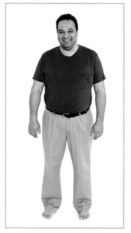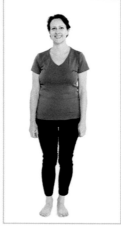

BEFORE

Richard and Suzanne M.

Travel and weight loss aren't exactly known for going hand in hand. And traveling to a place that's known for having some of the most delicious food in the world? *Fuggedaboutit.*

But that wasn't the case for Richard and Suzanne, who already had a vacation in Italy planned before they decided to start eating clean. Instead of just taking time off from their weight-loss goals, they decided that they'd enjoy themselves without letting their trip turn into a week-long pizza-and-pasta binge. And the proof is in the results they reaped by sticking with the program.

For breakfast, they'd usually stop at a local grocery store for some fresh fruit. "We never once missed having a big breakfast, and it allowed more time to get out and tour," says Suzanne. For lunches or dinners, they'd order what they wanted—but in a way that made it easy to keep their portions in check. "We didn't binge on pasta or bread. We tried to balance our meals," she says. Instead of ordering two appetizers and two pasta dishes, Suzanne would get a grilled vegetable dish and Richard would get pasta. Then, they'd split the two plates.

The couple also made trade-offs by skipping the stuff they didn't care about that much; that way, they had room for the foods they really loved. For instance, they'd always pass on the breadbasket at mealtimes. And since Richard and Suzanne aren't big drinkers, they didn't bother with wine or cocktails. But Suzanne, who's always loved sweets, *did* treat herself to delicious gelato made from high-quality ingredients.

In fact, after realizing how delicious simple meals made with fresh, quality ingredients could be, Suzanne was inspired to re-create at home many of the produce-centric dishes she and Richard enjoyed in Italy. These days, they're eating tasty foods sparked by their travel memories, like cabbage and bean soup, minestrone soup, and even homemade pasta with fresh sauces. "Now, eating clean just seems like common sense," Richard says.

Dr. Wendy Observes: Richard and Suzanne are a testament to the fact that travel can be exciting, delicious, and still supportive of your health. They turned what had been a potential obstacle to their weight-loss progress into a major success, complete with great food, memories, and even new recipe inspirations for their clean-eating lifestyle. It's proof of how much you can achieve in virtually any life situation—without deprivation!

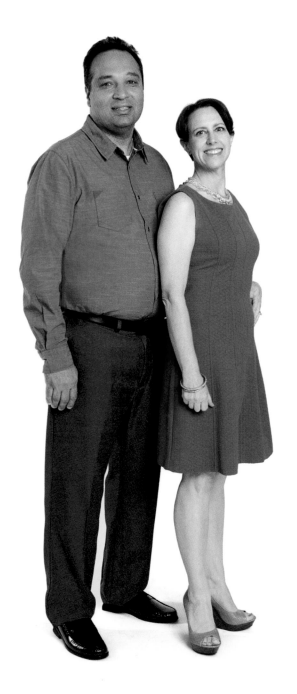

TOTAL POUNDS LOST

RICHARD

21 lbs

SUZANNE

4.5 lbs

TOTAL INCHES LOST

RICHARD

8.75

SUZANNE

4.25

MOST NOTABLE IMPROVEMENTS

Richard: His systolic blood pressure (the top number) dropped by 24 points and his diastolic blood pressure (the bottom number) dropped by 11 points, bringing both out of the high blood pressure range. His LDL ("bad") cholesterol dropped by 17 points, bringing him from borderline high to just 4 points outside of the desirable range.

Suzanne: She used to crave sugar on a daily basis, but now, her taste for sweets has started to disappear.

Is it possible to reframe social events and special occasions so you can have your cake (or in this case, your weight-loss success) and eat it, too? Yes—but it's important to answer these questions honestly first.

1. Do food splurges define what you call special?

2. Does eating whatever you want or as much as you want make or break the specialness of the occasion?

The answer to both is *probably not*. Remember, while the food is certainly fun, it usually isn't the sole reason you're gathering with others. In fact, it isn't even the *main* reason. So when an event comes up, think about why you're really there. Are you celebrating an important achievement? Getting an opportunity to spend time with people who matter to you, who you don't get to see very often? By shifting your attention to the true focus of your gathering or event, the food immediately takes second place—which is right where it should be.

dessert, or to a holiday event with the eggnog or special cinnamon bread that you look forward to every year? If you know that you'll have an opportunity to eat things that you really love, decide ahead of time what specific things you'll eat and how much of them you'll have. By planning your indulgence in advance, you're choosing to stay in control instead of letting your appetite or craving lure you on a whim. That way, you'll be able to enjoy a bit of your treat instead of feeling guilty that you caved to temptation.

And if it's a situation where you know the food isn't going to be that great? It's not worth the splurge if it's not truly delicious, so decide ahead of time to steer clear of the junky stuff. (Sorry, boring mini quiches that came from a box.) Fill a small plate with cleaner offerings, like crudités and hummus, shrimp cocktail, fresh fruit, and a few cubes of cheese, and call it a meal. Or skip the food entirely and enjoy a clean meal beforehand or afterward. Why eat unhealthy stuff that you don't even care about?

Notes from a Clean Eater

"When I go to the movies, I bring my own stuff with me, like a Kashi bar. When my friends cooked spaghetti and meatballs for dinner, I brought ingredients to make a salad. At a bar, I'll have seltzer with a splash of cranberry juice—just enough to change the color."—**Steve B.**

Have a no-fail excuse. Just because someone offers you a cupcake or a second helping of buttery mashed potatoes doesn't mean that you have to eat it. Still, bumbling over an excuse about how you're trying to lose weight or eat cleaner probably isn't enough to steer a well-meaning food pusher away from your plate. ("You're at a party! Live a little! You can get back to your diet tomorrow!") What to say instead? **"Thanks, that looks delicious! But I'm not hungry right now."** By complimenting the food and putting the blame on your full belly, you'll avoid hurting your host's feelings. And if you're full, you're full! Nobody can argue with that. More importantly, this tactic avoids an all-out rejection by implying that you *might* want some later when your appetite comes back. (Even if you know that isn't gonna happen.)

Be a little deceptive. You don't need a reason for not wanting to try the Swedish meatballs or the signature mojito—but some people might ask anyway. If you're uncomfortable fielding those kinds of questions (or you just don't feel like it), playing pretend can help. A high-ball glass of sparkling water with lime looks an awful lot like an alcoholic drink—and if you don't say otherwise, no one will be able to tell the difference.

Another option? You can always serve yourself a small helping of something, even if you don't actually plan to eat it. Sometimes, just having something on your plate is enough to stave off intrusive questions. Of course, this only works if you're really confident that you won't be tempted to take a bite. For added insurance, pick something you don't actually like very much instead of, say, your favorite thing ever.

Build a Cleaner Party Plate

How can you make smart choices when you're surrounded by pigs in blankets and deep-fried egg rolls? Keep these rules of thumb in mind the next time you're at a party or gathering.

I. Scan your surroundings. Take a look at all of the offerings, *then* start filling up your plate. When you know everything that's being served, you can be more strategic about what you do—and don't—serve yourself.

2. Go for the clean goods first, then pick a treat. Divvy up your plate into four imaginary quarters. Fill two of those quarters with clean fruit and vegetable dishes. (Think salad, fresh berries, or roasted or sautéed vegetables, rather than creamed spinach or cheesy stuffed mushrooms.) Fill another quarter with lean protein, like roasted turkey breast or shrimp cocktail. And save the last quarter for *whatever* yummy treat you want. Mac and cheese? Scalloped potatoes? You got it.

3. Savor every bite and move on. Enjoyed everything on your plate? Good job. (But remember, if it turns out you *don't* like something on your plate, you don't have to eat it!) Your hunger should now feel satisfied, so skip the line for seconds. Go catch up with your friend or hit the dance floor, instead.

Obstacle #5: Dealing with Saboteurs

You've told your family members, friends, and coworkers that you're trying to eat cleaner and lose some weight. Everyone seems enthusiastic about your decision—after all, you're taking steps to improve your health! So what's with your spouse still insisting on bringing home a bucket of fried chicken for dinner? And why is your best friend continuing to insist that you hit the local pancake joint on Sunday mornings instead of taking a power walk through the park?

There's no doubt that the people who care about you

Sometimes, *showing* can be more powerful than simply telling. If you've told a friend or family member repeatedly about your intentions to eat clean and they're still not supporting you in the way that you need, set the words aside for a while and start relying on your actions to get the message across. As they *see* you continually make clean choices, they'll start to understand that *yes*—you're serious about this!

don't want you to have to deal with obesity-related conditions like high blood pressure, high blood sugar, or high cholesterol. They also don't want your weight to hold you back from the things in life that you enjoy. But at the same time, some of them might not feel completely comfortable with your decision to eat cleaner. Picking the smoothie or oatmeal bowl, for instance, might serve to highlight the fact that your dining companion's biscuit, sausage, and gravy platter is a less-healthy option. It can even cause the other person to feel like she's being judged—even if you have no feelings at all about what she's eating. In order to avoid feeling like she's making a terrible choice, the other person might encourage you to stop eating bird food and treat yourself. Just like misery, indulgent eating loves company.

Tensions can run even higher at home. If you and your spouse used to love going out for ice cream after dinner or your family always made cheesy nachos on movie nights, your decision to opt out can feel, to them, like a rejection. What's more, they might feel worried that your next move is to take away *their* favorite junky foods. To stop that from happening and get things back to how they used to be, they might try to sway you back toward your old habits.

How can you navigate these kinds of situations without abandoning your weight-loss goals or making things uncomfortable between you and the people you care about? When someone tempts you to hop off the clean-eating bandwagon, the best thing to do is be straight with them: Remind them that you're working to lose weight, and you're making these changes in order to achieve that goal. You're getting leaner because you want to feel great, have more energy, and most importantly, be as healthy as possible for the long haul. When you're honest about your feelings, most people will try to respect them. Still, it might take a number of reminders before it really clicks. After all, if you've done something one way for a long time or tried other diets that didn't last long, others may not immediately be convinced that this time's for real. And if there's someone who continually tries to sabotage your efforts by not respecting your wishes, you may want to think about whether he or she is really worth your time.

Help! My partner is a junk-food addict. Does your dearly beloved *love* fatty fried foods, desserts, and sugary drinks? These smart strategies can help you keep your healthy habits going—and maybe even nudge your partner to make slightly cleaner choices without starting a fight.

❊ **When he wants pizza or burgers for dinner every single night . . .** Your partner might never be the kind of person who's going to crave brown rice and broccoli for dinner. So meet him halfway by showing him how delicious cleaner versions of his old standbys can be. Instead of ordering pizza, make it with whole wheat crust and top it with sauce, loads of veggies, and a smidge of cheese. Or make grilled fish tacos instead of pork carnitas. And if you always serve dinner with a salad, you've got your clean eating covered!

❋ **When she's constantly bringing junky snacks into the house . . .** Be up front with your feelings. Your partner might not understand how tempting or distracting it can actually be for you to have a gallon of ice cream or a giant bag of chips in the house, so tell her how having all that stuff around stresses you out. When she sees things from your point of view,

she'll probably want to do what she can to avoid upsetting you—such as not buying those foods, or storing them out of sight and eating them when you aren't around.

❋ **When you're legitimately concerned about what he's eating . . .** Yup, your partner went and ordered a slab of deep fried meat loaf with cheesy fries for dinner. You're cringing inside, but try to hold back on the judgment. Instead of starting a fight in the middle of your meal, wait until later to talk—and then be honest. State the facts about why his order was objectively bad for his health (in this case, loads of unhealthy fat and refined carbs). Then explain the *real* reason why it bothers you: You love your partner, and you want him to be around for a long time, too.

Taking the Focus Off Food

How can you stick to your clean-eating guns without putting up a fight—or making your eating plan the topic of conversation for the next 3 hours? First, remember that eating doesn't have to be the main event of every social gathering. Sure, food-centric traditions have their place—and no one's saying that you should serve fruit salad instead of pumpkin pie on Thanksgiving or insist that everyone eat tofu instead of hot dogs at the annual Fourth of July cookout. (In fact, we'd strongly recommend against it.)

But you also don't *have* to buy popcorn and candy just because you and your partner are seeing a movie. Or have cookies with your coffee every time your friend comes over to chat. Instead of meeting with your team

over lunch, why not try a walking meeting outside? By finding ways to keep food out of the social equation (or at least to make it a smaller part of it), you'll feel less tempted to abandon your eating goals. You'll also be less likely to come up against resistance from people who might try to sabotage your healthy habits. After all, the point of socializing is to connect with others—not spend the entire time with your mouths full!

Another option is to make an effort to compromise. If your gang wants to make dinner plans, chime in with a suggestion for a restaurant that offers some satisfying clean options for you in addition to the old standbys for them. When the neighbors invite you over for a cocktail party, ask if you can bring a snack to share with

Family Matters

We know–it isn't always easy to eat clean when you've got a gaggle of pint-size pizza and burger lovers to feed. But it's not impossible, either. Here are some smart tips that'll help you keep your sanity *without* breaking your diet.

❈ **Cook one dinner–for everyone.** Trying to cater to everyone's tastes is exhausting, so don't even bother. Instead, double or triple the Eat Clean, Stay Lean dinner recipes as needed so everyone can have what you're having. (If they're hungry, they'll eat it!)

❈ **Make meal prep a family event.** Still not sure your kids will be into eating salmon or grilled chicken for dinner? Enlist their help in the kitchen to make dinner together, and over time, those "yucky" foods will become a whole lot more appealing.

❈ **Stock up on (only) healthy snacks.** Sticking to clean foods is surprisingly easy if there's no junk around to tempt you. For the next few weeks, stock up on fresh fruit, veggies, nuts and seeds, and whole grain crackers and hummus instead of the usual junky chips and cookies.

Sure, the kids might complain, but they'll get over it.

❈ **Have fun without food.** For the next 3 weeks, try breaking the food-as-fun habit by planning family activities that don't involve eating—like a morning bike ride, a trip to the local bowling alley, or a predinner hike. Chances are, everyone will benefit.

everyone, such as hummus with fresh-cut vegetables for dipping. (*You'll* know it's clean, but everyone else will just see it as another delicious option.) If your family is begging for their favorite beef stir-fry, make it with half the meat and twice the vegetables, and make the sauce from scratch instead of using the packaged stuff with the artificial ingredients that you used to rely on. (Or pick a cleaner store-bought option.)

And when you can't beat them? Join them. Just be smart! The next time your dining companion absolutely *insists* on going to the place that only serves meatball subs or trying the new food truck known for its irresistible doughnuts, join in and have fun. Speaking up about your preferences and finding ways to meet your own needs is important. But once in a while, it's worth going with the flow. In those cases, find ways to keep your portions smaller without going hungry. Order a side of grilled vegetables so you can eat less of the poor quality entrée, or start your meal with a cup of broth-based vegetable soup.

Notes from a Clean Eater

"My brother-in-law, Alan F., lives next door. So he'd make two meals a week, and I'd make two meals a week, and we'd share. Doing it with somebody was huge. Not just for the emotional support, but because someone was making half the meals for me."—**Kathy C.**

When Jealousy Strikes

Once the pounds start melting off, the compliments will likely start flying. And if you were used to hiding your heavier body in baggy clothes, you might decide to start wearing outfits that are more flattering to your stronger, leaner shape. The kind words and awesome new reflection in the mirror are both great motivators to continue eating clean and working toward your weight-loss goals. But the newfound focus on your appearance could leave your partner or friends a little green-eyed—especially if they are on the heavier side.

Of course, if all that positive attention makes another person want to eat cleaner and lose weight too, great! If not? Your decision to get leaner is a good thing for both you and your loved ones—but it's about you, not them. And it's okay to remind them of that in a nice way. If your partner is prone to jealousy, diffuse the issue by stressing that you aren't trying to lose weight to impress others. You're doing it to feel better about yourself—both physically *and* mentally. Losing weight allows you to pursue a more active lifestyle—like meeting your friends for a round of tennis or taking that hiking vacation you've always talked about. It can increase your energy to help you be more productive during the day, and it can even reignite your sex life. Most importantly, though, losing weight improves your health so you have more healthy years to spend together.

When You "Mess Up"

Whether you overdo it on those irresistible cheese poppers at a party, eat an entire basket of chips at your favorite Tex-Mex spot, or even devour an entire pint of ice cream in front of the TV, remember: It's not the single wild splurge that throws your weight loss off track—it's how you deal with it *afterwards*. One poor choice isn't going to cause your pants to suddenly be too tight or make you gain 10 pounds. But dwelling on it might. That's because when you let yourself feel gross, guilty, or out of control over something you ate, you're usually driven to make more unhealthy choices. It might seem like the floodgates are open, so you may as well just keep on eating junk. Or maybe you get the idea in your head that you don't "deserve" to have a lean body, so you subconsciously start eating stuff that causes the pounds to pile back on.

But diving into more poor-quality food will only make you feel worse. And *everyone* deserves to have a strong, healthy body that they love. So instead of seeing the situation as proof that you're a failure at eating clean and wishing that it had never happened, use it as a chance to learn something new that can help you make better choices in the future. Did you devour all of the cheese snacks because you skipped lunch and showed up to the party starving? Next time, eat beforehand so you aren't ravenous when you arrive. Were your inhibitions

It's your weight-loss goal and you have to do the work, so why should you get others involved? Like with any challenging journey, strong support is key to success. In fact, findings show that dieters who embark on a weight-loss program with friends or family are more successful at maintaining their loss compared to dieters who go it alone.[3]

And support can come in many forms. There's emotional support from a friend who smiles with your successes and comforts you when you're frustrated. There's motivational support from your workout buddy who helps you find the get-up-and-go to lace up your sneakers. There's hands-on support from your spouse or family members who help shop for clean foods, keep tempting trigger foods out of sight, or watch your kids so you can steal some time for exercise or meal prep. There's even support-as-distraction from people who encourage new kinds of activities that don't center around eating, like taking a hike instead of meeting up for ice cream.

So be open about your feelings, ask for what you need, and be willing to accept help. You'll feel stronger, and chances are, you'll have an easier and more enjoyable time working toward your goals.

lowered at the restaurant because you'd had a little too much to drink? Make a mental note to sip your cocktail more slowly next time, or to stick with water. Did you reach for the ice cream because you were bored? Next time you have a free night, think about what you can do to stay busy so you're not tempted to snack.

No, making a plan for the future won't undo what happened in the past. But it *will* take your mind off the flub so you're not replaying it in your head and letting yourself feel terrible about it. And it'll give you a game plan for next time. Because you're not going to let one measly slipup stop you from eating clean and achieving your weight-loss goal. Nope—*no way*.

Notes from a Clean Eater

"On an extremely anxious day, I desperately needed a peanut butter and jelly fix. So I scratched that itch. I adjusted for it for the rest of the day, and then I moved on."—**Alan F.**

Putting It All Together

1 **Expect the unexpected.** All journeys, including weight-loss journeys, have speed bumps. By knowing where they might pop up, you can ride over them more smoothly.

2 **Know that you can eat clean *anywhere*.** Whether you're dining out, on vacation, or at a social event, it's almost always possible to make a healthier choice.

3 **Remember, honesty is the best policy.** If it seems like a friend or family member might be trying to sabotage your weight loss, give it to them straight and tell them why you want to get lean. When you're up front about what matters to you, they'll want to give their support—and you'll feel more motivated to stay on track, too.

4 **Don't let yourself get derailed.** Everyone overdoes it from time to time. So look at an unexpected splurge as a learning opportunity for next time.

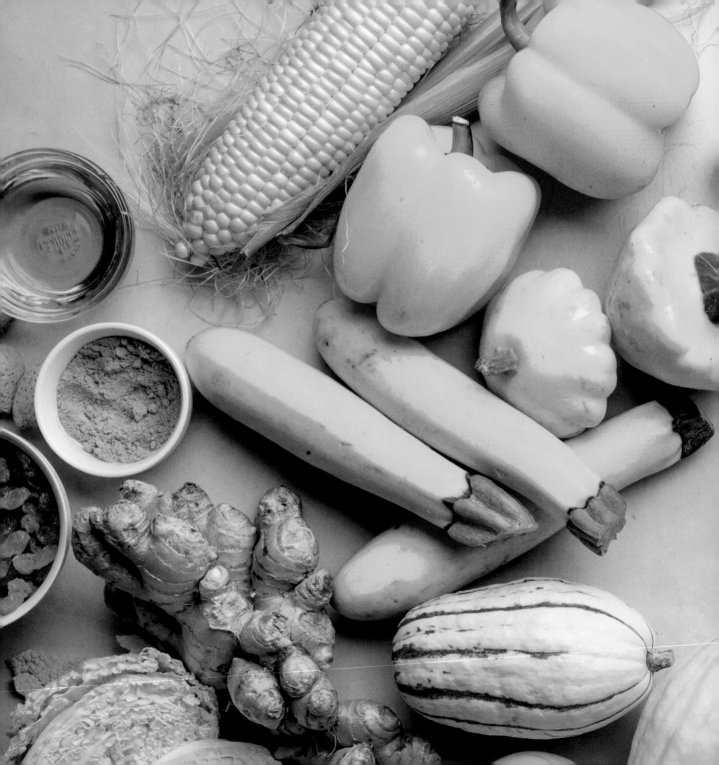

The Eat Clean, Stay Lean Weight-Loss Plan

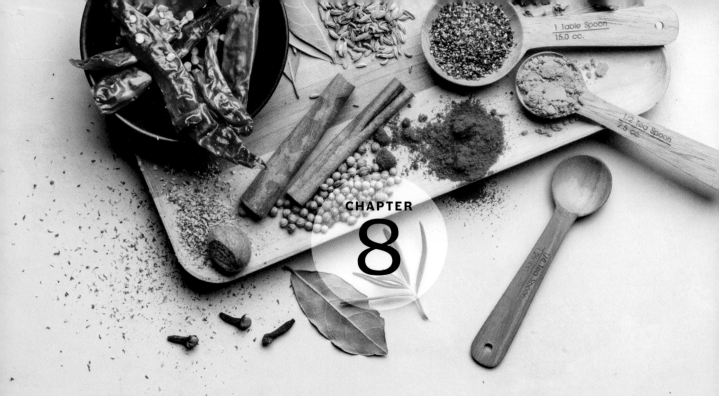

How to Make This Plan Work for You

Okay, you get it! Eating clean is the *best* way to get lean for life—and you're ready to get started. Following our 3-week plan will jump-start your weight loss—not to mention increase your energy levels, slash those tough-to-kick cravings, and take control of your health. Let's do this!

Why This Plan *Works*

The Eat Clean, Stay Lean weight-loss plan is designed for maximum weight loss. By utilizing nutrient-dense foods in the right ratios, it kicks your body's fat-burning engine into high gear—while helping you stay fuller, longer and keeping diet-derailing cravings at bay. Just as important, it's free of the stuff that can zap your energy, make you daydream about sugar, and prompt your body to store more fat.

Best of all? It's flexible—and it was designed for real life. Rather than having to work around a complicated, rigid program, you can enjoy our delicious, satisfying meals and snacks in the way that works for *you*. The weekly menus can be followed exactly as they are or be used as inspiration for building your own menus using our recipes and meal ideas. And the Get Lean Guidelines in the Breakfasts, Lunches and Dinners, and Snacks and Desserts chapters lay out everything you need to know to succeed at every single one of your daily eating occasions. So you don't just get the tools you need to lose weight *now*. You also learn how to build healthier eating habits to stay lean for life.

There's one essential thing to remember: **To achieve your best results, you've got to stick to the plan as closely as possible.** You can achieve some pretty significant changes in just 3 weeks—as long as you're willing to put in the work. But we know you can do it!

The Eat Clean, Stay Lean Focus Foods

What can you eat on this plan? By now, we bet you might already have a pretty good idea of what to expect: real, whole foods that are fresh or minimally processed and made without added chemicals or excess sugar or salt.

❋ **Fresh fruits and vegetables** at *every* meal and for at least one snack daily

❋ **Lean proteins,** such as chicken, turkey, pork, fish and seafood, lean beef, and eggs

❋ **Complex carbohydrates,** such as whole grains, and especially pulses and legumes (such as beans, split peas, and lentils)

Real People, Real Success

Here's more proof that when it comes to the Eat Clean, Stay Lean plan, losing weight is just the tip of the iceberg.

❋ "I still have sugar cravings, but they're definitely less often and less intense."—**Suzanne M.**

❋ "No heartburn. No trouble falling asleep. No fatigue."—**Steve B.**

❋ "I definitely have more energy. And my mood is better, too." —**Maryann L.**

❋ "Before, I didn't have a concept of portion size or when to say enough was enough. Now, I'm much more aware of how much I'm eating." —**Vimal P.**

* **Healthy fats,** such as nuts and seeds, olive oil, and avocados

* **Low-fat dairy,** such as low-fat plain Greek yogurt; low-fat milk; and some cheeses

* **No- or low-calorie beverages,** such as water (flat or bubbly), coffee, and tea

* **Flavorful condiments, and other clean add-ins,** such as vinegar, tamari, mustard, and salsa, and plant oils, such as olive oil, avocado oil, coconut oil, and organic canola oil (in moderation)

* **Fresh and dried herbs and spices,** such as fresh garlic, ginger, basil, and mint, as well as dried herbs and spices including oregano, thyme, rosemary, cinnamon, ginger, paprika, turmeric, and black pepper

Clean Eats, Big Results

By following this plan, you can expect to lose up to 10 pounds in just 21 days.

Men and those who are larger or more active will tend to lose more weight, while women and those who are smaller and less active may lose less. Remember, everybody is different when it comes to losing weight! Factors like your metabolism, body type, activity level, and even sleep can all play roles in how quickly the pounds come off. Regardless of the specific number of pounds you lose in that time, you're guaranteed to feel leaner, stronger, more energized—and all around better. You'll also experience fewer cravings and come away with the tools you need to keep eating clean and losing weight.

Steer Clear of These Foods!

This list likely won't come as a surprise—but we're reminding you anyway! Please, please, please avoid this stuff for the duration of the plan. Sure, it's tough, but the results will be worth it. (And you *can* do it.)

* **White sugar and added sugars,** unless they're called for in one of the Eat Clean, Stay Lean recipes
* **Enriched, refined flours,** such as all-purpose flour
* **Refined pasta, grains, or breads,** such as white pasta, white bread, or white rice

* **Baked goods or packaged sweets,** such as cookies, cakes, or ice creams
* **Packaged foods containing trans fats or artificial ingredients,** such as preservatives, colors, or flavors
* **Alcohol or soda,** including diet soda

* **Highly processed foods and packaged snacks,** which means anything with more than 10 ingredients, any unrecognizable ingredients or hyped-up health claims, and empty-calorie or poor-quality snacks. (For more on finding clean packaged foods, see Chapter 3.)

Using the Plan

The Eat Clean, Stay Lean plan is a 3-week program designed to jump-start your weight loss—and help you stay satisfied and energized while you do it. By planning out all of your meals and snacks ahead of time, you'll make it a cinch to stick with. And since you get to eat five or six times per day, you'll never have to worry about going hungry.

Notes from a Clean Eater

"Preparation and planning are key. And don't skip the snacks. You'll overeat at mealtime or eat so fast that you miss the goodness."—**Alan F.**

Getting Started

Ready to get this show on the road? Here's *exactly* how to do it.

Step 1: Map out your week of meals. What's on the menu for breakfasts, lunches, dinners, and snacks this week? It's up to you! Follow the weekly sample menus at the end of this chapter to the letter, if you'd like. Or use them as inspiration to design your own custom menus using the template on page 157 or at bazilians.com/ECSLdiet/extras. All of the meal and snack recipes on this plan are interchangeable, so as long as you stick with them, it works. What matters is that you have a plan.

Step 2: Determine your snack quota. If you're larger or more active, you may need more calories than someone who is smaller or more sedentary (even while you work to lose weight). Depending on your current weight, goal weight, and activity level, you should do one of the following:

❊ **Have three meals and two snacks** if you're a woman who exercises for 45 minutes or less on most days OR a man or woman who weighs less than 160 pounds.

❊ **Have three meals and three snacks** if you're a woman who exercises for 60 minutes or more on most days OR a man or woman who weighs more than 160 pounds OR you have 25 or more pounds to lose.

Step 3: Prep for success. With your weekly menu in place, it's time to make a grocery list and stock up on your ingredients. When you bring everything home, prep any meal or snack components that you know might be tough to tackle during the week. Wash and precut veggies. Whip up a batch of bean dip. Make the hearty salad that can sit in the fridge all week. The more you do ahead of time, the less likely you are to get thrown off if things suddenly get hectic later in the week.

Plan out your meals and snacks for the upcoming week on Thursday evening (or, at the latest, on Saturday morning), and make a shopping list. Both times tend to be quieter and more reliable than Friday, when you may be tired from a busy workweek or excited about the weekend.

With your shopping list in tow, hit the market on Saturday or during the first half of Sunday. You'll have fresh ingredients for the start of the week, and if you want to prep any of your meals or snacks beforehand, you'll have plenty of time to do so.

Step 4: Follow the Get Lean Guidelines in the Breakfasts, Lunches and Dinners, and Snacks and Desserts chapters. Different times of day come with different challenges (no time to make breakfast, last-minute dinner invitation, and so on), so we've laid out how to succeed at each separate eating occasion. Thoroughly review the Get Lean Guidelines, and you'll feel even more prepared to make clean choices at every meal, every day.

Step 5: Repeat—and lose big. Repeat this cycle for 2 more weeks, for a total of 3 weeks. Want to lose even more weight? Feel free to repeat the entire 3-week cycle, like our Clean Eaters did. You'll continue to lose weight—and reap all of the feel-good rewards of eating clean.

When Should I Weigh Myself?

Monday mornings. *That's* your day to weigh. Monday weigh-ins kick off your week with a motivated, enthusiastic start. Plus, you're more likely to stay on track over the weekend if you know that you have a weigh-in coming up first thing on Monday morning. If you're worried that you might be bleary-eyed and forget, set a recurring reminder on your phone.

As for the rest of the week, it's tempting, but resist the urge to hop on that scale at other times. Your weight fluctuates day by day—and even hour by hour, since we tend to retain more water as the day goes on. And just like the occasional bad hair day, there are days that if you were to hop on the scale, you might not see an accurate reflection of the progress that you're *really* making by following this program. That sort of up-and-down can spark a roller coaster of emotions that leave you overly optimistic (*Down 2 pounds. Maybe I can afford to splurge today?*) or completely defeated (*Up a pound—I'm a failure*). And neither of those is good for weight loss.

At 3 weeks long, this plan is more of a middle-distance race, not a sprint. Progress will happen faster than you might expect—but you won't see a difference every single day. That's just not how healthy weight-loss works. But if you stick with the plan, you *will* lose weight. And you'll feel better, too. Eventually, you'll get to your goal—and you'll find that staying there is your new, healthy norm.

Getting Set for Success

Losing weight takes hard work—so make yours go further. Put your get-lean pedal to the metal with these smart strategies.

Stick with the program. This plan was designed to jump-start your weight loss in just 3 to 6 weeks. And you can achieve big results—as long as you follow through! So stick to the meals and snacks on the program as closely as possible. Limit eating at restaurants, parties, or social functions as much as you can, and try to avoid nonessential travel. (Of course, it's possible to eat clean at all of these places, but it requires much more vigilance!) And temporarily part ways with your nightly glass of wine or your favorite dessert. Following the program and steering clear of extras might seem tough, but the results will be worth it. Remember, your favorites will still be there when you're done! And chances are, after seeing how great eating clean makes you feel, you'll be able to enjoy them in a healthier, more moderate way.

Remember, *always* plan ahead. How do you avoid ordering takeout when the fridge is practically empty when you get home late from work? Or making a beeline for the vending machine when your hunger gets the best of you in the middle of the afternoon? Plan, plan, *plan*. Even if you have to make an adjustment or two midweek, having a road map makes it easy to know which ingredients you need—and which you need to prepare in advance—in order to eat clean meals and snacks. Sure, it requires a little bit of extra work up front. But after a couple of weeks, you'll probably wonder how you ever got by any other way.

Do what's easiest for you. One of the best things

(continued on page 146)

Dr. Wendy Says . . .

If you're used to struggling with your weight, stepping on the scale might not be a pleasant experience. **And though it can sometimes be a little unnerving, research shows that people who have the most success with losing weight—and maintaining that loss—do use the scale as a tool.**

The key to weighing-in without letting it rule (or ruin) your day is to see the scale for what it really is. The scale isn't a living thing that's out to judge you or hurt your feelings. It's a simple machine that reads off a number. And that number is just *one* part of your story. Because remember, you're not just in this to lose weight—you're in this to build healthy habits for life, too. Keeping a journal where you record the foods you eat and your progress and patterns, stress levels, and sleep is just as important—and often, even more so—than merely tracking what the scale says.

And anyway, the physical benefits of eating clean go well beyond whatever that number might be. Even if your weight hasn't budged yet, you may already be losing inches and becoming more toned. Not to mention that you may have more energy, fewer cravings, clearer skin, and healthier digestion, just to name a few clean-eating benefits. So hop on the scale, look at the number, jot it down, and get on with your day.

Clean Eater

Melissa R.

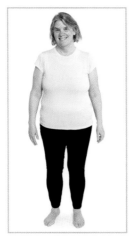

BEFORE

Melissa had always struggled with her weight. But after menopause and severe knee arthritis set in, her weight reached 302 pounds. At that point, walking a mere two blocks became a big deal.

Then, in July 2015, the 60-year-old decided it was time to get a knee replacement. An avid walker before her arthritis kicked in, Melissa gradually started building up to walking 11,000 steps per day—and the pounds started falling off. Before long, she had lost close to 75 pounds.

An emotional eater who struggled with cravings, Melissa soon found that heading outside for a stroll helped quell her desire to eat, especially when she felt stressed. So when she started eating clean to kick-start her progress again and lose some additional weight, Melissa stuck with what worked. "Cravings are like a siren call, and you're actively trying to find a buffer [to mute the call]. And it doesn't have to be a long walk. Just going around the block helps," she says.

But cravings were just a speed bump compared to the other challenges Melissa faced. Her sister had been dealing with a series of severe health issues, including multiple strokes and cancer, so Melissa flew down to her hometown of Oxford, Mississippi, to be with her. Despite the stress, she managed to make time to go food shopping so she could still eat clean meals, such as cereal and berries for breakfast or salad for lunch.

But dinners were more challenging in her sister's home, where Melissa's family would usually make something like fettuccine Alfredo. Without another option ready, Melissa would usually eat a small serving, using her new knowledge about portions to guide her. The experience taught her to be better prepared in the future—an important lesson she learned from looking at this challenge through her new clean-eating lens. "So next time I know that I have to do my own dinners. I can't hand my power over to them so I really do have to plan ahead," she says.

Dr. Wendy Observes: Melissa discovered that her weight-loss and health journey is truly hers alone and that only she has the power to make things happen. She also found out that despite life's many challenges and demands on her time, emotions, and energy, there are always ways to navigate toward success. It would have been easy for Melissa to fall into a pattern of eating whatever was convenient and quick, but she took steps to make clean eating convenient by stocking up on some simple staples while away from home.

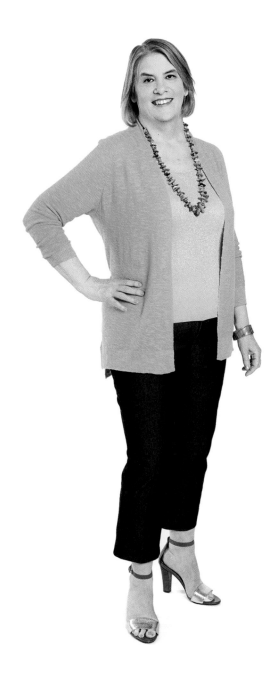

TOTAL POUNDS LOST

9.5 lbs

TOTAL INCHES LOST

11

MOST NOTABLE IMPROVEMENTS

Melissa's total cholesterol dropped by 8 points, her LDL ("bad") cholesterol fell by 9 points, and she lost more than 3 inches off her hips.

about the Eat Clean, Stay Lean plan is that you can tailor it to your needs. So take advantage! When planning your weekly menus, alternate more involved recipes with easy-assembly meals so you can spend less time in the kitchen. If you know you have a hard time packing lunches to take to work, double your dinner recipe and take the leftovers for lunch. And feel free to repeat stuff! Whether it's a single recipe or an entire weekly menu, if you love it and it works for your lifestyle, there's no reason why you can't make it over and over.

Track your progress. Success breeds motivation, so pay close attention to yours. Weigh yourself at the same time each week, and keep track as the pounds fall off. And if the scale hasn't budged yet? Don't let that discourage you. Everybody is different, and factors like age, size, body type, and even how much water you might be retaining all have an impact on how quickly or slowly you lose weight. So even if you don't see changes right away, they *will* come.

Count *every* victory. Remember, pounds lost aren't

What If I . . .

. . . AM INVITED TO A RESTAURANT OR SOCIAL EVENT?

Sorry, we strongly recommend eating only the meals in the plan, and that means not eating out. It might seem strict—but if you want to see real weight-loss results in just 3 weeks, it's important to buckle down. In the end, it'll be worth it! Of course, skipping restaurant meals doesn't mean that you have to stop socializing. Instead of meeting friends for dinner or drinks, try a nonfood activity. Go for a hike, see a movie, or meet them at a café for a cup of coffee or pot of tea.

What if there's something you really can't get out of, like an important work event or a family gathering? If you have to do it, you have to do it. But try to eat as clean as possible: Stick to lean protein and fruits and vegetables—and eat until you're satisfied, not stuffed. Stick to water or tea instead of alcohol or soda, and skip grains, refined carbs (like bread), and dessert. For more tips on eating clean while dining out, see Chapter 7.

. . . REALLY WANT A GLASS OF WINE OR DESSERT?

The clean snacks and treats built into the plan are designed to satisfy your sweet tooth without sacrificing your weight loss. Take the time to enjoy them!

Aside from those, remember: You'll lose the most weight by sticking to the plan exactly as it was designed. That means no booze and no desserts that aren't part of the plan. The alcohol in just one drink can make it harder to lose weight by slowing down your metabolism and causing your blood sugar to fluctuate. Alcohol also lowers your inhibitions, which makes it harder to stay on track and make smart choices. So please, please, steer clear!

. . . AM STILL HUNGRY?

The meals and snacks on the plan combine protein, fiber, and healthy fats to help you stay satisfied, so it's unlikely that you'll still feel hungry after you finish eating. (But remember, it's *normal* to start feeling hungry in the hour

the only markers of success when you're eating clean. Do your clothes fit more comfortably? Are you sleeping better at night or feeling more energetic during the day? Do you find your moods to be more stable? Are you craving less sugar? *All* of these are signs that you're making significant, positive changes to your health. Celebrate them!

Making Modifications

Got questions about how to modify the plan to meet your specific needs? We've got answers.

If you're vegetarian or vegan . . . You can adapt this plan to make it work for you by swapping meat proteins

or two leading up to a meal or snack.) It might be tough, but try to avoid nibbling on things that aren't a part of your weekly menu. Even clean, healthy foods have calories, and going over your calorie budget can slow your weight loss. If you need something to take the edge off, have a glass of water or sip a cup of herbal tea, then wait 20 minutes. Still feel like eating? Think about whether you'd be satisfied with fruit or raw vegetables. If the answer is yes, go ahead and have some. (Stick to one piece of fruit or a cup of raw veggies.) If the answer is no, you're probably just in the throes of a craving. Try to ride it out!

. . . CAN'T EAT ALL ORGANIC?

We know, organic options aren't always easy to find—and they tend to be more expensive than their conventional counterparts. Organic foods can help you fuel your body with the nutrients it needs—which is key to losing weight and feeling your best. But that doesn't necessarily mean that you need to go organic 100 percent of the time. Differ-ent fruits and vegetables contain different levels of pesticide residues (even after being washed), so it makes sense to go organic when possible. It's also a good idea to strive for organic if you're buying canola oil and foods containing corn or soy. (For more on why organic matters and which fruits and vegetables you should buy organic whenever possible, see Chapter 3.) Still, the benefits of eating conventional fruits and vegetables are significant, so don't skip something just because it isn't organic. Buy organic when you can, but never pass up an abundance of *any* fruits and vegetables on your journey toward a leaner you.

. . . SLIP UP?

Nobody's perfect! One flub won't completely wreck your weight loss—but how you deal with it can have a big impact. So if you cave and have a cookie or a slice of pizza, don't throw in the towel and eat more junk. Instead, accept your mistake and get right back on track with your next meal or snack. That's how you lose weight and keep it off for good.

for whole, plant-based alternatives: Think tofu, tempeh, lentils, beans and peas, nuts and seeds, and high-quality protein powders like those made from peas, hemp, or brown rice. (Skip the meat analogues, which tend to be highly processed and contain fillers and lots of belly-bloating sodium.) You may get more complex carbohydrates and less protein with these substitutions, which means that you might not lose as much weight as fast as someone who eats meat. But in the end, you will lose as much and more: Research shows that those who follow plant-based or vegetarian diets tend to be leaner than omnivores overall. And you'll still reap all of the benefits that come with eating a clean, nutrient-dense diet and keeping your calories in check.

If you can't eat gluten . . . No worries. The majority of the recipes in this plan are gluten-free, and those that aren't can easily be modified.

✳ **Swap gluten-containing grains like farro for gluten-free grains like quinoa or brown rice.**

✳ **Swap wheat bread or tortillas for gluten-free bread or gluten-free tortillas made from whole grains, nuts, seeds, or legumes.** Avoid gluten-free bread or tortillas made with refined flours or starches.

✳ **If a recipe calls for a packaged ingredient, such as oats, always check to confirm that the ingredient you buy is labeled gluten-free.**

If you have a food allergy . . . If you have an allergy or an intolerance to an ingredient in a recipe, please don't use it! Stick to recipes with ingredients that are safe for you to eat, or try modifying the recipe to meet your needs. For instance, swap peanuts or tree nuts for seeds, or sub shellfish for another lean protein.

Eat Clean, Stay Lean Sample Menu Plans

Follow these meal plans on the following pages exactly, or use them as a reference and tweak to your liking. Love one week? Fond of a particular breakfast or lunch option? Feel free to repeat it. Sticking with meals and snacks that you find delicious—and that easily fit your lifestyle—is key to losing weight and keeping it off.

When you see . . .

Eat Clean, Stay Lean

Find the full recipes for these meals and snacks beginning on page 220.

Clean and Simple

Find quick steps for these looser, easy-to-assemble meals and snacks right in the Breakfasts, Lunches and Dinners, and Snacks and Desserts chapters.

Week 1

MONDAY	
Breakfast	2 tablespoons *Eat Clean, Stay Lean PB&J Granola* (page 282) with ¾ cup low-fat plain regular OR Greek yogurt (or ¾ cup low-fat, low-sodium cottage cheese) AND one of the following: ¾ cup berries, mango, or pineapple OR ½ banana
Lunch	*Eat Clean, Stay Lean Turkey Cuban Wrap with Zesty Black Bean Salad* (page 238)
Dinner	**Clean and Simple Fish** (page 187) OR 4 ounces clean canned tuna mixed with 2 tablespoons Greek yogurt, 1 teaspoon mustard, chopped celery, and your favorite herbs or spices AND *Eat Clean, Stay Lean Roasted Broccoli with Chile and Lemon* (page 277)
Snack 1	1 small apple with 1 tablespoon almond butter
Snack 2	3 small whole grain crackers with 1 ounce (about 2 tablespoons) goat cheese
Snack 3	1 snack from the snack list (page 197) OR piece of fruit (optional)
TUESDAY	
Breakfast	*Eat Clean, Stay Lean Overnight Steel-Cut Oatmeal* (page 226)
Lunch	*Eat Clean, Stay Lean Black Bean Sweet Potato Sherry Soup* (page 263) AND 1 large piece of fruit OR 1 cup mixed fruit
Dinner	*Eat Clean, Stay Lean Cuban Avocado and Pineapple Salad* (page 269) AND **Clean and Simple Grilled Chicken** (page 187) AND 1 piece of fruit OR ¾ cup berries
Snack 1	1 medium orange (or 3 clementines) with 8 almonds
Snack 2	*Eat Clean, Stay Lean Curry Butternut Squash Soup* (page 262)
Snack 3	1 snack from the snack list (page 197) OR piece of fruit (optional)
WEDNESDAY	
Breakfast	*Eat Clean, Stay Lean Overnight Steel-Cut Oatmeal* (page 226)
Lunch	*Eat Clean, Stay Lean Turkey Cuban Wrap with Zesty Black Bean Salad* (page 238)
Dinner	**Clean and Simple Entrée Salad with Tuna, Veggies, and Fruit** (page 179) AND ½ cup fresh fruit salad OR small piece of fruit AND ½ whole wheat pita, 1 corn tortilla (5- or 6-inch) OR 5 or 6 whole grain crackers
Snack 1	1 small apple with 1 tablespoon almond butter
Snack 2	3 small whole grain crackers with 1 ounce (about 2 tablespoons) goat cheese
Snack 3	1 snack from the snack list (page 197) OR piece of fruit (optional)

Week 1 (cont.)

THURSDAY	
Breakfast	2 tablespoons *Eat Clean, Stay Lean PB&J Granola* (page 282) with ¾ cup low-fat plain regular or Greek yogurt OR ¾ cup low-fat, low-sodium cottage cheese AND ¾ cup berries, mango, or pineapple OR ½ banana
Lunch	*Eat Clean, Stay Lean Black Bean Sweet Potato Sherry Soup* (page 263) AND I large piece of fruit OR I cup mixed fruit
Dinner	*Eat Clean, Stay Lean Tuna and Cannellini Salad* (page 233)
Snack I	I *Eat Clean, Stay Lean Pumpkin-Cranberry-Cherry Breakfast Ball* (page 229)
Snack 2	I medium orange (or 3 clementines) with 8 almonds
Snack 3	I snack from the snack list (page 197) OR piece of fruit (optional)
FRIDAY	
Breakfast	*Eat Clean, Stay Lean Overnight Steel-Cut Oatmeal* (page 226)
Lunch	*Eat Clean, Stay Lean Tuna and Cannellini Salad* (page 233)
Dinner	*Eat Clean, Stay Lean Shrimp Scampi over Garlicky Greens* (page 246) AND ½ baked sweet potato
Snack I	I small apple with I tablespoon almond butter
Snack 2	I *Eat Clean, Stay Lean Pumpkin-Cranberry-Cherry Breakfast Ball* (page 229)
Snack 3	I snack from the snack list (page 197) OR piece of fruit (optional)
SATURDAY	
Breakfast	*Eat Clean, Stay Lean Avocado Tostadas with Huevos Rancheros* (page 223)
Lunch	**Clean and Simple Stuffed Veggie Pitas** (page 182)
Dinner	*Eat Clean, Stay Lean Maple Mustard Glazed Pork Tenderloin with Roasted Vegetables and Apples* (page 256)
Snack I	I small apple with I tablespoon almond butter
Snack 2	*Eat Clean, Stay Lean Curry Butternut Squash Soup* (page 262)
Snack 3	I snack from the snack list (page 197) OR piece of fruit (optional)

(continued)

Week 1 (cont.)

	SUNDAY
Breakfast	*Eat Clean, Stay Lean Avocado Tostadas with Huevos Rancheros* (page 223)
Lunch	*Eat Clean, Stay Lean Creamy Chicken, Green Grape, and Farro Salad* (page 237)
Dinner	*Eat Clean, Stay Lean Cuban Avocado and Pineapple Salad* (page 269) AND 4 ounces grilled salmon or chicken AND I piece fruit OR ¾ cup berries
Snack I	I *Eat Clean, Stay Lean Pumpkin-Cranberry-Cherry Breakfast Ball* (page 229)
Snack 2	3 cups *Eat Clean, Stay Lean Gremolata Parmesan Popcorn* (page 279)
Snack 3	I snack from the snack list (page 197) OR piece of fruit (optional)

Week 2

	MONDAY
Breakfast	**Clean and Simple Cereal and Fruit** (page 171)
Lunch	**Clean and Simple Stuffed Veggie Pitas** (page 182)
Dinner	*Eat Clean, Stay Lean Turkey Roulade* (page 251) AND I cup steamed broccoli with lemon
Snack I	2 tablespoons dried cherries with 5 walnut halves
Snack 2	¾ cup organic non-GMO steamed edamame (in pods)
Snack 3	I snack from the snack list (page 197) OR piece of fruit (optional)
	TUESDAY
Breakfast	*Eat Clean, Stay Lean Green Ginger Smoothie* (page 232) blended with I scoop clean protein powder
Lunch	*Eat Clean, Stay Lean Turkey Roulade* (page 251) AND I cup steamed broccoli with lemon
Dinner	*Eat Clean, Stay Lean Chickpea Curry–Stuffed Squash* (page 255)
Snack I	I hard-boiled egg with 5 whole grain crackers
Snack 2	2 tablespoons dried cherries with 5 walnut halves
Snack 3	I snack from the snack list (page 197) OR piece of fruit (optional)

Week 2 (cont.)

WEDNESDAY	
Breakfast	**Clean and Simple Cereal and Fruit** (page 171)
Lunch	**Clean and Simple Stuffed Veggie Pitas** (page 182)
Dinner	*Eat Clean, Stay Lean Summer Roll Salad with Peanut Dipping Sauce* (page 270) AND *Eat Clean, Stay Lean Cauliflower Rice Pilaf* (page 278)
Snack 1	1 hard-boiled egg with 5 whole grain crackers
Snack 2	¾ cup organic, non-GMO steamed edamame (in pods)
Snack 3	1 snack from the snack list (page 197) OR piece of fruit (optional)

THURSDAY	
Breakfast	*Eat Clean, Stay Lean Green Ginger Smoothie* (page 232) blended with 1 scoop protein powder
Lunch	*Eat Clean, Stay Lean Chickpea Curry–Stuffed Squash* (page 255)
Dinner	**Clean and Simple Soup Combo** (page 185) AND a small side salad
Snack 1	2 tablespoons dried cherries with 5 walnut halves
Snack 2	1 large celery stalk with 1 tablespoon peanut butter
Snack 3	1 snack from the snack list (page 197) OR piece of fruit (optional)

FRIDAY	
Breakfast	**Clean and Simple Cereal and Fruit** (page 171)
Lunch	*Eat Clean, Stay Lean Hearty Lentil Mushroom Soup* (page 265) AND ¾ cup low-fat Greek yogurt with ½ cup berries
Dinner	*Eat Clean, Stay Lean Israeli Couscous Salad with Salmon* (page 245)
Snack 1	1 clean granola or protein par
Snack 2	¾ cup organic, non-GMO steamed edamame (in pods)
Snack 3	1 snack from the snack list (page 197) OR piece of fruit (optional)

(continued)

Week 2 (cont.)

SATURDAY	
Breakfast	*Eat Clean, Stay Lean Easy Buckwheat Crepes* (any variety; page 227)
Lunch	*Eat Clean, Stay Lean Israeli Couscous Salad with Salmon* (page 245)
Dinner	*Eat Clean, Stay Lean Slow Cooker BBQ Pulled Chicken Flatbreads* (page 248)
Snack 1	1 large celery stalk with 1 tablespoon peanut butter
Snack 2	2 tablespoons dried cherries with 5 walnut halves
Snack 3	1 snack from the snack list (page 197) OR piece of fruit (optional)
SUNDAY	
Breakfast	*Eat Clean, Stay Lean Easy Buckwheat Crepes* (any variety; page 227)
Lunch	*Eat Clean, Stay Lean Israeli Couscous Salad with Salmon* (page 245)
Dinner	*Eat Clean, Stay Lean Kale Quesadillas* (page 235)
Snack 1	1 hard-boiled egg with 15 grapes
Snack 2	1 clean granola or protein bar
Snack 3	1 snack from the snack list (page 197) OR piece of fruit

Week 3

MONDAY	
Breakfast	*Eat Clean, Stay Lean Dried Tart Cherry Chia Jam and Ricotta on Toast* (page 285) AND 1 hard-boiled egg OR 5 or 6 walnut halves
Lunch	*Eat Clean, Stay Lean Hearty Chicken Panzanella* (page 241)
Dinner	*Eat Clean, Stay Lean Beef Scallion Roll-Ups* (page 242)
Snack 1	1 organic string cheese and piece of fruit
Snack 2	2 tablespoons *Eat Clean, Stay Lean Lemony Rosemary White Bean Dip* (page 286) AND 1 cup assorted raw vegetables
Snack 3	1 snack from the snack list (page 197) OR piece of fruit (optional)

Week 3 (cont.)

	TUESDAY
Breakfast	**Clean and Simple Oatmeal with Berries and Nuts** (page 168)
Lunch	***Eat Clean, Stay Lean Beef Scallion Roll-Ups*** (page 242)
Dinner	***Eat Clean, Stay Lean Kale Quesadillas*** (page 235)
Snack 1	3 dried apricots with 20 pistachios
Snack 2	2 tablespoons ***Eat Clean, Stay Lean Lemony Rosemary White Bean Dip*** (page 286) AND 1 cup assorted raw vegetables
Snack 3	1 snack from the snack list (page 197) OR piece of fruit (optional)
	WEDNESDAY
Breakfast	***Eat Clean, Stay Lean Dried Tart Cherry Chia Jam and Ricotta on Toast*** (page 285) AND 1 hard-boiled egg OR 25 pistachios
Lunch	**Clean and Simple Sliced Apple and Peanut Butter "Sandwich"** (page 182) AND 8 carrot sticks (1 large or 2 medium sliced carrots) with ¼ cup hummus
Dinner	***Eat Clean, Stay Lean Tuna and Cannellini Salad*** (page 233)
Snack 1	1 ***Eat Clean, Stay Lean Pumpkin-Cranberry-Cherry Breakfast Ball*** (page 229)
Snack 2	1 organic string cheese with piece of fruit
Snack 3	1 snack from the snack list (page 197) OR piece of fruit (optional)
	THURSDAY
Breakfast	**Clean and Simple Oatmeal with Berries and Nuts** (page 168)
Lunch	***Eat Clean, Stay Lean Tuna and Cannellini Salad*** (page 233)
Dinner	***Eat Clean, Stay Lean Fiesta Quinoa with Shrimp*** (page 273)
Snack 1	1 hard-boiled egg with piece of fruit
Snack 2	2 tablespoons ***Eat Clean, Stay Lean Lemony Rosemary White Bean Dip*** (page 286) AND 1 cup assorted raw vegetables
Snack 3	1 snack from the snack list (page 197) OR piece of fruit

(continued)

Week 3 (cont.)

	FRIDAY
Breakfast	***Eat Clean, Stay Lean Dried Tart Cherry Chia Jam and Ricotta on Toast*** (page 285) AND I hard-boiled egg OR 10 almonds
Lunch	***Eat Clean, Stay Lean Fiesta Quinoa with Shrimp*** (page 273)
Dinner	***Eat Clean, Stay Lean Israeli Couscous Salad with Salmon*** (page 245)
Snack I	I hard-boiled egg with piece of fruit
Snack 2	3 dried apricots with 20 pistachios
Snack 3	I snack from the snack list (page 197) OR piece of fruit (optional)

	SATURDAY
Breakfast	***Eat Clean, Stay Lean Mini Spinach Mushroom Quiche*** (page 224)
Lunch	***Eat Clean, Stay Lean Israeli Couscous Salad with Salmon*** (page 245)
Dinner	***Eat Clean, Stay Lean White Gazpacho with Grapes and Almonds*** (page 264) AND ***Eat Clean, Stay Lean Summer Roll Salad with Peanut Dipping Sauce*** (page 270)
Snack I	3 dried apricots with 20 pistachios
Snack 2	I ***Eat Clean, Stay Lean Pumpkin-Cranberry-Cherry Breakfast Ball*** (page 229)
Snack 3	I snack from the snack list (page 197) OR piece of fruit

	SUNDAY
Breakfast	***Eat Clean, Stay Lean Mini Spinach Mushroom Quiche*** (page 224)
Lunch	***Eat Clean, Stay Lean White Gazpacho with Grapes and Almonds*** (page 264) AND ***Eat Clean, Stay Lean Summer Roll Salad with Peanut Dipping Sauce*** (page 270)
Dinner	**Clean and Simple Fish, Poultry, or Lean Meat** (page 187) AND ***Eat Clean, Stay Lean Roasted Citrus-and-Herb Sweet Potatoes*** (page 276)
Snack I	I organic string cheese with piece of fruit
Snack 2	2 tablespoons ***Eat Clean, Stay Lean Lemony Rosemary White Bean Dip*** (page 286) AND I cup assorted raw vegetables
Snack 3	I snack from the snack list (page 197) OR piece of fruit (optional)

Make-Your-Own Weekly Menu Template

Prefer to build your own weekly menus? Go for it! Choose from any of the breakfasts, lunches, dinners, and snacks in the following chapters, and write your picks in the spots provided. And feel free to repeat meals as often as you like to make planning, shopping, and prepping easier. Make copies of this template for future weeks, or find a printable version at bazilians.com/ECSLdiet/extras.

MONDAY	
Breakfast	
Lunch	
Dinner	
Snack 1	
Snack 2	
Snack 3	I snack from the snack list (page 197) OR piece of fruit (optional)
TUESDAY	
Breakfast	
Lunch	
Dinner	
Snack 1	
Snack 2	
Snack 3	I snack from the snack list (page 197) OR piece of fruit (optional)
WEDNESDAY	
Breakfast	
Lunch	
Dinner	
Snack 1	
Snack 2	
Snack 3	I snack from the snack list (page 197) OR piece of fruit (optional)

(continued)

Make-Your-Own Weekly Menu Template (cont.)

THURSDAY	
Breakfast	
Lunch	
Dinner	
Snack I	
Snack 2	
Snack 3	I snack from the snack list (page I97) OR piece of fruit (optional)

FRIDAY	
Breakfast	
Lunch	
Dinner	
Snack I	
Snack 2	
Snack 3	I snack from the snack list (page I97) OR piece of fruit (optional)

SATURDAY	
Breakfast	
Lunch	
Dinner	
Snack I	
Snack 2	
Snack 3	I snack from the snack list (page I97) OR piece of fruit (optional)

SUNDAY	
Breakfast	
Lunch	
Dinner	
Snack I	
Snack 2	
Snack 3	I snack from the snack list (page I97) OR piece of fruit (optional)

Putting It All Together

1 **Focus on nutrient-dense foods to get lean—fast.** Eating the right foods can kick your body's fat-burning engine into high gear, helping you lose up to 10 pounds in just 21 days.

2 **Stick to the plan as much as possible.** The closer you follow it, the more successful your weight-loss efforts will be. Yup, it'll take some commitment. But you can do it!

3 **Map out your weekly meals and plan ahead.** Follow the sample menus or build your own using our template. Just make sure you stick with the meals and snacks as outlined earlier, and plan ahead so you're always prepared.

4 **Make it work for you.** If you follow a gluten-free, vegan, or vegetarian eating style, or if you have a food allergy, tweak the menus and recipes to fit your needs. You'll still lose weight and make big improvements to your health!

5 **Stay positive.** Everyone loses weight at different rates, and nobody eats perfectly 100 percent of the time. Just stick with eating clean, and if you slip up, accept it and move on. The pounds *will* come off.

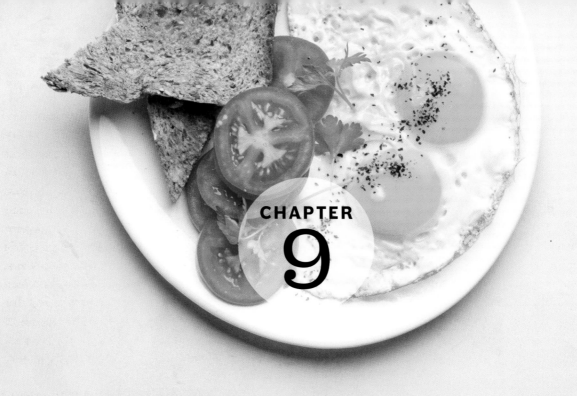

Breakfasts

It's the most important meal of the day, especially when it comes to getting lean. And yet, many of us are perpetually guilty of giving breakfast the brush-off. So let's stop the morning madness: These tasty meal ideas and smart strategies will help you make clean breakfasts a delicious—and *doable*—part of your a.m. routine.

Be a Breakfast Buff

I don't have time! I'm not hungry right now! I'll pick something up on the way to work! No matter what your excuse for skipping breakfast, it's time to set it aside. **When it comes to losing weight, breakfast really *is* the most important meal of the day.** In fact, 78 percent of people who have lost weight—and kept it off—say that they eat breakfast *every day*. If you're serious about slimming down, it's time to join their ranks.

What makes breakfast so special? For starters, a clean morning meal sets the tone for making smart food moves throughout the rest of the day. You feel good when you kick things off with a bowl of Greek yogurt and fresh fruit or scrambled eggs with vegetables—and that clean-eating high can motivate you to make another awesome choice at lunch, and again at dinner. From personal experience, you may have already learned that a greasy breakfast sandwich or sugary muffin doesn't exactly have the same effect.

More importantly, breakfast ensures that your blood sugar stays steady, which means you won't suddenly find yourself starving at 10:30 a.m. and struggling with an urge to scrounge around the break room for a doughnut. (In fact, findings suggest that eating a balanced breakfast can actually help stave off junky cravings *all day long*.[1]) There's also the fact that breakfast wakes up your metabolism—kind of like putting a fresh log on the fire when the flames start to die down. And of course, breakfast gives you fuel to be active. You're way more likely to want to walk the kids to school rather than drive them, or to take the steps instead of the elevator, if you have something in your belly. Add it all up, and it's easy to see why making a habit of eating in the a.m. is a no-brainer.

So what exactly should you eat, and is there anything else you can do to make your morning meal a success? Right this way—we've got some delicious answers.

Dr. Wendy Says . . .

True, plenty of us struggle to find the time or energy for breakfast amid the morning mayhem. But there's a better group to be a part of, instead: the thousands of people belonging to the National Weight Control Registry. These inspiring folks haven't just lost a significant amount of weight—they've *maintained* that loss for many years. And the majority of them have one very important daily behavior in common: *They eat breakfast.*[2]

Still, not every morning meal needs to be a set-the-table-and-sit-down affair. And if you know you rarely have the time for that, planning grab-and-go breakfasts can help set you up for a.m. eating success. Build easy, eat-and-run meals into your breakfast menu, and you'll know exactly what to prep or reach for before you head out the door. Some smart, simple options include:

❋ **Clean and Simple Scramble (page 164).** Fold your toast in half to make a sandwich.

❋ **Clean and Simple Fruit on the Bottom Yogurt (page 166).** Top it with slivered almonds.

❋ **Clean and Simple Almond Butter and Banana Toast (page 170).** Sprinkle this easy open-faced sandwich with cinnamon, if you'd like.

Get Lean Guidelines: Breakfast

There are an awful lot of things that can get in the way of a healthy breakfast—and we're not just talking about the toaster pastries staring you down when you open your pantry. Mornings are hectic, after all. Still, a little bit of a.m. craziness doesn't have to stop you. No matter what's going on, you can set yourself up for triumph at the breakfast table (or in the car, or at your desk) every morning of the week. Here's exactly how to do it.

❋ **Plan out your meals.** Plan your breakfasts at the same time that you plan the rest of your meals for the week—either by following the weekly menu or by using the template or an app to create your own. Take time to think about what you'll be in the mood to eat and what will work best with your schedule. (Is it supposed to be chilly? Maybe oatmeal would be satisfying. Know you won't have much time for meal prep? Greek yogurt with fruit and nuts only takes 2 minutes to prep.) Then write it down. Having a plan doesn't just mean that you'll know what's for breakfast and know what you need to do to prepare it. It also sets the *intention* of eating a clean breakfast, which in itself can be a powerful motivator.

❋ **Be a repeat offender.** When planning your weekly breakfast menu, choose at least two different options, but no more than three. Trying new recipes is great, and it's fun to experiment when you have time. (That's what weekends are for, right?) But keeping things simple, especially on busy weekday mornings, boosts your likeli-hood of actually following through. How about alternating eggs on Monday, Wednesday, and Friday with smoothies on Tuesday and Thursday, and enjoying crepes on the weekend?

❋ **Always have a fruit or vegetable.** Fruits and vegetables are essential to eating clean, so don't skip out! Stir fresh berries into your cottage cheese, or have some sliced tomato alongside your scrambled eggs. Following the meal ideas in this chapter? You're all set. Each one delivers at least one serving of fruits or vegetables—and often, even more.

❋ **Remember, don't wait *too* long.** You don't have to eat the minute you wake up, but try to get something in your stomach within an hour or two. When you wait too long, your metabolism starts to slow down in an effort to conserve fuel.

❋ **Take notes on your meal.** Have your preplanned menu handy when you sit down to eat, and jot down your thoughts. Did you need to make any changes—like scrambling your eggs instead of hard-cooking them because you were short on time? What were your hunger, energy, and stress levels like? These sorts of notes can serve as a record for what works and what doesn't at breakfast time—so you can troubleshoot and plan more efficiently in the future. Jot your notes directly on your weekly menu or write them in a separate notebook.

❋ ***Do not* skip breakfast! No matter what, eat breakfast every day.** You're building a healthy habit, so stick with it!

Let's Eat!

If you've tried to lose weight in the past, your breakfast may have consisted of bars or shakes, plain fruit, or rubbery egg whites. But a clean morning meal can also be a delicious one—and making it doesn't have to be time-consuming. So what's on the menu? Here's *exactly* what you need to know in order to make a clean breakfast, plus delicious meals that can help you get lean fast.

Building a Clean Breakfast

What separates a satisfying breakfast that delivers lasting energy from one that leaves you feeling sluggish, prone to cravings, and possibly hungry again by 10:30 a.m.? The happy combo of lean protein, high-fiber carbs, and healthy fats. All of the meal ideas and recipes in this book serve up the right balance of all three—so if you choose to add them to your morning menu, just prepare and enjoy. Rather try building your own, instead? Go for it! Just keep these simple rules in mind.

❖ **Start with a shot of protein.** Aim for 15 to 20 grams, which will help you stay full for longer, keep your blood sugar steady, and blunt cravings. Think one or two eggs; 3/4 cup of low-fat plain regular or Greek yogurt; 3 ounces of poultry, fish, or meat; 2 tablespoons of nuts or nut butter; 1/2 cup of beans; or 1 scoop of clean protein powder.

❖ **Pick some produce.** It's not a well-rounded meal without fruits or vegetables, so be sure to include 3/4 cup of fruit or at least 1 cup of vegetables.

❖ **Go with the whole grain.** You don't have to include a grain as part of your breakfast. But if you do, make sure it's a whole grain that's high in belly-filling fiber. A slice of whole grain toast (80 to 100 calories per slice), 1/3 cup of dry oats (2/3 cup cooked), or a 5- to 6-inch corn tortilla all work.

❖ **Finish with fat.** Healthy fats don't just make your breakfast taste better, they also give the meal some

---

Dr. Wendy Says . . .

Enjoy your morning joe! Coffee is loaded with phytonutrients, and the caffeine can give your metabolism an extra boost. And while a splash of milk and a teaspoon or two of sugar is perfectly fine, more than that can start to derail your weight-loss progress—especially if you're drinking multiple cups. As for fancy drinks like lattes or cappuccinos, feel free to enjoy them unsweetened—but account for the calories and where they fit into your day. A 12-ounce latte made with 2% milk has about 150 calories, which is about the same as a snack. So if you have one occasionally in addition to your breakfast, cut out one of your snacks for the day.

staying power in your stomach. Of course, calories do add up, so be choosy. Limit your fats to those that are built into whole foods, such as eggs, avocados, nuts and seeds, or nut butters. If you're adding extra fat, such as olive oil, keep it to 2 teaspoons, maximum.

Eat Clean, Stay Lean Breakfasts

You can find all of the full Eat Clean, Stay Lean recipes in Chapter 13. Clean and Simple recipes are meant to be looser, easy-assembly, mix-and-match sorts of meals—so we've included quick steps for making those right here.

EGGS

Eat Clean, Stay Lean Avocado Tostadas with Huevos Rancheros (page 223)

Eat Clean, Stay Lean Mini Spinach Mushroom Quiche (page 224)

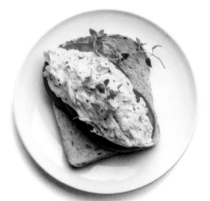

Clean and Simple Scramble

Top 1 slice whole grain toast
with 1 scrambled egg.
Serve with 1 medium sliced tomato
OR ¾ cup fruit.

Clean and Simple Cheddar Cheese, Egg, and Tomato Toast

Top one slice whole grain bread with 1 whole egg (poached or scrambled), 1 medium sliced tomato, and 2 tablespoons grated sharp Cheddar cheese. Toast until the bread is toasted and the cheese is melted.

and

A medium apple, a medium orange,
OR ¾ cup berries

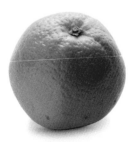

YOGURT AND COTTAGE CHEESE

2 tablespoons Eat Clean, Stay Lean PB&J Granola (page 282)

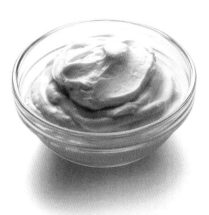

and

¾ cup low-fat plain regular or Greek yogurt OR
¾ cup low-fat, low-sodium cottage cheese

and

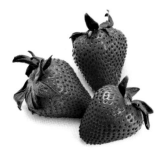

¾ cup berries, mango, or pineapple OR ½ banana

Shop Clean Checklist: Whole Grain Bread and Pita

LOOK FOR:

* A whole grain as the first ingredient (like "whole wheat")
* Five or fewer ingredients (ideally): Whole grain flour (may be more than one type), water, yeast, salt, and natural sweetener such as honey, maple syrup, molasses, cane sugar, date paste, or raisin paste
* Up to 100 calories and at least 2 g of fiber per serving
* Less than 200 mg of sodium per serving
* Little or no added sugar. (If there is sugar, it should be a clean ingredient and not one of the first four ingredients.)

EAT CLEAN, STAY LEAN PICKS:

* Rudi's Organic Bakery breads and English muffins (regular and gluten-free)
* Food for Life Ezekiel 4:9 breads— 7 Sprouted Grains, Sesame, and Cinnamon Raisin
* Manna Organics breads and gluten-free breads
* Milton's Craft Bakers 100% Whole Wheat, Seeds and Grains, and Healthy Multi-Grain Plus breads
* Trader Joe's Gluten Free Whole Grain Bread
* The Julian Bakery Paleo Bread (gluten-free varieties)
* Trader Joe's Whole Wheat Pita Bread (½ pita = 1 serving)
* Against the Grain Gourmet Lebanese-Style Pita Bread (½ pita = 1 serving)

Clean and Simple Yogurt, Berry, and Nut Parfait

Layer ¾ cup nonfat plain regular or Greek yogurt with ½ medium sliced banana, I cup sliced strawberries OR ½ cup blueberries or raspberries, and 2 tablespoons chopped nuts or seeds. Drizzle with I teaspoon honey.

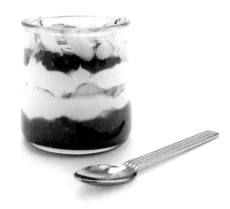

Clean and Simple Fruit on the Bottom Yogurt

Layer 2 tablespoons Eat Clean, Stay Lean Dried Tart Cherry Chia Jam (page 285) with I cup low-fat plain regular or Greek yogurt.

and one of the following:

2 tablespoons slivered almonds, sprinkled on the yogurt OR
¾ cup whole grain cereal, sprinkled on the yogurt OR I hard-boiled egg, on the side

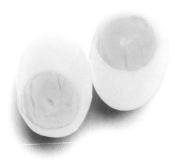

Clean and Simple Baked Apple with Yogurt and Nuts

Heat the oven to 350°F. Core an apple and place it in a shallow baking dish. Fill the dish with ¼" of water and sprinkle cinnamon into the cored area. Bake for 30 minutes, or until tender. Top the baked apple with I cup nonfat or low-fat plain regular or Greek yogurt (or ¾ cup no-salt-added nonfat cottage cheese), and 2 tablespoons ground flaxseeds OR 2 tablespoons chopped nuts.

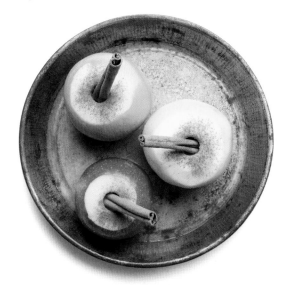

Shop Clean Checklist: Jam

LOOK FOR:

❋ Fruit as the first ingredient
❋ Ideally, jams made with all fruit (plus pectin, a natural thickener)
❋ No more than 8 g of sugar per serving

❋ If a jam has added sugars, the sugars should be natural, such as fruit juice, honey, or cane sugar
❋ Zero artificial sweeteners

EAT CLEAN, STAY LEAN PICKS:

❋ Trader Joe's Organic Reduced Sugar Preserves
❋ Polaner All Fruit spreads
❋ St. Dalfour I00% Fruit spreads

❋ Crofter's Premium Spread
❋ Bionaturae Organic Fruit Spread

OATMEAL

Eat Clean, Stay Lean Overnight Steel-Cut Oatmeal (page 226)

Eat Clean, Stay Lean Pumpkin-Cranberry-Cherry Breakfast Balls (page 229)

Clean and Simple Oatmeal with Berries and Nuts

Cook 1 ounce dry (1 packet or ⅓ cup) oats with ¾ cup low-fat milk, plant-based milk alternative, or water according to package directions. Top with ¾ cup berries, 1 tablespoon nuts or 1½ tablespoons ground flaxseed, and ¼ teaspoon cinnamon. If cooking the oats with water, add 2 teaspoons of honey, if desired. (Omit the honey if cooking the oats with milk or milk alternative.)

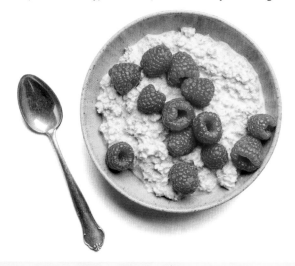

Over Oatmeal?

A bowl of oats might be the usual choice for a whole grain breakfast, but it certainly isn't the only one. In fact, you can turn almost *any* whole grain into a hearty porridge just by simmering it in milk instead of water and adding in your favorite toppings. A few flavorful combos:

❊ Per serving, use: ⅓ cup dried grains, 1 cup fruit or vegetables, ½ teaspoon dried herbs or spices, 2 tablespoons nuts, and 1 to 2 tablespoons dried fruit.

❊ Quinoa + strawberries + toasted almonds + vanilla bean (remove vanilla bean after cooking)

❊ Polenta + fresh raspberries + cinnamon + chopped dried figs

❊ Brown rice + steamed spinach + chopped scallions + low-sodium tamari

❊ Barley + sautéed mushrooms + dried thyme + soft-boiled egg

❊ Buckwheat + chopped pears + chopped walnuts + ground ginger

TOAST, TOSTADAS, AND CREPES

Eat Clean, Stay Lean Dried Tart Cherry Chia Jam and Ricotta on Toast (page 285)

and

1 hard-boiled egg OR 5 or 6 walnut halves, 10 almonds, or 25 pistachios

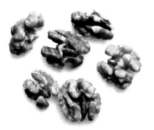

Eat Clean, Stay Lean Avocado Tostadas with Huevos Rancheros (page 223)

Eat Clean, Stay Lean Easy Buckwheat Crepes (page 227) (savory or sweet!)

SAVORY FILLINGS

❋ **Spinach, tomato, olive, and feta**

❋ **Ham, pear, and arugula**

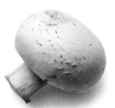

❋ **Black bean, cumin, and cilantro**

❋ **Asparagus and mushroom**

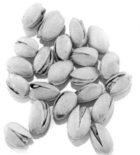

SWEET FILLINGS

❋ **Strawberry and ricotta**

❋ **Grapefruit and pistachio**

Clean and Simple Cheddar Cheese, Avocado, and Tomato Toast

Top I slice whole grain bread with I whole egg (poached or scrambled), I medium sliced tomato, 2 tablespoons mashed avocado, and 2 tablespoons grated sharp Cheddar cheese. Toast until the bread is toasted and the cheese is melted, and sprinkle with crushed red pepper flakes (optional).

and one of the following:

A medium apple, a medium orange, OR ¾ cup berries

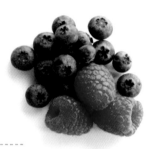

Clean and Simple Almond Butter and Banana Toast

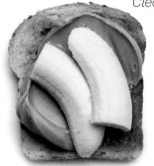

Spread I½ tablespoons almond or peanut butter on whole grain toast.
Top with ½ medium sliced banana.
Enjoy open-faced or folded as a half sandwich.

Clean and Simple Cheddar Cheese, Egg, and Tomato Toast (see page 164)

Want to Do Nondairy?

Simply choose a higher-protein option, such as organic soymilk. Or, if you prefer to choose a lower-protein nondairy milk, such as coconut milk, almond milk, or hemp milk, add I hard-boiled egg, I scoop of clean protein powder, or 2 tablespoons of sliced almonds to your breakfast. **And always, always choose unsweetened milk alternatives.** (The "original" flavor is frequently sweetened.)

CEREAL

- -

Clean and Simple Cereal and Fruit

Top I serving whole grain cereal with I cup low-fat milk, ¾ cup whole milk, or I cup clean milk alternative. Enjoy with ¾ cup berries, I small banana (or ½ large banana), or other fruit.

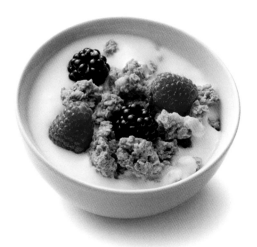

Shop Clean Checklist: Whole Grain Cereal

LOOK FOR:

❋ A whole grain as the first ingredient (like "whole wheat")
❋ Organic, when possible
❋ I0 g or less of sugar per serving

❋ At least 5 g of protein and 5 g of fiber per serving (8 g of fiber or more is even better)

EAT CLEAN, STAY LEAN PICKS:

❋ Kashi Organic Promise Sprouted Grains, Kashi Organic Promise Sweet Potato Sunshine, and Kashi Autumn Wheat
❋ Barbara's Honey Rice Puffins (gluten-free) and Barbara's Shredded Wheat
❋ Arrowhead Mills Maple Buckwheat Flakes (gluten-free),

Arrowhead Mills Organic Sprouted Corn Flakes (gluten-free), and Arrowhead Mills Amaranth Flakes (wheat-free)
❋ Nature's Path organic Heritage Flakes and Nature's Path organic Mesa Sunrise

SMOOTHIES

Eat Clean, Stay Lean Horchata Smoothie (page 231),
with 1 scoop of a clean protein powder
(15 g protein) added before blending

Eat Clean, Stay Lean Green Ginger Smoothie (page 232),
with 1 scoop of a clean protein powder (15 g protein) added before blending

- -

Create-Your-Own Clean and Simple Smoothie

In a blender, combine and blend until smooth:

2 servings fresh or frozen fruit like berries, mangos, or banana (or a combination)

and

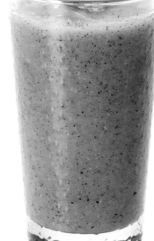

1 handful leafy greens like baby spinach or kale

and

1 scoop clean protein powder (15 g protein) OR
¾ cup low-fat Greek or regular yogurt

and

1 serving healthy fat, such as
1 tablespoon almond butter, ground flaxseeds,
or hemp hearts, OR 2 tablespoons ripe avocado, OR
2 teaspoons liquid oil, such as coconut, pumpkin seed,
or avocado oil

and

3/4 cup liquid, such as milk OR
unsweetened plant milk (almond, hemp, or organic soy) OR
coconut water OR half water
and half 100 percent juice

Shop Clean Checklist: Protein Powder

❋ Whey, egg white, hemp, non-GMO soy, brown rice, or pea proteins

❋ Clean, simple ingredients and no hormones, artificial ingredients, or additives

❋ 100 to 120 calories and 15 to 20 g of protein per servingNo sugar added (preferably), but less than 10 g of natural sugar added if you choose a sweetened variety

EAT CLEAN, STAY LEAN PICKS:

❋ NOW Sports organic and non-GMO protein powders (whey, egg white, sprouted brown rice, organic pea, and non-GMO soy)

❋ Nutiva Organic Hemp Protein

❋ NutriBiotic Raw Organic Rice ProteinSunwarrior plant-based proteins

❋ Vega Protein & Greens

Putting It All Together

1 **Become a regular breakfast eater.** Eating a morning meal sets the tone for eating clean for the rest of the day. Plus it stokes your metabolism, helps stave off sugary cravings—in the morning and throughout the day—and gives you fuel to power through your morning, all of which can help you get lean.

2 **Plan your breakfasts—and keep them simple.** Having a plan means that you always know what's on the menu, even on busy mornings. And sticking with easy meals means that you're more likely to achieve breakfast success.

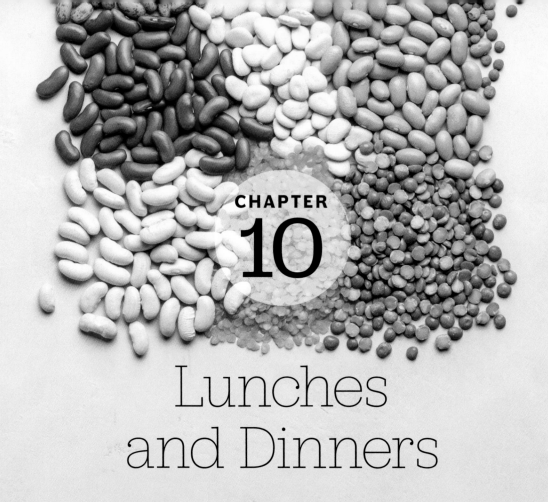

CHAPTER 10

Lunches and Dinners

Sure, they're two different meals eaten at two different times of day. But when it comes to losing weight, lunch and dinner have more in common than you might think. If breakfast is all about kicking things off with a clean start, the goal of both your midday and evening meals is to keep that good momentum going. Which—we know—is often easier said than done, no matter how motivated you might be to slim down! But when you've got a strong lineup of good-for-you meals in your back pocket, along with smart strategies for minimizing surprises (and dealing with them when they *do* strike), you can make it happen. We'll show you how.

174

Double Trouble

Let's be honest: When it comes to lunch and dinnertime, the clean-eating cards aren't always stacked in your favor. The morning rush limits—or altogether erases—the time you have to pack a midday meal, which means you're often stuck scrounging for sustenance at the closest sandwich shop or take-out joint. Or worse, you end up skipping out on eating altogether. Plus, both work obligations and social invitations tend to revolve around dining out—which usually means an endless stream of appetizers, alcohol, gigantic entrées, and desserts. The thought alone can be enough to make your stomach churn!

And when you *do* have the luxury of enjoying a quiet dinner at home? Chances are, you stumble in after work or activities with a growling belly and little idea of what you can throw together that's fast, tasty, and reasonably good for you. And after you're done eating, all you really want to do is crash on the couch for a little while before you go to sleep. As for packing a clean lunch for tomorrow? It's pretty much the last thing on your mind—and understandably so. And that means there's a good chance that you'll end up repeating this whole cycle again the next day.

Still, that doesn't mean you can't reshuffle the deck to stack the odds in your favor. **By taking steps to plan ahead and make meal prep as simple and straightforward as possible, you can set yourself up to eat clean lunches and dinners every day—and achieve your weight-loss goals.**

Double Duty

You might have certain ideas about what counts as an appropriate lunch and what makes sense for dinner. But guess what? There's no rule saying you have to have a sandwich or salad in the middle of the day and a piece of fish or chicken with vegetables at night.

As a matter of fact, losing that mind-set can make eating clean a lot more manageable. When you only have 15 minutes to get dinner on the table, assembling a simple salad or heating up a batch of soup might be more realistic than trying to turn out a protein and two sides from scratch. And when you *do* have the time to make a full entrée, it makes a heck of a lot more sense to save some of those leftovers for lunch the next day instead of spending *more* time brown bagging an entirely different meal. Get what we're saying?

That's why, in the name of ultimate clean-eating convenience, *all* of the meal ideas and recipes you'll find here are designed to be eaten at lunch *or* dinner. So go ahead and bring leftover grilled salmon and asparagus to eat on your lunch break. (Preferably in the cafeteria or break room, or even outside. Whatever you do, don't eat at your desk, if possible, since it's tough to eat mindfully while you're working!) Have a turkey wrap when you get home from work, if you don't feel like cooking! It doesn't matter if you flip-flop traditional lunch meals for dinner meals or vice versa, as long as you stick with the meals that are part of this plan. And you will, because they're easy to make *and* delicious to eat.

Get Lean Guidelines: Lunch and Dinner

Time to get down to the nitty-gritty. What are the secrets to eating clean lunches and dinners every day without tearing your hair out? They're right here. To achieve maximum weight-loss success, review these guidelines and stick with them. They'll help you get leaner, faster—*and* build healthy lunch and dinnertime habits that you can use for life.

✳ **Cook at home as much as possible.** We know, going out to eat is fun (not to mention convenient). But you'll see greater success when you prep your meals at home, since the nutrient combinations in these recipes are designed to help maximize your metabolism and weight loss. If you *do* choose to dine out, be sure to review the rules for success at the end of this chapter. (For even more tips on eating clean while dining out, head back to Chapter 7.)

✳ **Plan out your meals.** Having a weekly menu for lunches and dinners means that your clean meals are already laid out. All you have to do is follow along! Follow one of the weekly guides (see page 150), or use the template (see page 157) or an app to create your own delicious meals. Remember, having a plan doesn't just mean that you'll know what's for lunch and dinner. It also helps you set the *intention* of eating clean lunches and dinners all week long. Think of it as your road map to clean-eating victory.

✳ **Keep it simple—and interesting.** Many fad diet plans ask you to make entirely different meals every single day. That might be fun for your taste buds, but it can be tough to actually find the time to do. Instead of planning a different lunch and dinner every single day, consider sticking with just three or four different meals. You'll have enough variety to keep from getting bored, but you won't end up driving yourself crazy with meal prep. Plus, getting familiar with the recipes means that they're more likely to become part of your permanent clean-eating routine. And who doesn't love a go-to meal?

✳ **Think about repurposing a dinner into a lunch the next day.** The recipes in this chapter were designed to be eaten for lunch *or* dinner, which helps make meal prep as simple as possible. So plan to double your dinner recipes and take the leftovers for lunch the next day. This is a *huge* time-saver—and you'll never find yourself scrambling to pack a sandwich at 7:30 in the morning while you're trying to run out the door.

✳ Do one soup or salad every day. Both deliver loads of vegetables, but more importantly, soups and salads both have a high water content, which means you can eat more for fewer calories. Start building the one-soup-or-salad-a-day habit now, and it'll feel like second nature by the time you finish the plan and are ready to strike out on your own.

✳ Always have a fruit or vegetable. All of the meals in this chapter include a fruit or vegetable (or both). Don't skip them! They fill you up for fewer calories than other foods and offer tons of nutrients. And, just as important, following the fruit or vegetable rule of thumb during the plan helps you build another good clean-eating habit that'll help you stay lean for the long haul.

✳ Take notes on your meal. Same as with breakfast, folks! During your meal or afterward, pull out your preplanned menu and write down your thoughts. Do you need to make menu changes for next time? What were your hunger, energy, and stress levels like? These notes can serve as a record for what works and what doesn't so you can troubleshoot and plan more efficiently in the future. Jot your notes directly on your weekly menu or write them in a separate notebook.

✳ Don't skip meals. Even if you're insanely busy. Even if you can't pull together a picture-perfect meal because you're at a restaurant or a cocktail party. Always eat lunch, and always eat dinner! Skipping meals will backfire by slowing down your metabolism and leaving you ravenous later on.

Let's Eat!

If you've tried to lose weight before and are still haunted by the memories of tasteless diet recipes or dull pre-packaged meals, please accept our apologies. The recipes and meal ideas *here* are none of those things. Of course they have the right balance of proteins, complex carbs, and healthy fats—plus loads of vegetables and fruits that'll kick your metabolism into high gear and turn you into a lean, fat-burning machine. But in terms

Dr. Wendy Says . . .

Find yourself nearing lunch or dinner-time without a plan—or the necessary ingredients? Don't sweat it. **You can always have breakfast, take two!**

Head back to Chapter 9, look through the breakfast options, and choose one that's satisfying and easy to make. Cheddar, avocado, and tomato toast?

Oatmeal with blueberries and walnuts? A fresh fruit smoothie? It's your call!

of tastiness, they're downright craveworthy. And they won't leave you hungry again in 2 hours. *Promise.*

Remember, sticking with the plan as much as possible will help you lose more weight. But if you *have* to dine out, the guidelines at the end of the chapter should act as your road map for picking a clean option.

Eat Clean, Stay Lean Lunches and Dinners

Use these meals to build your lunch and dinner menus for the entire program. Find all of the full Eat Clean, Stay Lean recipes starting on page 220. Clean and Simple recipes are meant to be looser, easy-assemble, mix-and-match sorts of meals, so you'll find quick steps for making those right here. If a meal says to add something, such as a side dish or a piece of fruit, do so. If it doesn't, you're all set! It's a complete meal as is.

Shop Clean Checklist: Canned or Boxed Fish, Shrimp, and Chicken

LOOK FOR:

* ❊ Plain and packed in water or in clean, natural sauces like olive oil, citrus, or tomato
* ❊ BPA-free cans, cartons, or vacuum-sealed bags
* ❊ For salmon: Wild salmon
* ❊ For tuna: Chunk light or sustainably caught albacore or skipjack
* ❊ For chicken: Preferably organic

EAT CLEAN, STAY LEAN PICKS:

* ❊ Wild Planet tuna, wild salmon, sardines, mackerel, yellowtail, shrimp, and organic roasted chicken breast
* ❊ Safe Catch tuna
* ❊ Vital Choice anchovies, sardines, and other wild fish
* ❊ Crown Prince baby clams, tuna, oysters, and sardines
* ❊ Valley Fresh organic white chicken

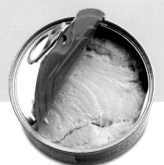

ENTRÉE SALADS

Eat Clean, Stay Lean Tuna and Cannellini Salad (page 233)

Eat Clean, Stay Lean Creamy Chicken, Green Grape, and Farro Salad (page 237)

Eat Clean, Stay Lean Hearty Chicken Panzanella (page 241)

Eat Clean, Stay Lean Fiesta Quinoa with Shrimp (page 273)

Clean and Simple Entrée Salad with Tuna, Veggies, and Fruit

Toss 2 cups mixed greens with ¼ cup shredded carrots; ½ cup diced tomatoes; 3 ounces flaked clean, water-packed tuna (drained); and ½ cup mandarin orange slices or sliced strawberries. Top with I tablespoon vinaigrette (or I teaspoon olive oil and 2 teaspoons balsamic vinegar).

and

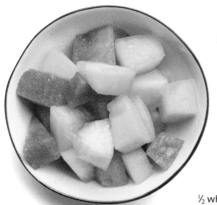

½ cup fruit salad OR small piece of fruit
(in addition to the fruit in the salad)

and

½ whole wheat pita, I corn tortilla (6 inches), OR
5 or 6 whole grain crackers

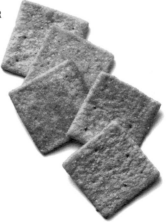

SALAD COMBOS

Eat Clean, Stay Lean Cuban Avocado and Pineapple Salad (page 269)

and

4 ounces Clean and Simple Salmon or Chicken (page 187)
(or grilled leftovers from another dinner, or store-bought from a quality prepared foods deli counter)

and

I piece fruit or ¾ cup berries (in addition to the fruit in the salad)

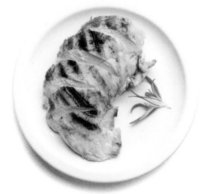
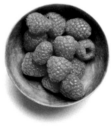

Shop Clean Checklist: Beans and Legumes

LOOK FOR:

❊ Less than 150 mg of sodium per serving (always drain and rinse beans before using to wash off excess)

❊ BPA-free cans or cartons

EAT CLEAN, STAY LEAN PICKS:

❊ Eden Organic
❊ Whole Foods Market 365 Everyday Value
❊ Trader Joe's Wild Harvest

❊ Pacific
❊ Amy's Organic Light in Sodium varieties

Eat Clean, Stay Lean Summer Roll Salad with Peanut Dipping Sauce (page 270)

and one of the following:

Eat Clean, Stay Lean Roasted Citrus-and-Herb Sweet Potatoes (page 276)
Eat Clean, Stay Lean Roasted Broccoli with Chile and Lemon (page 277)
Eat Clean, Stay Lean Cauliflower Rice Pilaf (page 278)
Eat Clean, Stay Lean Peanut Butter Banana Blondie (page 290)

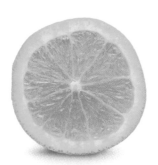

A large orange or apple,
or a medium banana

½ cup low-fat Greek yogurt
with ¼ cup berries

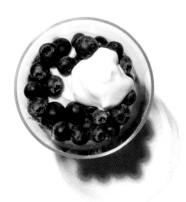

Shop Clean Checklist: Boxed Crackers

LOOK FOR:

❋ At least 2 g of fiber and no more than 200 mg of sodium per serving

❋ A whole grain as the first ingredient (like "whole wheat")

EAT CLEAN, STAY LEAN PICKS:

❋ Mary's Gone Crackers (assorted varieties, all are gluten-free)
❋ Kashi Original 7 Grain Snack Crackers and Pita Crisps
❋ Doctor Kracker (assorted varieties)
❋ Van's Simply Delicious The Perfect 10 Crackers (gluten-free)
❋ Wasa (assorted varieties)

❋ Kavli All Natural Whole Grain Crispbread and Hearty Thick Crispbread
❋ Finn Crisp (assorted varieties)
❋ Whole Foods Market 365 Everyday Value Woven Wheats
❋ Trader Joe's Woven Wheats Wafers

WRAPS, TORTILLAS, AND SANDWICH-STYLE MEALS

Eat Clean, Stay Lean Turkey Cuban Wrap with Zesty Black Bean Salad (page 238)

Eat Clean, Stay Lean Beef Scallion Roll-Ups (page 242)

Eat Clean, Stay Lean Kale Quesadillas (page 235)

Eat Clean, Stay Lean Slow Cooker BBQ Pulled Chicken Flatbreads (page 248)

Clean and Simple Sliced Apple and Peanut Butter "Sandwich"

Core and slice a large apple crosswise into ½-inch-thick rings. Using the two largest rings as your "bread" slices, top one slice with 1½ tablespoons nut butter, and 2 tablespoons granola (either the Eat Clean, Stay Lean PB&J Granola on page 282 or another clean variety, such as KIND clusters). Top your "sandwich" with the second large ring. Enjoy the rest of the apple rings on the side.

and one of the following:

¾ cup low-fat milk
(or ½ cup whole milk) or milk alternative

8 carrot sticks
(1 large or 2 medium carrots, sliced)
with ¼ cup hummus

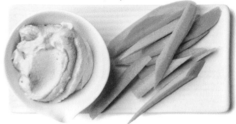

Clean and Simple Stuffed Veggie Pitas

Toss 1 cup spinach or other salad greens with ⅛ cup shredded carrots, 1 tablespoon crumbled feta or goat cheese, 1 tablespoon chopped walnuts, ½ chopped fruit (such as pear, apple, or peach), and 2 tablespoons vinaigrette dressing. Stuff the mixture into half of a whole wheat pita.

and

¾ cup berries or piece of fruit

SOUPS AND SOUP/SALAD COMBOS

Eat Clean, Stay Lean Black Bean Sweet Potato Sherry Soup (page 263)

and one of the following:

Eat Clean, Stay Lean Shaved Salad (page 266)
Eat Clean, Stay Lean Clean Coleslaw (page 275)
Eat Clean, Stay Lean Roasted Broccoli with Chile and Lemon (page 277)
Eat Clean, Stay Lean Cauliflower Rice Pilaf (page 278)

Large piece of fruit or
I cup mixed fruit

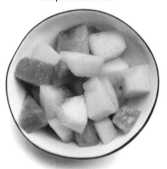

Shop Clean Checklist: Salad Dressings

LOOK FOR:

✽ Oil- and vinegar-based, not cream-based
✽ No more than 300 mg of sodium and 4 g of natural sugar per 2-tablespoon serving

✽ 40 to 60 calories per 2-tablespoon serving
✽ Organic, when possible

EAT CLEAN, STAY LEAN PICKS:

✽ Annie's Naturals Lite Gingerly Vinaigrette, Lite Italian, Lite Honey Mustard Vinaigrette, Lite Goddess, and Lite Raspberry Vinaigrette
✽ Bragg Organic Fat Free Hawaiian Dressing & Marinade and Organic Fat Free Braggberry Dressing & Marinade

✽ Newman's Own Zesty Italian, Lite Italian, Sesame Ginger, Lite Balsamic Vinaigrette, Lite Caesar, Sun Dried Tomato Lite Vinaigrette

Eat Clean, Stay Lean Hearty Lentil Mushroom Soup (page 265)

and one of the following:

Eat Clean, Stay Lean Shaved Salad (page 266)

Eat Clean, Stay Lean Roasted Broccoli with Chile and Lemon (page 277)

Eat Clean, Stay Lean Cauliflower Rice Pilaf (page 278)

¾ cup low-fat Greek yogurt

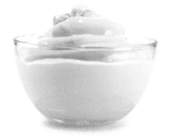

Eat Clean, Stay Lean White Gazpacho with Grapes and Almonds (page 264)

and

Eat Clean, Stay Lean Summer Roll Salad with Peanut Dipping Sauce (page 270)

Eat Clean, Stay Lean Cuban Avocado and Pineapple Salad (page 269)

and

1½ cups clean canned or boxed organic, low-sodium soup,
like lentil vegetable, split pea, or minestrone, OR 1 cup chili

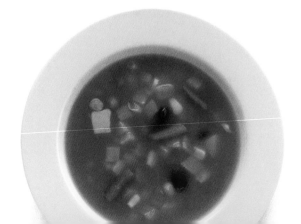

Clean and Simple Soup Combo

1½ cups clean canned or boxed bean-, poultry-, or fish-based soup OR 1 cup chili

and one of the following:

¾ cup low-fat Greek yogurt and ½ cup berries

1 apple or orange and 5 walnut halves,
8 almonds, or 15 pistachios

2 tablespoons dried cherries or raisins and 5 walnuts halves,
8 almonds, or 15 pistachios

Small side salad: 1 cup greens with 5 cherry tomatoes,
¼ cup grated carrot, and 1½ tablespoons vinaigrette
(2 teaspoons extra-virgin olive oil mixed with
1 to 2 teaspoons balsamic vinegar or
fresh lemon or lime juice)

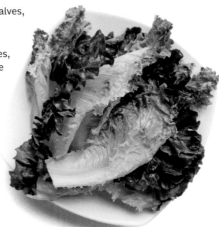

Vive la (Homemade) Vinaigrette!

It's perfectly fine to buy a clean bottled salad dressing. But making your own vinaigrette is a cinch—and the result is worlds fresher and tastier than what you'd get from the store. To make your own, just combine 1 part oil, 1 to 2 parts vinegar or freshly squeezed citrus juice, and fresh or dried herbs or spices (to taste) in a jar, and shake well to combine. Here are a few fantastic flavor combos for you to try.

❋ Extra-virgin olive oil + balsamic vinegar + fresh chopped basil + Italian seasoning blend

❋ Extra-virgin olive oil + red wine vinegar + dried oregano
❋ Organic canola oil + rice wine vinegar + sesame seeds + fresh chopped scallions
❋ Avocado oil + freshly squeezed lime juice + chili powder
❋ Organic canola oil + freshly squeezed orange juice + fresh grated ginger
❋ Avocado oil + white balsamic vinegar + cumin + black pepper
❋ Extra-virgin olive oil + balsamic vinegar + garlic powder + thyme

DINNER ENTRÉES

Eat Clean, Stay Lean Slow Cooker BBQ Pulled Chicken Flatbreads (page 248)

Eat Clean, Stay Lean Florentine Chicken Meatballs with Spaghetti Squash and Salsa Cruda (page 252)

Eat Clean, Stay Lean Chickpea Curry–Stuffed Squash (page 255)

Eat Clean, Stay Lean Maple Mustard Glazed Pork Tenderloin with Roasted Vegetables and Apples (page 256)

Eat Clean, Stay Lean Israeli Couscous Salad with Salmon (page 245)

Eat Clean, Stay Lean Shrimp Scampi over Garlicky Greens (page 246)

and one of the following:

½ baked sweet potato

Eat Clean, Stay Lean Honey-Glazed Radishes (page 275)

Shop Clean Checklist: Boxed or Canned Soups and Chilis

LOOK FOR:

❋ BPA-free cans, cartons, or cups
❋ Higher protein bean-, lentil-, meat-, or poultry-based soups for meals; simple broth-based soups for sides and snacks
❋ 250 to 325 calories per serving for meals, 100 to 175 calories per serving for snacks

❋ Less than 2 g of saturated fat per serving
❋ Low sodium, light in sodium, no salt added (less than 480 mg sodium per serving is a good goal; less than 350 mg sodium per serving is ideal)

EAT CLEAN, STAY LEAN PICKS:

❋ Amy's Light in Sodium Organic Soups: Lentil, Butternut Squash, Lentil Vegetable, Minestrone, Chunky Tomato Bisque, and Split Pea
❋ Healthy Valley Organic, No Salt Added Soups: Chicken Noodle, Lentil, Tomato, Mushroom Barley, Split Pea, Vegetable, Minestrone, Potato Leek, and Chicken Rice
❋ Amy's Light in Sodium Organic Chili: Medium and Spicy

❋ Imagine Organic Light in Sodium soups: Creamy Butternut Squash, Creamy Garden Tomato, and Creamy Harvest Corn
❋ Dr. McDougall's Lower Sodium soups: Split Pea, Lentil, and Garden Vegetable
❋ Frontier Soups mixes: chicken noodle, tortilla, potato leek, tomato basil, and red pepper corn chowder (substitute milk where directions indicate cream)

Eat Clean, Stay Lean Cauliflower Rice Pilaf (page 278)

Eat Clean, Stay Lean Turkey Roulade (page 251)

and one of the following:

I cup steamed broccoli with lemon

I cup steamed spinach

Clean and Simple Fish, Poultry, or Lean Meat

Marinate 5 to 6 ounces (raw weight) fish, chicken, turkey, or lean meat. (See "Marinate *This*," below.) Grill, bake, or broil until desired doneness.

and one of the following:

Eat Clean, Stay Lean Clean Coleslaw (page 274)

Eat Clean, Stay Lean Honey-Glazed Radishes (page 275)

Eat Clean, Stay Lean Roasted Citrus-and-Herb Sweet Potatoes (page 276)

Eat Clean, Stay Lean Roasted Broccoli with Chile and Lemon (page 277)

Eat Clean, Stay Lean Cauliflower Rice Pilaf (page 278)

Eat Clean, Stay Lean Cuban Avocado and Pineapple Salad (page 269)

Marinate *This*

Firing up the grill or broiler? Whip up a clean, flavor-packed marinade with this simple formula. It makes enough for a pound of chicken, fish, beef, vegetables, or *whatever.*

✳ 6 tablespoons freshly squeezed citrus juice, such as orange, lemon, or lime

✳ I½ tablespoons clean oil, such as olive, avocado, or organic canola

✳ 2 tablespoons chopped fresh herbs (or I tablespoon dried herbs or spices), such as:
  - Italian seasoning
  - Garlic powder + cinnamon + ginger
  - Rosemary + thyme + oregano + garlic powder
  - Smoked paprika + garlic powder + thyme + black pepper

Clean and Simple Salmon with Yogurt Dill Sauce

Grill a 5-ounce (raw weight) salmon filet. Whisk 3 tablespoons nonfat plain yogurt with I teaspoon fresh minced dill (½ teaspoon dried) and ¼ to ½ teaspoon horseradish. Top the salmon with sauce.

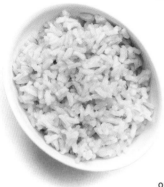

and

⅔ cup cooked brown rice

and

I cup steamed broccoli with lemon

and

¾ cup berries with ½ cup low-fat yogurt OR
one Eat Clean, Stay Lean Peanut Butter Banana Blondie (page 290)

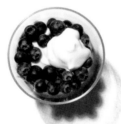

Dr. Wendy Says . . .

Herbs and spices are some of the easiest, most delicious ingredients you can use to liven up simple protein, vegetable, or grain dishes. And with loads of beneficial phytonutrients and practically zero calories, they're also some of the cleanest! Consider giving these globally inspired flavor combos a go.

Asian

❊ Chinese five-spice: Star anise, peppercorns, cloves, fennel, cinnamon, and coriander seeds (optional, to make it 6)

❊ Fresh or ground ginger, sesame seeds, and dried onions or fresh scallions

Indian

❊ Curry powder: Turmeric, ginger, coriander, and cumin

❊ Garam masala: Cinnamon, cardamom, and cumin

Italian or Mediterranean

❊ Oregano, thyme, rosemary, parsley, and garlic

❊ Cumin, cinnamon, paprika, coriander, cloves, and black pepper

Mexican, Latin America, or Caribbean

❊ Cumin, oregano, and chili powder

❊ Jerk spice blend: Thyme, cinnamon, garlic powder, allspice, and ground red and black pepper

Clean and Simple Tofu Veggie Stir-Fry

Sauté ½ cup sliced white onion, I teaspoon fresh crushed garlic, and 3 ounces cubed firm organic tofu* in 2 teaspoons olive oil or organic canola oil. Add 2 cups cut, nonstarchy vegetables (such as asparagus, zucchini, green or red bell peppers, broccoli, tomato, spinach, or snow peas) and ¼ cup water. Cook 4 to 6 minutes, until the tofu is golden and the vegetables are crisp-tender.

and

½ cup whole wheat couscous or brown rice

and

Eat Clean, Stay Lean Broccoli Leek Soup (page 262) OR
Tomato Basil or Sherry Mushroom Soup (page 262) OR
Eat Clean, Stay Lean Roasted Strawberries with Dark Chocolate Sauce (page 288)

*For firmer, chewier tofu, freeze and defrost it before cubing and sautéing, if you have time.

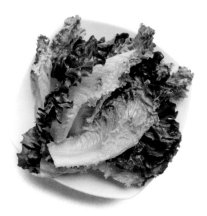

Clean and Simple Pasta Primavera

Steam I medium carrot, thinly sliced; I rib celery, thinly sliced; ¼ red bell pepper, thinly sliced; and ¼ cup snow peas. Toss with ¾ cup clean marinara sauce (warmed), ½ cup cooked whole wheat or gluten-free penne or ziti, I teaspoon fresh chopped basil, and 2 teaspoons freshly grated Parmesan cheese.

and

I cup salad greens and mixed veggies with I tablespoon vinaigrette

Shop Clean Checklist: Tomatoes, Sauces, and Salsas

LOOK FOR:

* BPA-free cans or cartons, or glass jars
* Less than 60 calories and 300 mg of sodium per ½-cup serving for tomatoes and sauce; less than 15 calories and 200 mg of sodium per 2-tablespoon serving for salsa

* Less than 6 g natural sugar per serving (and preferably no sugar added)

EAT CLEAN, STAY LEAN PICKS:

PASTA SAUCE

* Organico Bello Tomato Basil, Kale Tomato Basil, Marinara, and Spicy Marinara
* Muir Glen Organic Cabernet Marinara, Tomato Basil, Portobello Mushroom, and Italian Herb

* Sprouts No Salt Added Marinara

TOMATOES

* Muir Glen Organic (assorted varieties)
* Full Circle Organic Diced Tomatoes, No Salt

* Hunt's No Salt Added Tomato Sauce, Diced, or Stewed Tomatoes
* S&W Premium Tomatoes, Diced with No Salt Added

SALSA

* Amy's Black Bean and Corn and Medium
* Muir Glen Organic (assorted varieties)
* Newman's Own Mild

* Frontera Gourmet Mexican Tomatillo, Mango Key Lime, and Chipotle
* La Victoria Salsa in Thick 'n Chunky and Salsa Victoria

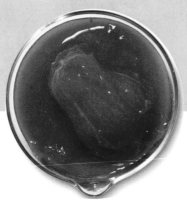

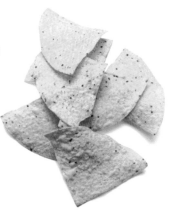

Clean and Simple Beans and Rice

In a bowl, assemble ½ cup cooked brown rice with ½ cup low-sodium, BPA-free canned black beans (drained, rinsed, and warmed); ¼ teaspoon cumin; ⅛ avocado, diced; ¾ cup chopped lettuce; and ½ cup diced tomato. Top with 3 tablespoons clean chunky salsa.

and one of the following:

One 5- or 6-inch corn tortilla, cut into wedges and toasted

I apple or ¾ cup berries

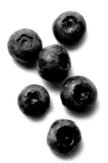

Clean and Simple Frozen Entrées

Frozen entrée that meets the Shop Clean criteria below

and one of the following:

I apple, IO carrot sticks, I cup salad greens, ¾ cup berries

Shop Clean Checklist: Frozen Entrées

LOOK FOR:

❋ 300 to 400 calories, IO to 25 g of protein, and at least 5 g of fiber per serving

❋ Less than 600 mg of sodium per serving

❋ Made with clean, whole foods like whole grains, lean proteins, vegetables, and fruit and free of ingredients that you wouldn't add to a recipe if you were making it at home

EAT CLEAN, STAY LEAN PICKS:

❋ Kashi entrées

❋ Luvo entrées and breakfasts

❋ Amy's regular and gluten-free entrées

❋ Evol Single Serve Meals

❋ Tandoor Chef entrées

❋ Saffron Road frozen entrées

Eating Clean Anywhere, Anytime

Whether you're picking something up at the deli or grocery store for a fast lunch or are headed to a restaurant for dinner (or the other way around!), you can *still* make clean choices. Remember, in order to lose the maximum amount of weight while you're following the plan, it's worth cooking as many of your meals at home as possible. But if and when that just can't happen, these guidelines can help.

At delis, grab-and-go spots, or grocery stores with prepared foods . . . Pick a whole grain carbohydrate, a simple protein, and two servings of vegetables or a serving of vegetables and a serving of fruit. Steer clear of premade salads with cheese or mayonnaise, not because they're bad, but because you can't control how much cheese or mayo went into them.

TRY THESE:

❋ A small (tennis ball–size) baked sweet potato with ¼ pound grilled salmon and 1 cup of spinach salad with vegetables

❋ A small turkey wrap on a 5-inch whole grain tortilla and 1 cup of berries or other fruit

❋ ½ cup of quinoa salad with ¼ pound grilled chicken and 1 cup of steamed broccoli

❋ ½ cup of wild rice salad with ¼ pound sliced roast turkey and 1 cup of diced Greek salad (cucumbers, tomatoes, and feta)

❋ ¾ cup of roasted potatoes (about 3 small) with 3 ounces of teriyaki tofu and 1 cup of kale and apple salad

At restaurants . . . Enjoy a grilled or baked protein (such as fish, chicken, lean meat, or beans) with two servings of vegetables and a serving of fruit (or three servings of vegetables and no fruit). And pass on the starchy carbs, including bread, pasta, rice, other grains, or potatoes.

TRY THESE:

❋ Grilled chicken or fish with a small green salad, steamed broccoli, and a bowl of fresh berries

❋ Entrée salad with greens, vegetables, and flaked chunk light tuna, with a sliced orange

❋ Jumbo shrimp cocktail with a mixed greens and vegetables salad and a poached pear

❋ Mussels (cooked in broth) with a mixed greens and strawberry salad

❋ Grilled salmon with steamed spinach and a bowl of fresh berries

❋ Three pieces of sashimi with miso soup, seaweed salad, and a sliced orange

Everywhere . . . *Always* be portion smart. Remember, too much of any foods—even clean ones—can stall your weight loss. And whether you're picking up a sandwich at the corner store or ordering an entrée at a fancy steakhouse, chances are you'll be getting way more food than you need. To keep your meal the right size (instead of oversize), use these simple guidelines to eyeball your servings. Push the rest to the side of your plate and take it home for tomorrow!

❋ A serving of protein (3 to 4 ounces) or beans (¾ cup) = the size of your palm or smartphone

❋ A serving of vegetables = the size of your fist

❋ A serving of fruit = the size of your fist

❋ A serving of whole grains or a sweet potato = the size of a tennis ball

❋ A serving of whole grain bread or pita = ½ of an 8-inch pita or an 80- to 100-calorie slice

Need more? For lots more tips on how to eat clean at parties, restaurants, and while you travel, head back to Chapter 7.

Putting It All Together

1 **Plan ahead—and keep it simple.** Like with breakfast, mapping out your lunches and dinners in advance ensures that you will always have a clean meal on the horizon. And while you might enjoy making more elaborate meals when you have the time, don't feel pressured to churn out fancy dishes on a regular basis. When you aim for simple, you'll be more likely to succeed.

2 **Don't be afraid of leftovers.** It's a great idea to save some of tonight's dinner for tomorrow's lunch, or vice versa. Letting your meals do double duty saves time on meal prep, so you're more likely to always have a clean option ready to eat when you need it.

3 **Learn how to roll with the punches.** Whether it's a social invitation or just a matter of not having the time or energy to cook, at some point, dining out happens. When it does, be prepared to make a clean choice that supports your weight-loss efforts so you finish your meal feeling great.

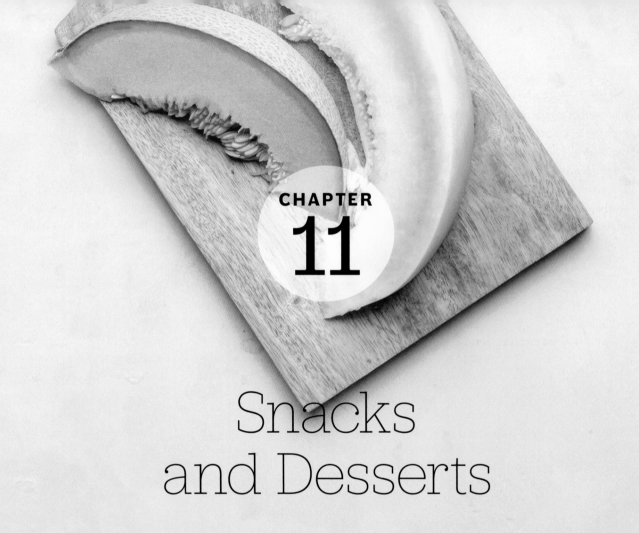

Snacks and Desserts

When it comes to getting lean, snacks can be your best allies—or your biggest stumbling blocks. A clean, well-planned snack can help you resist diet-derailing temptations, stave off the overly hungry feeling that drives you to raid the refrigerator the minute you walk in the door, and keep your body's fat-burning drive in high gear. As for a not-so-clean impulse snack that's scarfed down mindlessly? Well, let's just say that you want to avoid those as much as possible. So how can you build a snacking strategy that's smart, sustainable, and satisfying? Get ready—you're about to find out.

Snacks Made Smart

We do it in the car, on the train, in front of the TV, on the phone, and even in bed. For most of us, snacking has become so automatic that our brains barely register the hand-to-mouth motion. And unsurprisingly, all of those between-meal bites are bad news, weight-wise. As the number of calories we take in from snacks has increased, so too have our waistlines. We're eating twice as many snacks as we were in the 1970s.[1] At the same time, obesity rates among US adults have more than doubled. Coincidence? Not likely.[2]

But isn't that because we're eating junky snacks instead of healthy ones? It's true that the majority of Americans snack on processed, empty-calorie foods like chips, pretzels, cookies, and the like. Or we eat stuff that *pretends* to be healthy, like sugary granola bars or cereals. And of course, making any of those foods mainstays of your diet practically guarantees that you'll throw yourself into a vicious cycle of nonstop cravings and sluggishness as those numbers on the scale steadily creep up. Sure enough, you'll find that your body is in full-on fat-storage mode, and your favorite pants no longer fit. Of course, clean snacks like fruits and vegetables, nuts and seeds, hummus, and plain yogurt or cottage cheese are worlds better for you than all that packaged grub. But you can *still* eat too much of them. It's just basic math. All food contains calories. **And if you eat too many calories—from anything!—you'll have a hard time losing weight or maintaining your weight loss.**

And yet, snacking plays an important role when you're on the path to getting lean. The right snacks can keep you energized and satisfied between meals, making you less tempted to hit the vending machine or buy a cookie to go with your afternoon cup of coffee. Eating every few hours keeps your metabolism revved, too, so you burn more fat and slim down faster. Plus, snacks are fun!

The key to making it all work? Pick clean foods to snack on—and snack at preplanned times rather than eating, well, whenever. It's easier than you think! And after a few weeks, you might start to wonder how the heck you ever snacked any other way.

Get Lean Guidelines: Snacks

What separates smart, clean snacking from mindless munching? Make these rules of thumb your ultimate get-lean snacking strategy.

❖ **Set your daily snack number.** Remember, the number of snacks you should eat each day depends on your size and activity level.

● **Have three meals and two snacks if . . .** You're a woman who exercises for 45 minutes or less on most days OR a man or woman who weighs less than 160 pounds.

● **Have three meals and three snacks if . . .** You're a woman who exercises for 60 minutes or more on most days OR a man or woman who weighs more than 160 pounds OR you have 25 or more pounds to lose.

❈ **Plan your weekly menu.** Pick two to four options to rotate throughout the week, and add them to your weekly menu. This sweet spot gives you enough variety so you don't get bored but doesn't make things overly complicated. More importantly, prep your snacks ahead of time! Whether you're following a recipe or going with something simple, such as a handful of nuts, portion and package your snacks in individual bags or containers so they're easy to grab when you're heading out the door.

❈ **Have a fruit or vegetable with at least one of your daily snacks.** You knew this one was coming, right? You should have a fruit and/or vegetable almost every time you eat—including snacks. Have an apple or an orange along with that piece of string cheese. Dunk carrot sticks and red bell pepper slices into your hummus. You'll load up on nutrition and stay fuller for longer, and your metabolism will be more efficient, too.

❈ **Pick out your snack times—and stick to them.** Setting a snacking schedule not only minimizes mindless munching, it also gives you something to look forward to, which can go a long way toward helping you resist junky temptations. After all, it's a lot easier to pass on that cake for your coworker's birthday if you know that you're having yogurt and fruit in an hour.

❈ *But,* **learn to be a little flexible.** If there's a change to your usual routine, let your eating schedule change with it. Usually have lunch at 12:00, a snack at 3:00, and dinner at 6:00? On nights when you know you'll be eating dinner later, try to hold off on lunch until 1:00 or 2:00, and save your snack until 4:00 or 5:00. That way, you won't be starving for hours before your evening meal. The key is to push both your meal *and* your snack a little later so the number of hours between the two stays about the same and you don't end up too hungry.

❈ **Be a snack tracker.** Just like at mealtimes, have your preplanned menu nearby and jot down your thoughts after you snack. Did you stick with the plan? Did the snack satisfy your hunger? How did

58%

That's the percentage of Americans who say that most of their snacks are completely unplanned, according to a recent survey by Nielsen.[3] If you're among them, join the minority of plan-ahead snackers and prepare to reap the weight-loss benefits.

you feel while you ate? And would you make any changes to this snack the next time you eat it? It might sound like a lot to consider for a measly between-meal bite, but keeping a record can help you become a smarter snacker. Jot your notes directly on your weekly menu or write them in a separate notebook.

❋ **Always eat your snacks!** You might think you're being "good" by skipping your snacks, but that move will most likely backfire. Passing on a snack sets you up for feeling ravenous when mealtime rolls around, which can lead to overeating. Plus, eating every few hours keeps your metabolism running at full speed, helping you burn as much fat as possible.

Let's Eat!

What counts as a clean snack? Whether your taste buds veer toward sweet and creamy or salty and savory, we've got *plenty* of easy, delicious options that'll help you stay satisfied between meals—and get lean faster. Take your pick!

Eat Clean, Stay Lean Snacks

YOGURT AND COTTAGE CHEESE

❋ ¾ cup low-fat plain Greek yogurt with ¾ cup raspberries

❋ ¾ cup low-fat plain Greek yogurt with ½ cup seedless grapes

❋ ½ cup low-fat plain Greek yogurt with 2 tablespoons *Eat Clean, Stay Lean PB&J Granola* (page 282)

❋ 6-ounce container clean flavored yogurt

When Should I Snack?

What's the best time to eat your snacks? That depends on your lifestyle and when you normally have breakfast, lunch, and dinner. Take a few minutes to think about your daily routine and decide which snacking schedule works better for you.

❋ **Be an early snacker if . . .**
You have 5 or more hours between your usual breakfast and lunch. In that case, have one snack between breakfast and lunch and a second snack between lunch and dinner.

❋ **Be a later snacker if . . .**
You only have 3 to 4 hours between your usual breakfast and lunch but a longer stretch between lunch and dinner. (Think 7 or more hours.) In that case, have one snack midafternoon and a second snack around 5:30.

* ½ cup organic low-fat cottage cheese with ½ cup blueberries

* ½ cup organic low-fat cottage cheese with 1 cup sliced strawberries

* ¾ cup organic low-fat cottage cheese with 1 cup cherry tomatoes

NUTS AND NUT BUTTERS

* DIY Trail Mix: 2 tablespoons dried fruit (such as dried cherries, raisins, or 3 small apricots) with 2 tablespoons nuts or seeds (such as walnuts, almonds, or 20 pistachios)

* 1 large stalk celery with 1 tablespoon peanut butter

* 1 small apple with 1 tablespoon almond butter

* 1 medium orange (or 3 clementines) with 8 almonds

SAVORY OR SALTY

Tend to get hit with cravings for salty chips or pretzels? These savory bites are the right snacks for you.

* 3 cups *Eat Clean, Stay Lean Gremolata Parmesan Popcorn* (page 279)

* ⅛ cup *Eat Clean, Stay Lean Lemony Rosemary White Bean Dip* (page 286) with 5 or 6 whole grain crackers OR 1 cup assorted raw vegetables

* ¾ cup organic, non-GMO steamed edamame (in pods)

* ¼ cup hummus with 1 cup assorted raw vegetables

* 2 ounces tuna, sardines, or salmon with 5 whole grain crackers

Shop Clean Checklist: Flavored Yogurt and Kefir

LOOK FOR:

* Less than 150 calories and at least 12 g of protein per serving

* Ideally less than 11 g (and no more than 18 g) of sugar
* No artificial flavors, sweeteners, or thickeners

EAT CLEAN, STAY LEAN PICKS:

* Siggi's (various flavors)*
* Dreaming Cow Grass-Fed Cream Top (various flavors)*
* Oikos Triple Zero*
* Chobani Fruit on the Bottom
* Stonyfield Organic Whole Milk Greek, 100% Grassfed, or Greek and Chia

* Fage 0% and 2% Split Cups
* Lifeway Organic ProBugs Kefir (various flavors, slightly lower in protein than yogurt)*
* Green Valley Organics Green Apple–Kale Kefir (slightly lower in protein than yogurt)

*Lowest sugar options

* 1 hard-boiled egg with 15 grapes

* 1 hard-boiled egg with 5 whole grain crackers

* 2 small whole grain crackers with 1 ounce (2 tablespoons) goat cheese

* 4 ounces organic oven-roasted turkey breast (4 thick or 8 thin slices) with 1 medium carrot

* 1 piece string cheese with 4 green olives

SWEET OR FRUITY

Sometimes you're just in the mood for something sweet. These snacks are sure to satisfy!

* 1 serving *Eat Clean, Stay Lean Dried Tart Cherry Chia Jam and Ricotta on Toast* (page 285)

* 1 small apple with 1 tablespoon almond butter

* 1 medium orange (or 3 clementines) with 8 almonds

* 1 piece string cheese with piece of fruit

* 1 *Eat Clean, Stay Lean Peanut Butter Banana Blondie* (page 290) (no more than two times a week)

SMOOTHIES

Make a full-size breakfast smoothie and save the other half for later! It's just as tasty the next day.

* ½ *Eat Clean, Stay Lean Horchata Smoothie* (page 231) blended with 1 scoop clean protein powder

* ½ *Eat Clean, Stay Lean Green Ginger Smoothie* (page 232) blended with 1 scoop clean protein powder

* ½ Create-Your-Own Clean and Simple Smoothie (page 172)

Shop Clean Checklist: Bottled Smoothies

LOOK FOR:

* 100 to 200 calories per serving for a snack (half bottle), or 200 to 400 calories per serving for a meal (full bottle)

* At least 15 g of protein for the entire bottleNo added sugars (just natural sugars from fruit and fruit juices)

EAT CLEAN, STAY LEAN PICKS:

* Bolthouse Farms Protein PLUS Mango
* Columbia Gorge Organic CoGo Protein
* Naked Protein Zone and Protein Double Berry
* Odwalla Strawberry Protein, Original Super Protein, and Mango Protein

* Stonyfield Farms OP (Organic Protein) Strawberry, Vanilla, and Chocolate
* Suja Elements Spiced Chai Protein (vegan, but slightly lower in protein)

SOUPS

Soup for a snack? Try it! Soups are nutritious, flavor-packed, and super filling. For on-the-go snacking, just pour your soup into a thermos.

❈ 1 serving *Eat Clean, Stay Lean White Gazpacho with Grapes and Almonds* (page 264)

❈ 1 serving *Eat Clean, Stay Lean Broccoli Leek Soup* (page 262)

❈ 1 serving *Eat Clean, Stay Lean Sherry Mushroom Soup* (page 262)

❈ 1 serving *Eat Clean, Stay Lean Curry Butternut Squash Soup* (page 262)

❈ 1 serving *Eat Clean, Stay Lean Smoked Paprika Cauliflower Soup* (page 262)

❈ 2 servings *Eat Clean, Stay Lean Tomato Basil Soup* (page 262)

BARS AND CLUSTERS

Store-bought bars and clusters can vary widely in terms of calories, sugar, and ingredients. Stick with one of our picks (try any flavor you like!), or use the Shop Clean checklist (opposite) to find another good option.

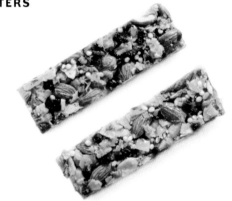

❈ 5 NOW Real Food Crunchy Clusters

❈ 1 Go Raw Sprouted Bite

❈ 1 Health Warrior Chia Bar

❈ 1 Kashi granola bar

❈ 1 Kind bar

Dr. Wendy Says . . .

Beware of snack traps! Planning out your weekly menu is key to staving off mindless snacking. But despite those good intentions, it can still be dangerously easy to find yourself sneaking extra bites—sometimes without even realizing it. And it doesn't take long for those nibbles to start adding up—and stall your weight loss. So keep a sharp eye out for times when you'd normally snack without thinking, like when you grab the leftovers off of your child's plate or take a few too many "tastes" of a dish while you're cooking. When you notice yourself about to snack, hit the pause button and take a step back and a deep breath. Of course, it's normal to have a few slip-ups at first. Old habits die hard! But rest assured: Over time, you'll get better at catching yourself *before* you put that mindless and meaningless something in your mouth.

LEFTOVERS AND SIDES

If you loved them as part of a meal, why not have them again as a snack?

❋ 1 serving *Eat Clean, Stay Lean Cuban Avocado and Pineapple Salad* (page 269)

❋ 1 serving *Eat Clean, Stay Lean Clean Coleslaw* (page 274)

❋ 1 serving *Eat Clean, Stay Lean Roasted Broccoli with Chile and Lemon* (page 277)

❋ 2 servings *Eat Clean, Stay Lean Honey-Glazed Radishes* (page 275)

Shop Clean Checklist: Bars and Clusters

LOOK FOR:

❋ 100 to 190 calories and at least 5 g of protein per serving
❋ Less than 10 g of sugar per serving
❋ No protein isolates, added sugar, or artificial ingredients

❋ 10 or fewer mostly whole food ingredients (like fruit, nuts, whole grains, and protein concentrates)

EAT CLEAN, STAY LEAN PICKS:

❋ Kashi Organic Crunchy Granola and Seed and, GoLean Bars
❋ NOW Real Food Crunchy Clusters
❋ Go Raw Sprouted Bites and Sprouted Bars

❋ Health Warrior Chia Bars
❋ KIND Nuts & Spices bars and Fruit and Nut bars
❋ Oatmega Vanilla Almond Crisp, Chocolate Coconut Crisp, and Lemon Chia Crisp (gluten-free and soy-free)

What's for Dessert?

By this point, you understand how eating foods made with lots of sugar and refined carbs tends to wreak havoc on your metabolism and blood sugar and ultimately makes it harder to lose weight. (If you need a refresher, just head back to Part I.) So yeah, we'd probably all be better off, health-wise, if we cut out desserts altogether. But that's not exactly realistic, is it?

When it comes to enjoying dessert on the Eat Clean, Stay Lean plan, there's some good news and some bad news. The good news is that you *can* still enjoy sweet treats. (Yay!) The bad news is that if you want to lose weight in just 3 weeks, you'll have to be pretty choosy about which desserts you eat—and how often you have them. Here's how to have your cake—figuratively!—and eat it, too.

❊ **Stick to Eat Clean, Stay Lean desserts.** The desserts on this plan are made from real-food ingredients and don't pack insane amounts of sugar, so you can indulge your sweet tooth without sabotaging your weight loss. We know—resisting the siren call of a fresh bakery cookie or a scoop of ice cream isn't easy! But the results will be worth it. And once the plan is over, you can go back to enjoying your favorite desserts; that is, in moderation, if you'd like. (For more information on how that works, check out Chapter 12.)

❊ **Enjoy them up to twice a week.** But try not to decide to eat dessert on the fly. Rather than give in to impulses or cravings, you want to get into the habit of making deliberate choices about the foods you eat—and following through. Plan your desserts as part of your weekly menu so you can look forward to them, and stick with the schedule you set.

❊ **Substitute your dessert for a snack.** Sadly, dessert doesn't come free. So when you opt to indulge in a treat, have it in lieu of one of your regular snacks that day.

Eat Clean, Stay Lean Desserts

Eat Clean, Stay Lean Roasted Strawberries with Dark Chocolate Sauce (page 288)

Eat Clean, Stay Lean Peanut Butter Banana Blondies (page 290)

Clean and Simple Dark Chocolate

1 ounce 80 percent or higher dark chocolate (⅓ of a 3-ounce chocolate bar)
OR 54 dark chocolate chips
OR 3 individually packaged Ghirardelli squares

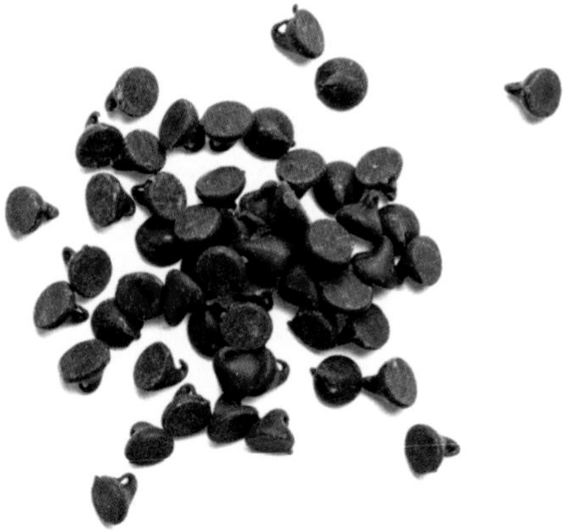

Clean and Simple Sweet Berries and Cream Bowl

Top ¾ cup berries with ½ cup low-fat plain yogurt,
and drizzle with I teaspoon honey or maple syrup (optional).

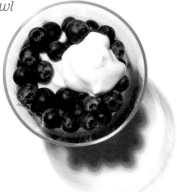

Clean and Simple Baked Apples

Heat the oven to 350°F. Place cored apples in a shallow baking dish. Fill the dish with ¼" water and sprinkle cinnamon into the cored areas. Bake for 30 minutes, or until the apples are tender. Enjoy one apple as a dessert; save additional apples for breakfasts or snacks.

Putting It All Together

1 **Say yes to snacking.** Clean, well-planned snacks can make you less tempted to snack on salt, sugar, and fat traps. And snacks keep you satisfied, so you're less likely to be starving and prone to overeating at mealtimes.

2 **Snack mindfully.** The right snacks can be powerful weight-loss allies. But too much of *any* foods, even clean ones, can work against you on the scale. Enjoy your planned, portioned snacks, but avoid adding in extra bites between meals. Even clean calories add up!

3 **Be flexible with your snack schedule.** Sticking to a regular schedule can help you avoid mindless eating. But it's also a good idea to shift your snacks as needed to make them work for you. For instance, if you know that you're having a later-than-usual lunch or dinner, push your snack a little bit later, too. That can help you stay more satisfied until it's mealtime.

4 **Treat yourself mindfully.** Stick to Eat Clean, Stay Lean desserts during the plan, and indulge up to twice per week. You'll satisfy your sweet tooth but without sacrificing your weight-loss progress.

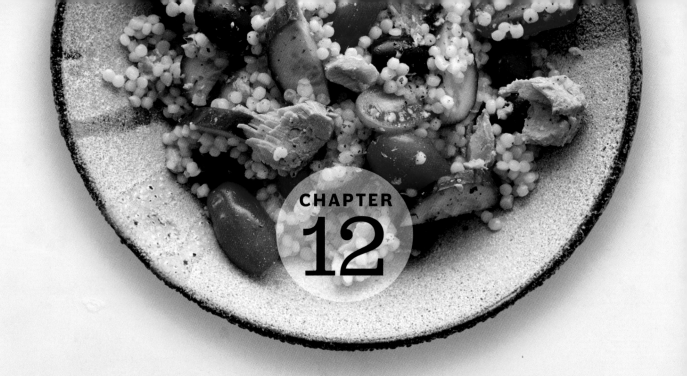

Staying Clean, For Life

Congratulations, you made it! You learned how to eat clean, made major changes to your diet, and jump-started your weight loss. Now it's time for the training wheels to come off. So how can you keep on applying what you've learned from *Eat Clean, Stay Lean* once you're no longer following the plan? If you're trying to lose more weight, how can you deal with the dreaded plateau? And most importantly, how can you maintain your momentum once the initial enthusiasm of eating clean wears off?

Eating Clean *Your* Way

Maybe you've already reached your goal weight by following the Eat Clean, Stay Lean plan and are looking to maintain that loss. Or maybe the plan was more of a kick-starter to help you lose those first 10 or 20 pounds quickly, and now you're ready to continue losing weight at a more moderate pace. Regardless of what your plans for the future might be, you've learned the skills you need to eat clean and are ready to try doing it on your own.

Which, sure, might seem a little scary. Without a set of expert-designed menus and meals to guide you, who's to say that you'll be able to keep eating clean? Who's to say that you won't cave to an intense craving that throws you off the wagon for the rest of the day—or even longer? Worst of all, who's to say that you won't regain the weight you worked so hard to lose—and then some?

Well, *you*, of course! *You* strove to learn all of the ins and outs of eating clean. *You* made the effort to plan your weekly menus. *You* dedicated the time to shopping for groceries and preparing all of your meals and snacks. *You* sought to understand the difference between true hunger and a craving. *You* put strategies in place to surround yourself with support, resist temptations, and make clean choices even when the situation was less than ideal.

You cleaned up your diet, took control of your health, and lost the weight. Nobody did it for you! So give yourself the credit you deserve, and start practicing a little bit of self-trust. You've already proven that you're a pro at eating clean and getting lean. And as long as you keep on planning, cooking, eating, and moving by those same principles, things won't suddenly change just because you're flying solo. And that's good news!

What's Next?

If you've ever lost weight on a diet only to regain it almost as soon as the diet was over, you might be wondering whether this time will actually be any different. It will, and here's why: Eating clean is a lifestyle based around the very simple—but very powerful—principle of choosing real, nutrient-dense foods over processed, empty-calorie fare. When you eat clean, you give your body what it needs to feel energized and what *you* need to feel satisfied. To fight stress, boost your mood, and sleep well. And most importantly, to keep the (majority of) your cravings at bay. In short, eating clean makes you feel really, really good. And when you *feel* good, you want to *do* good. You're motivated to keep choosing clean foods. To pay closer attention to your body's hunger and fullness cues so that you don't get up from the table feeling uncomfortably full. To enjoy your favorite treats in a moderate way that leaves you feeling happy, not guilty. To make physical activity a regular part of your life. To take responsibility for your weight—and your health.

Yes, the meals, snacks, and menus on this plan were calorie-controlled to help you lose the most weight you could as quickly as possible. If you want to get lean quickly, you have to make a strategic effort to cut back. But now that you've moved past the jump-start phase, it's time to shift your focus more toward maintaining your healthy habits. Of course, that doesn't mean that calories no longer count at all. When you consistently take in more energy than you need—whether it's from chocolate ice cream or chicken breast—you end up gaining weight. But as you might have learned from trying to diet in the past, keeping track of all those numbers day in and day out isn't sustainable.

What is sustainable? Committing to eating clean, paying attention to your hunger and emotions, and employing other behaviors that set you up for success. Healthy choices beget more healthy choices. Now it's time to put the core principles that you've learned from *Eat Clean, Stay Lean* to work in your everyday life and let them act as both your motivator and your guide.

Pledge to Be a Planner

Planning ahead is, hands down, *the* number one step you can take to set yourself up for clean-eating success, whether you're following a weight-loss plan or not. When you plan ahead, you give yourself the time and space to make a clean choice—and figure out exactly what you need to do in order to follow through. You can have all the good intentions in the world to eat clean. But when you get home after work and realize that the only thing in your fridge is leftover mac and cheese, or you're ravenous and are stuck with whatever's in the office vending machine because you forgot to pack a clean snack, the obstacle to actually making a clean choice becomes considerably more difficult to overcome.

The good news? You already know how to build your weekly menus and plan ahead. And because you've been doing it for weeks and taking notes along the way, you have a good idea of what works for you and what doesn't. Maybe you've learned that yogurt and fruit for breakfast helps you stay fuller than a smoothie does. Or that you should time your afternoon snack so that you have something healthy to nibble on when the office manager brings in that mouthwatering pastry tray like clockwork every Friday afternoon. Or perhaps that it's essential to rely on easy-assembly meals on nights when you get home later, because they let you get dinner on the table sooner and feel less tempted to snack on junk. Whatever it is, you've dedicated the time to getting to know yourself better—and you've reaped the healthy benefits.

So even though you're finished with *Eat Clean, Stay Lean*, commit to being a habitual planner. Print out a year's worth of weekly menu templates and stick them in a binder so you always have a fresh one handy—and so you can refer to menus from the past. Make a spreadsheet. Download a meal-planning app. Use a simple notebook and pen. *How* you make your plan doesn't matter, as long as you keep on doing it. Not sure you'll remember? Schedule weekly reminders in your calendar or phone.

Use Your Go-Tos

Do you love having scrambled eggs, toast, and tomatoes every morning for breakfast? Look forward to that afternoon apple and peanut butter more than any other snack? Go ahead and enjoy! Having a core group of meals and snacks that are delicious, satisfying, and above all easy to prep makes clean menu planning a breeze. Plus, on those rare occasions when you don't have a plan, you can turn to one of these old favorites rather than trying to figure out something totally new on the fly.

And remember, this holds for all the meals and snacks you ate on the Eat Clean, Stay Lean plan. If there were certain recipes that you kept coming back to over and over again during these last 3 or 6 weeks, make them mainstays on your future menus, too.

Dr. Wendy Says . . .

Sticking with your go-to meals makes clean meal prep a cinch. But you also know that variety is the spice of life—and good health! So when you can, find ways to make simple, low-stress swaps while keeping things familiar. Alternate between berries and chopped pear in your yogurt. Instead of the usual carrots, dunk red pepper strips in your hummus. Make a batch of quinoa for your dinner side one week, then do brown rice the next week. Different foods contain different nutrients, and switching things up ensures that you regularly hit all of your bases. And by keeping your taste buds engaged, you'll also keep your cravings for sugary, salty, or fatty processed fare at bay.

Pay Attention to Portions

Weighing and measuring every single thing you eat is pretty unrealistic. (Imagine bringing a measuring cup to the swanky restaurant downtown. Silly, right?) Still, making an effort to keep your portions in check is key to maintaining your weight loss or continuing to lose more. So how can you keep on being portion smart when you're not eating Eat Clean, Stay Lean recipes? Keep these tactics in mind.

❋ **Measure healthy fats.** Tasty foods like olive oil, avocados, and nuts and nut butters are crazy good for you. But they're also pretty calorie-dense, so it's important to pay attention to how much you're eating. When you're cooking, measure out these higher-fat ingredients (as well as butter and cheese) instead of adding them willy-nilly. When snacking on nuts, count them out or measure them with a measuring cup instead of just grabbing a big handful. (Measure those snacks in advance for easy grab-and-go options—and to make it easy to resist the temptation to mindlessly reach for a second handful.)

✳ **Sleuth out the serving size.** For packaged foods, get into the habit of checking the nutrition label to see what *actually* counts as a serving. If the label offers a specific number, like 8 crackers or 10 tortilla chips, count them out. If it gives a measurement, like 1 cup of yogurt or ¾ cup of cereal, measure out your portion so you know exactly how much you're eating.

✳ **Rely on your eyes.** After 3 weeks of following the recipes on this plan, you've probably developed a sharper sense of what an appropriate serving size is, versus what's way too big. When you're dining out or are away from home, try to stick with the same sizes that you've learned to serve yourself at home.

✳ **Check the recipe yield.** You might be surprised to find out that the pasta salad or chili recipe you usually whip up for your family of four is actually meant to serve six or eight. So always check to see how many servings a recipe is *supposed* to make—and divvy it up accordingly. And trust your senses. If a recipe seems to yield unusually large serving sizes compared to the Eat Clean, Stay Lean recipes you've been making, the portions are probably too big. Trust your gut and make adjustments. Remember that the recipe yields are just suggestions from the cookbook author. *You* are in charge of figuring out the best portion size for your energy levels, weight, and health goals—so serve yourself accordingly!

✳ **When in doubt, veg out.** Loading up your plate with vegetables automatically leaves less room for the heavier stuff. Whether you're at home, ordering off a restaurant menu, or enjoying a meal at a party or gathering, fill half of your plate with nonstarchy picks like leafy greens, broccoli, cauliflower, Brussels sprouts, tomatoes, string beans, asparagus, mushrooms, or peppers.

Notes from a Clean Eater

"A lot of times, I'd rely on my eye to serve myself the right portion. But then I'd put it on the scale and see that it was a little heavy. It's a good reminder to check yourself with that."—**Mary Pat S.**

Focus on Hunger and Fullness

Remember, food is meant to give your body energy—not entertain you when you're bored, distract you when you're stressed, or keep you company when you're lonely. By now, you've had some practice at paying attention to your hunger and fullness cues, as well as uncovering some of the emotional triggers that send you straight to the pantry or fridge. And chances are, you're getting pretty good at eating only when your stomach is grumbling and stopping when it's satisfied (instead of stuffed). If that's the case, keep it up! If you could use some more practice or feel like you could use a refresher course before striking out on your own, head back to Chapter 4 for some helpful practices and exercises.

Find Ways to Indulge Mindfully

We told you that eating clean meant that you could still enjoy the treats you love—and we meant it. And now that you've made it through the plan and jump-started your weight loss, you're ready to reincorporate some of your old favorites. (Or cleaner versions of them, at least. For more on that, see "Old Favorites, Made Cleaner" on page 213.) Here's how to do treats without *over*doing them.

❋ **Make them occasional, not everyday.** Whether your indulgence of choice is a mint chocolate chip ice cream cone, a plate of cheesy nachos, or a glorious glass of wine, *you can have it.* Just remember that these are once-in-a-while foods and drinks, not everyday ones. Go ahead and enjoy up to two of your favorite treats in reasonable portions every week. That's often enough to leave you feeling satisfied and like you're not missing out—but not so often that eating them becomes a habit or you end up regaining lost weight.

❋ **Look forward to them.** Sure, it's fine for your treats to sometimes be spontaneous—like when your neighbor stops by with a fresh batch of your favorite cookies or your family makes an executive decision that tonight *needs* to be fried chicken night. But in general, make an effort to plan your treats when you plan your weekly menu. Having that homemade chocolate cake or margarita to look forward to all week will make your treat that much more enjoyable. Anticipation is part of the fun, and more importantly, deciding on your splurge before-hand means that you're less likely to feel guilty after you indulge.

❋ **Have one helping.** If you've decided that you're going to have one slice of pie or a cookie, have one slice of pie or a cookie. We know—easier said than done! If you struggle with knowing when it's time to stop, make it harder to keep on munching. Buy a single pastry from the best bakery in town instead

(continued on page 212)

Do This Now!

We're willing to bet that following the Eat Clean, Stay Lean plan has helped you sharpen your mindful eating skills in a major way. But why not check your progress for yourself? Flip to page 65 and revisit the mindful-eating checklist you filled out back before you started getting lean. How many of your answers have changed?

Clean Eater

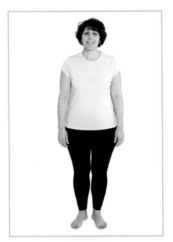

BEFORE

Kathy C.

Kathy had always been the kind of person who thought about what she ate. The problem was, she didn't pay much attention to *how much*. Sure, she'd reach for dried fruit–and nut-filled trail mix for an afternoon snack. But instead of serving herself a quarter cup, she'd pour herself a full cup.

Committing to eating clean meant scaling way back on her portions. But because she was eating whole, nutrient-dense foods, she found that her new, smaller serving sizes were still plenty satisfying. "It's surprising how little food you need," says the 50-year-old. "My snack would be 10 walnuts and 3 dried apricots. Before, I would've said that wouldn't have done anything for me. But it really did."

Of course, choosing clean foods was easier some times than others. A mom to teenage athletes, Kathy's schedule—and therefore, her food—is sometimes dictated by her kids' sporting events. If the gang was headed off to a tournament for the day, Kathy would bring along an easy-to-pack option like the Turkey Cuban Wrap (page 238). "I'd just eat it as a simple wrap so it wouldn't have to be heated," she says.

And when the kids had a sports banquet, she resolved to do what she could to eat as cleanly as possible by eating salad and chicken instead of bread or pasta. And because the piece of chicken was clearly too big, she only ate half. "I was really proud of myself because that's not what I typically would have done," she shares.

Kathy enjoyed walking for exercise before she started eating clean. And while she continued to do so afterwards, she admitted that she didn't make an effort to walk any *more* than she had been, which means that her impressive weight loss was largely the result of being more mindful about her portions. "Just the little bit of food that I *really* needed to eat to not be hungry was pretty amazing to me," she happily says.

Dr. Wendy Observes: Portions matter even when we're eating clean. But the thing that Kathy really realized was that smaller portions were plenty satisfying! Experimenting with eating a bit less food can sometimes be challenging, so I always tell clients to try it for just a few days. I always assure them that it's enough and that they'll be satisfied and energized, but they have to prove it to themselves. Kathy did!

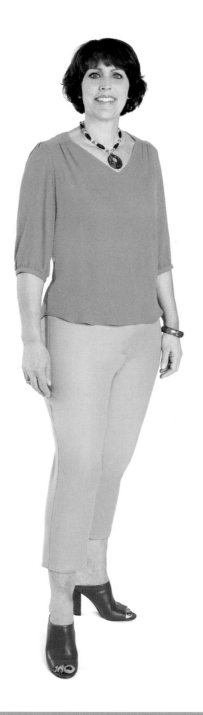

TOTAL POUNDS LOST

16 lbs

TOTAL INCHES LOST

13

MOST NOTABLE IMPROVEMENTS
After eating clean, **Kathy** became significantly more aware of how much food it actually took to fill herself up—and she was satisfied with less.

of an entire box from the grocery store. If you make something yourself, bring the extras to a friend or neighbor. When you order an indulgent meal, pass on bringing home that doggie bag, or give it to someone else. If it's not around, you can't keep eating it.

✳ **Be social.** Make it a point to have your treats in the company of others instead of eating them alone. Eating socially can help you stick with your intentions regarding how much and how often you have

dessert. And anyway, food is just more fun when the experience of eating it is shared.

✳ **Enjoy it—and move on.** Put your treat on a plate or in a glass. Sit down at the table. Savor every bite or sip. And when you're finished? Close your eyes, smile, and say to yourself, *That was wonderful.* Sure, it sounds a little cheesy. But taking the time to acknowledge how much you enjoyed something makes you feel good and appreciative—not guilty or like you need to have more.

Dealing with Plateaus

You made major changes to your diet and followed the Eat Clean, Stay Lean plan to a T. You moved more—both through traditional exercise and by building more activity into your day. And for a while, the number on the scale was inching downward. All of your hard work was really paying off. But now, your weight loss seems to have stalled.

Of course, you're still doing your part to lose weight. So why isn't your body holding up its end of the deal? Plateaus are insanely frustrating, and they might leave you feeling like you're suddenly doing something wrong. You're not—you just need to shake things up. Here's how to push on through.

Why You Hit a Wall

This might make you feel a little better—or it might make you feel a little worse. Either way, plateaus are completely normal. At some point or another, the vast majority of dieters find that their weight loss starts to drastically slow down or stop altogether. But don't worry—it's temporary!

What's more, hitting a plateau is actually a sign that you've been doing an awesome job of getting lean. When you clean up your diet, eat less, and move more, you lose weight. (Of course!) But here's the catch: As your body

gets smaller, it needs less food to function. So the amount that you needed to eat when you were 10 or 20 or 30 pounds heavier might be more than what your lighter frame needs now.

Plus, because you've been exercising, your fitness has likely improved by leaps and bounds. But if that workout you've been doing for weeks or even months feels a heck of a lot easier than it used to, your body isn't pushing itself as hard as it was when you were first starting out. As a result, even though you're walking

Old Favorites, Made Cleaner

That whole thing about choosing real, whole foods over processed, artificial ingredient–laden stuff?
It applies to your treats, too! Next time you're thinking about indulging, keep these clean swaps in mind.

- **Instead of:** A processed or packaged baked good or ice cream
- **Have:** A homemade baked good or a treat made by real people (like one from a local bakery, ice cream parlor, or farmers' market)

- **Instead of:** Movie theater popcorn or microwave popcorn with artificial flavors
- **Have:** Organic, non-GMO bagged popcorn or popcorn you pop yourself and flavor with real ingredients, such as smoked paprika or Parmesan cheese

- **Instead of:** A fruity cocktail made from a mix that includes artificial colors or artificial sweeteners
- **Have:** A glass of wine or a cocktail made with real ingredients, such as fresh fruit or real sugar, and a splash of sparkling water for some bubbles and to cut the calories a little bit, if you'd like

- **Instead of:** A conventional candy bar
- **Have:** An organic candy bar, chocolate bar, or peanut butter cup made from real-food ingredients, or dark chocolate with dried fruit

- **Instead of:** Conventional chips
- **Have:** Organic, non-GMO baked chips (potato chips are fine, but sweet potato, corn, or bean chips are even better), or homemade tortilla chips (made by slicing and baking a corn tortilla or whole wheat pita)

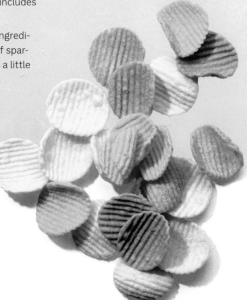

the same 10,000 steps or bicycling for the same hour as before, you're burning fewer calories while you do it.

If it sounds kind of unfair, well, we won't argue with you on that. Hitting a plateau can sometimes feel like the weight-loss gods (or even your body itself) are actively working against you. And that sort of frustration can drive you to take extreme or counterintuitive measures that might end up backfiring. You might be tempted to skip meals or drastically cut back your portions, which can leave you hungry, miserable, and prone to cravings. Or you might think about jumping ship altogether and heading to your favorite burger joint or ice cream parlor—which is a guaranteed recipe for feeling worse, not better. So instead of doing *either* of those things, stay calm. It's time to start thinking about some real, effective ways to get your weight loss moving again.

How to Beat a Weight-Loss Block

Ready to push through that plateau? We won't lie—you'll have to put in some more work to get things moving again. But you've already lost weight, and with these plateau-busting tactics, you can keep on losing more.

Be Honest About Whether You've Let Your Habits Slide

You probably felt energized and enthusiastic when you first started eating clean, and you followed your weight-loss plan to the letter. Of course, that kind of gung ho attitude is great—and it helped you get to where you are today. But it's tough to maintain that type of vigilance forever. Maybe after a month or two, you realized that you missed having a glass of wine with dinner, so you added that back in. Or you got into the habit of grabbing a dark chocolate square from your coworker's desk every time you went to talk to her.

Enjoying the occasional splurge isn't a bad thing. Always having to say no isn't fun, and treating yourself once in a while can strengthen your commitment to eating clean and keep you from feeling deprived. The thing is, it's easy to let even small indulgences go from something you have every so often to something you have all the time—especially once you've lost weight and feel like you have some wiggle room.

Stopping Your Habit Slide

Start by taking a look at your weekly food record. *Have you been getting a little bit looser with your splurges?* Are you still planning all of your meals and snacks, or have you started sometimes ordering takeout or relying on less healthy midday nibbles from the office break room? Are you stealing an extra couple of bites at dinner? If the answer to any of these questions is yes, make an effort to tighten up. And if you've stopped recording the foods you eat, get back to it! Writing everything down will give you insight into what you're actually eating.

✳ **Eat a little bit less.** Think small changes, not skipping meals or trying to eat like a bird. If you're having two or three snacks a day, can you cut back to just one or two? How about serving yourself slightly smaller portions at mealtimes, having raw vegetables instead of crackers with your bean dip, or making an open-faced sandwich with one instead of two slices of bread? Everyone's "little bit less" is a little bit different, and the key is finding tweaks that you're comfortable with and that don't leave you hungry. So start by trying one or two small changes for a few weeks to see whether they're enough to make a difference. If those don't seem to be enough, you can decide whether you feel comfortable making some other adjustments to your eating pattern.

✳ **Fire up your workout.** If you're meeting your daily movement goal, give yourself a pat on the back. By exercising regularly, you're already worlds ahead of most people—and you're doing great things for your health. Still, it might be time to think about kicking things up a notch. Can you increase your daily step count by a few thousand steps? Or ramp up the intensity of your exercise routine by adding in intervals or

strength-training sessions? Remember, your body has gotten pretty comfortable with whatever you're doing now. Find a way to shake things up!

✳ **Get more sleep.** Think that extra hour or two spent watching Netflix or scrolling through your phone couldn't possibly have *that* much of an effect on your weight loss? Sorry, think again. Remember, getting enough nightly shut-eye gives you more energy to make healthy choices and keeps your hunger hormones and blood sugar levels in check. You might even burn more fat *while you sleep.* Dieters who got less than 6 hours of sleep a night lost as much as 55 percent less fat while they snoozed than those who got a healthy 8½, according to one *Annals of Internal Medicine* study.[1] If you're not getting a full night's rest on the regular, it's time to start.

✳ **Get serious about lowering your stress levels.** Is the mere thought of hitting a plateau leaving you anxious? Heightened stress levels can nudge you to nibble on junk, so find a way to calm down that doesn't involve a sugary snack-fest. One option to consider is meditation. Sure, it might sound a little woo-woo.

Dr. Wendy Says . . .

It's human nature to want to let loose a little bit on the weekends. But make a conscious effort to keep that desire from thwarting your weight loss! **Research shows that dieters tend to eat more calories on Fridays, Saturdays, and Sundays than they do during the workweek.**[2] Rather than reward yourself with food on the weekend, think about other ways that you can relax and treat yourself. Can you book a massage or a manicure? Enjoy some much-needed time outdoors? Curl up with a great book or go see a movie? How about taking a luxurious afternoon nap? When you dedicate more time to self-care and activities you enjoy, you might find that you're less likely to want to splurge on extra food.

But in a recent review that looked at meditation's effect on eating behaviors, a whopping 86 percent of studies found that the practice improved behaviors including binge eating, emotional eating, or eating in response to external cues (such as sight, smell, or taste) instead of in response to physical hunger.[3] Can you take 5 minutes to pause, breathe, and let that busy brain clear out a little bit? You might find that afterwards, you feel a whole lot more optimistic about your ability to reignite your weight loss.

Maintaining Your Momentum

Anyone who's resolved to lose weight before knows that you can be crazy enthusiastic about a diet or plan in the beginning. But after a few weeks or months, all of the excitement is pretty much gone. You'd rather chill and watch TV than take time to plan out another weekly menu or—even worse—actually get up and exercise. You're bored with eating the same stuff all of the time. You sometimes start to wonder whether you can really keep getting leaner and whether eating clean is something you can actually do for the rest of your life.

All of these thoughts are completely and totally normal. You can even spend a few minutes letting yourself worry about them, if you really want to. But after that, you have to set them aside and find a way to regain some of that lost zest so that you can keep on keeping on. And happily, doing that might be easier than you think. After all, the impressive clean-eating efforts you've already made are proof of how far you've already come!

❊ **Set another goal.** Maybe you set out to lose 5, 10, or 25 pounds on the Eat Clean, Stay Lean plan. These are all admirable goals—but now what? Even though you'll no longer be following a formal diet plan, you still need to have an idea of what the next step in your weight-loss journey will be. Having a goal in mind gives you an endpoint to actively work toward and encourages you to lay out specific steps to get there. More importantly, it offers you a clear-cut way to measure your success so you can savor the pride and satisfaction of achieving what you set out to do.

Losing more weight or getting healthier might be your overall goal. But what, specifically, do you want to achieve next—and by when do you want to reach that mark? Do you want to lose 10 more pounds over the next 2 months? Fit into smaller jeans by the time your high school reunion rolls around? Lower your cholesterol, blood pressure, or blood sugar numbers by a certain amount in time for your next doctor's visit? Maybe you're happy with the amount of weight that you lost, and you just want to focus on strengthening your healthy habits. Perhaps you want to become a person who walks for a full hour, 5 days a week. Or you want to ramp up your vegetable intake from five servings a day to seven or eight. Virtually *any* health or weight-loss goal is a good one, as long as it's realistic (read: not, "I will lose 50 pounds in a month") and it keeps you committed to eating clean.

❋ **Try new things.** When it comes to losing weight, routines can be a really good thing. Knowing that you'll wake up to exercise at 6:30 every morning or make chicken-and-vegetable fajitas for dinner every Friday frees up your brain from having to make those decisions every day or every week, so you have the energy to deal with more important stuff. Still, it's no secret that too much predictability can lead to boredom. And when you're bored, your motivation can start to dwindle fast.

This means that in order to keep your eye on the weight-loss prize, you've gotta find ways to keep the doldrums at bay. Don't worry, your brain gets excited about almost *any* new thing; that's why we're compelled to constantly check our phones, in-boxes, and social media feeds for messages. So you don't have to make sweeping gestures or overhaul your entire daily groove. Just pick a few small ways to change things up. Chances are, that slight shift in course will go a long way toward keeping you committed to eating clean and getting lean.

Ready for a Change?

Wondering how to inject some excitement into your weight-loss routine? Whenever you sense yourself starting to get antsy, try one of these easy tweaks.

❋ **Find fresh recipe inspiration.** Scroll through Pinterest, swap clean recipes with a friend, or pick up a new cookbook. Or how about experimenting with a new-to-you herb or spice combination?

❋ **Eat somewhere new.** Can you take your lunch to the park? Plan an indoor picnic in your living room on a rainy day? Bring dinner to a place where you can watch a fantastic sunset? Indulge in breakfast in bed?

❋ **Hit the farmers' market.** Chances are, seeing all of those piles of just-picked, peak-freshness produce will spark some serious culinary inspiration. You might even find a brand new fruit or vegetable to add to your repertoire.

❋ **Change your route.** Walk, jog, or bike a different path than usual when you exercise. Or throw in some speedy intervals to keep your metabolism firing optimally on all cylinders.

❋ **Listen to a new playlist or podcast.** Been working out to the same 10 songs for who knows how long? Switch up that mix!

❋ **Update your workout wardrobe.** Because let's face it: Nothing gets you more excited about lacing up your sneakers than a brand new outfit.

Be Kind to Yourself

You probably don't need us to tell you that losing weight is hard work. But it's worth repeating because it's something every clean eater should keep in mind when he or she is having a rough day. Losing weight is hard work! But it's also *good* work. And remember: You're doing a great job.

If you step on the scale and don't see the number that you were hoping for, or you buy a sugary, processed candy bar during a momentary lapse of judgment, or you wake up one morning and just can't deal with the thought of exercising, instead of putting yourself down or allowing yourself to feel like a failure, remember this: *Losing weight is hard—but good!—work.*

Of course, the fact that it's hard doesn't mean that you can't do it. You can, and you *are*. But a little bit of self-kindness can go a long way toward convincing yourself that getting lean is a journey that's worth continuing—even when you're feeling tired or burntout. If a friend who was trying to slim down told you that she was having a hard time staying motivated, you wouldn't tell her that she was a failure. You'd listen, then you'd acknowledge her struggle. *Losing weight is hard—but good!—work.* Maybe you'd even commiserate for a few minutes or swap stories about your own challenges with your weight. But after that, you'd encourage her to keep at it—not to abandon her goal just because of one bad day. You'd tell her to start looking on the bright side by feeling good about all of the things she's achieved so far. You'd tell her that she's *already* succeeded! And so will you.

When the going gets tough, treat yourself exactly how you'd treat that friend. Don't beat yourself up. Don't fill your brain with negative talk. Be kind, and acknowledge all of the effort you've made so far—and all of the effort you'll continue to make in the name of taking control of your health and feeling great. **Losing weight is hard—but good!—work. And I know you can do it.**

Putting It All Together

1 **Put your new skills to use.** You've learned how to plan your menus effectively, be smart about portions, and pay attention to your hunger and fullness signals. Now that you're striking out on your own, use these skills! They'll go a long way toward helping you continue to eat clean and get lean.

2 **Renew your relationship with treats.** As you reincorporate some of your old favorites, such as dessert or alcohol, commit to enjoying them moderately and mindfully. You can do it!

3 **Power through plateaus.** If your weight loss is stalled, you can make changes to get unstuck.

4 **Eat clean to stay lean.** When your motivation wanes, set new goals and experiment with trying new things to reignite your energy. And above all, be kind to yourself. You deserve it.

Eat Clean, Stay Lean Recipes

KEY GF = Gluten-Free; LO = Lacto-Ovo Vegetarian; V = Vegan; U30 = Under 30 minutes

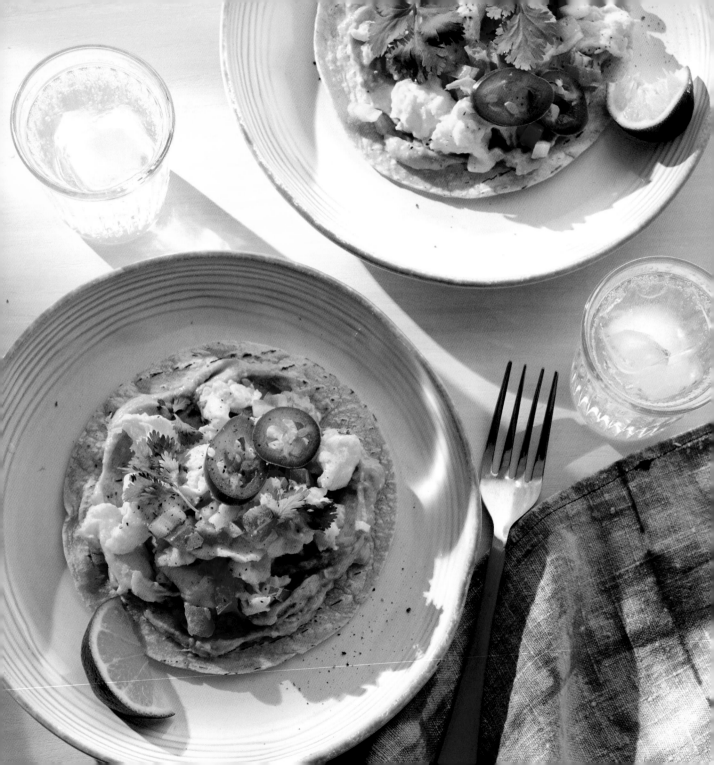

Avocado Tostadas with Huevos Rancheros

This Tex-Mex-inspired scramble, served over crispy corn tortillas and mashed avocado, is an easy, flavor-packed way to start your day. In a rush? Warm the tortillas in the microwave for 30 seconds instead of toasting them and fold the avocado and egg mixture inside to make mini tacos that you can eat on the go.

Active Time: 10 minutes
Total Time: 10 minutes
Makes 2 servings

- 2 corn tortillas (5" diameter)
- ½ medium avocado, mashed
- ¼ teaspoon ground cumin
- 1 teaspoon fresh lime juice
- ⅛ teaspoon sea salt
- ⅛ teaspoon freshly ground black pepper

- 4 large eggs, beaten
- 2 plum tomatoes, diced
- ½ cup diced red onion
- 2 tablespoons chopped fresh cilantro
- Pickled or fresh jalapeño slices (optional)

1. Heat the oven to 350°F or set the toaster oven on the medium cycle. Toast the tortillas in the oven or toaster until they're crisp around the edges. In a medium bowl, combine the avocado, cumin, lime juice, a pinch of the salt, and a pinch of the pepper. Spread the mixture over the tortillas.

2. In a medium nonstick skillet over medium heat, combine the eggs, tomatoes, onion, the remaining salt, and the remaining pepper. Cook, stirring constantly, for about 4 minutes, or until large, soft curds form. Divide the egg mixture between the 2 tortillas.

3. Top with the cilantro and jalapeños, if using.

Mini Spinach Mushroom Quiche

Served alongside fresh seasonal fruit, these right-sized, veggie-filled quiches are ideal for brunch. Got leftovers? Save them for fast weekday breakfasts.

Active Time: 15 minutes
Total Time: 40 minutes
Makes 12 (4 servings)

2 teaspoons extra-virgin olive oil

4 ounces lean ham, diced

2 cups diced mushrooms

½ cup diced onion

½ cup diced red bell pepper

2 cloves garlic, minced

Pinch of sea salt plus ¼ teaspoon

4 cups baby spinach

5 large whole eggs

3 large egg whites

¼ cup 2% milk

Pinch of ground red pepper

4 ounces shredded part-skim mozzarella cheese

1. Heat the oven to 375°F. Coat a 12-cup muffin tin with cooking spray.

2. In a medium nonstick skillet over medium heat, warm the oil. Add the ham and cook for 2 minutes, or until it begins to brown. Add the mushrooms, onion, bell pepper, garlic, and a pinch of salt, and cook, stirring, for 5 minutes, or until the vegetables have softened. Fold in the spinach and cook for 3 minutes more, or until wilted. Set aside to cool slightly.

3. In a medium bowl, whisk together the eggs, egg whites, milk, ground red pepper, and ¼ teaspoon salt.

4. Divide the vegetables among all of the cups. Pour the egg mixture over the vegetables until it's ¼" below the rim of each cup. Sprinkle the cheese over the top of each cup and bake for 25 minutes, or until the quiches are puffed and set in the center.

Make it ahead! The quiches can be made and refrigerated for up to 4 days or frozen for up to 1 month. Reheat a serving in the microwave at 50 percent power for 2 minutes.

Change it up! To make these vegetarian, leave out the ham and double the mushrooms.

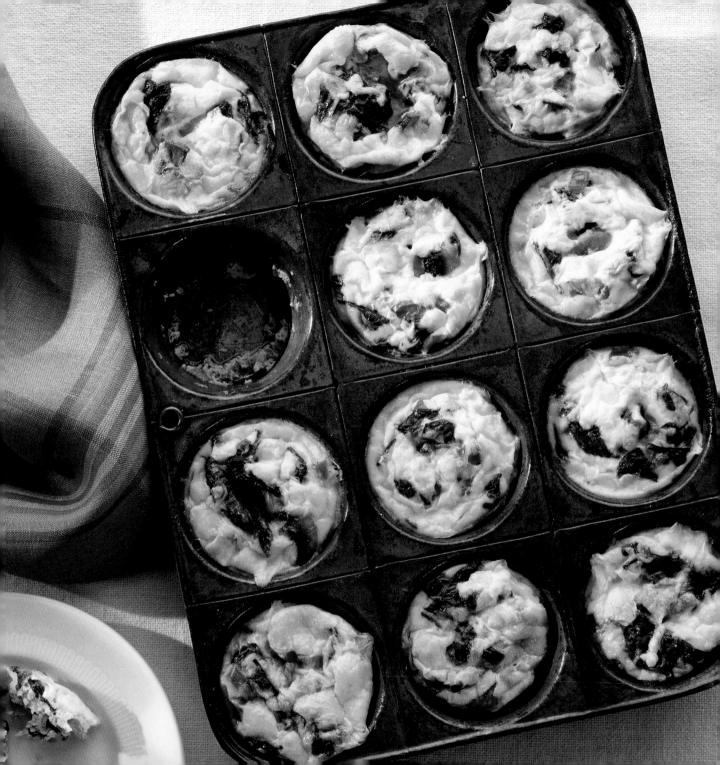

Overnight Steel-Cut Oatmeal

Packed with fiber, antioxidants, and a toothsome chew, these hearty fruit-and-nut-flecked oats are sweet and satisfying. Soaking the oats overnight cuts your cooking time in half the next morning.

Active Time: 15 minutes
Total Time: 8 hours
Makes 2 servings (about 1 cup each)

1½ cups water

½ cup steel-cut oats

2 tablespoons hemp seeds

Pinch of sea salt

1 cup fresh blueberries, raspberries, or blackberries

2 tablespoons chopped almonds

½ teaspoon ground cinnamon

1. In a medium saucepan over high heat, bring the water, oats, hemp seeds, and salt to a light simmer for 1 minute. (The top of the water will be cloudy, with minimal bubbles.) Cover, remove from the heat, and let the oats soak unrefrigerated overnight.

2. In the morning, cook the oats over medium-low heat for 10 minutes, or until creamy. (Alternatively, cook, covered, in the microwave, for about 3 minutes, stirring every 30 seconds.) Stir in or top with the berries, almonds, and cinnamon. Serve hot or cold.

Make it ahead! Make a double batch and transfer the cooked and cooled portions into jars. Top with the fruit, nuts, and seeds and refrigerate for fast grab-and-go breakfasts all week long.

Change it up! Swap out the berries for chopped apricots, pears, apples, or sliced bananas; swap the cinnamon with ground ginger or cardamom or fresh chopped mint; and swap the almonds for walnuts, pecans, hazelnuts, or unsweetened coconut flakes. You can also swap out the water for unsweetened almond or coconut milk.

Easy Buckwheat Crepes

This gluten-free, high-protein crepe batter is simple to whip up for Sunday brunch, and the crepes make easy wraps for on-the-go breakfasts or snacks. Take your pick of savory or sweet fillings!

Active Time: 25 minutes
Total Time: 25 minutes
Makes about 12 (6 servings)

I cup buckwheat flour

2 cups 2% milk

3 eggs

¼ cup ground flaxseeds

3 tablespoons organic canola oil or melted butter

¼ teaspoon sea salt

1. In a large bowl, whisk together the flour, milk, eggs, flaxseeds, oil or butter, and salt until mostly smooth. (A few lumps are okay.) Coat a medium nonstick skillet or crepe pan with cooking spray and place it over medium heat.

2. Pour ¼ cup of the batter into the skillet, swirling to evenly coat the bottom. Cook for about 1 minute, or until the edges appear set. Run a spatula around the edges to help release the crepe, flip, and cook for 30 seconds more. Transfer the crepe to a plate and repeat with the remaining batter.

3. Fill the crepes with your desired filling (see page 228). You can either put a crepe on a plate, fill half, and fold the other half over so you can eat it with a knife and fork, or you can put the filling in the center and roll it up like a burrito. Serve warm or at room temperature.

Make it ahead! Crepes can be made up to 5 days ahead and refrigerated, covered, with sheets of waxed paper between them. To reheat, wrap the crepes in foil and put them in a 300°F oven for 10 minutes; put them on a dish, cover with a damp paper towel, and microwave for 20 seconds; or return each crepe to a skillet over medium-low heat for 1 to 2 minutes, or until warmed on both sides.

(continued)

Savory Variations: Add ¼ cup of chopped fresh herbs (such as parsley, chives, basil, or cilantro) to the batter, if desired, and fill with one of the following:

1. **Spinach, tomato, olive, and feta–**In a large skillet over medium heat, cook 5 ounces of rinsed baby spinach with 1 chopped clove of garlic for 5 minutes, or until the spinach is wilted. Stir in 1 chopped tomato, 2 tablespoons of crumbled feta or chopped kalamata olives, and a healthy squeeze of lemon. Divide among 4 crepes. MAKES 2 SERVINGS. LO

2. **Ham, pear, and arugula–**Divide the following among 4 crepes: 2 ounces of sliced organic uncured ham, 1 cup of arugula, and 1 small pear, sliced. Sprinkle ½ ounce of grated, aged Cheddar or Gruyère evenly over all 4 crepes and serve. MAKES 2 SERVINGS. LO

3. **Black bean, cumin, and cilantro–**In a medium skillet or saucepan, heat 1 cup of rinsed and drained low-sodium black beans with ½ chopped tomato, ½ teaspoon of ground cumin, and a pinch of ground red pepper or chili powder. Stir occasionally for 2 to 3 minutes. Stir in 2 tablespoons of chopped cilantro and a healthy squeeze of lime. Divide among 4 crepes. Top each with ½ tablespoon of shredded Cheddar, if desired. MAKES 2 SERVINGS. LO

4. **Asparagus and mushroom–**Heat the oven to 400°F. Trim and chop ½ bunch of asparagus. Toss the asparagus on a baking sheet with 4 ounces of sliced cremini mushrooms, ½ sliced shallot, 2 teaspoons of tamari, ½ tablespoon of olive oil, and ¼ teaspoon of freshly ground black pepper. Roast for 20 to 25 minutes, or until the asparagus is tender and browned. Divide among 4 crepes. MAKES 2 SERVINGS. LO

Sweet Variations: Add the zest of 1 orange or lemon to the batter, if desired, and fill with one of the following:

1. **Strawberry and ricotta–**In a small bowl, mix 1 cup of sliced strawberries, 1 teaspoon of lemon zest, 1 teaspoon of lemon juice, and either 1 tablespoon of chopped fresh mint or ½ teaspoon of ground cinnamon. Spread each crepe with 1½ tablespoons of part-skim ricotta and divide the strawberry mixture among 4 crepes. MAKES 2 SERVINGS. LO

2. **Grapefruit and pistachio–**Segment 1 grapefruit and thinly slice ½ of a banana. Divide the fruit among 4 crepes. Top each crepe with 1 teaspoon of chopped unsalted pistachios and ¼ teaspoon of unsweetened cocoa powder. MAKES 2 SERVINGS. LO

Pumpkin-Cranberry-Cherry Breakfast Balls

Ever wished you could have cookies for breakfast? Now you can! These no-bake bites are low in sugar, high in fiber, and studded with nuts and seeds for extra protein. Take two for a grab-and-go breakfast, or enjoy one as a snack.

Active Time: 20 minutes
Total Time: 35 minutes
Makes 12 (2 per serving for breakfast; 1 per serving for a snack)

1¾ cups old-fashioned rolled oats

½ cup chopped almonds or pecans

¾ cup canned pure pumpkin puree (canned pure pumpkin)

⅓ cup unsweetened dried cranberries, dried tart cherries, or mixture of both, chopped

⅓ cup toasted, salted pumpkin seeds (pepitas), roughly chopped

⅓ cup hemp seeds

¼ cup pure maple syrup

2 tablespoons grape-seed oil

½ teaspoon ground cinnamon

¼ teaspoon ground ginger

¼ teaspoon sea salt

1. Heat the oven to 350°F.

2. Scatter the oats and almonds or pecans on a baking sheet. Bake for 10 to 12 minutes, or until toasted and very fragrant. Transfer to a large bowl.

3. Add the pumpkin, cranberries or cherries, pumpkin seeds, hemp seeds, syrup, oil, cinnamon, ginger, and salt to the oats mixture. Stir to evenly combine.

4. Scoop the mixture into golf ball–size portions and roll it firmly into balls. Set the balls on a tray or baking sheet and refrigerate for about 15 minutes, or until firm. Transfer them to a covered container and refrigerate or freeze until you're ready to eat them. (They'll keep for up to a week in the fridge or a month in the freezer.)

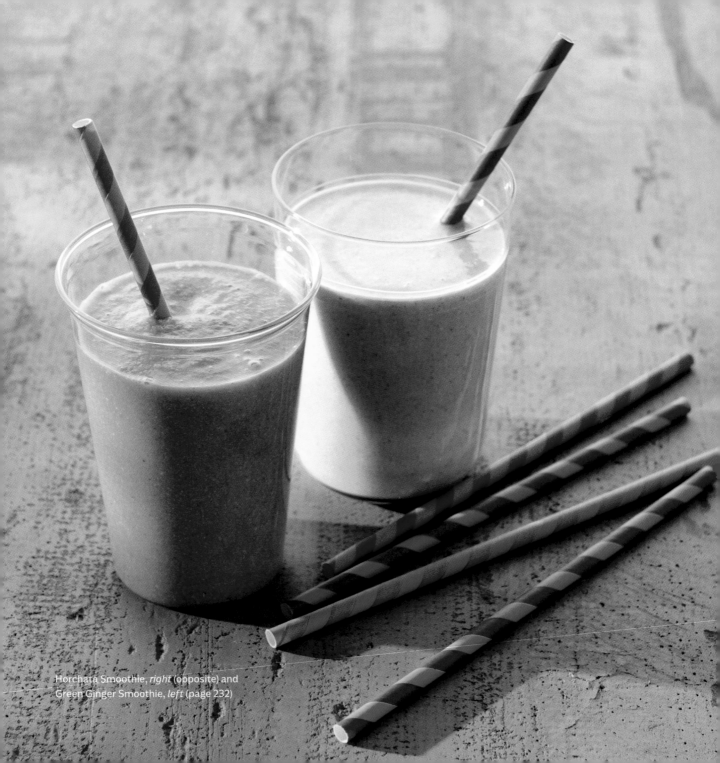

Horchata Smoothie, *right* (opposite) and
Green Ginger Smoothie, *left* (page 232)

Horchata Smoothie

Horchata is a Mexican milky beverage made from almonds, rice, and cinnamon. Add a frozen banana and a handful of rolled oats, and this refreshing drink transforms into a silky, satisfying smoothie. Have the full smoothie for breakfast or enjoy half as a snack. Just shake the leftovers in a sealed container or give them a quick whirl in the blender, and you're all set!

Active Time: 5 minutes
Total Time: 2 hours
Makes I serving (about 2 cups)

2 tablespoons raw almonds

2 tablespoons brown rice, uncooked

1½ cups water

I medium frozen banana, cut into chunks

I teaspoon pure vanilla extract

½ teaspoon ground cinnamon

¼ cup old-fashioned rolled oats

I. Soak the almonds and rice in the water for at least 2 hours or as long as overnight.

2. Transfer the almonds, rice, and water to a blender and blend until most of the almonds and rice are broken up. Strain, reserving the liquid. (You should have about I cup.)

3. Return the liquid to the blender with the banana, vanilla, cinnamon, and oats. Blend until smooth.

Tip: If you're low on time, skip steps 1 and 2 substitute 1 cup of plain unsweetened rice milk and/or almond milk for 1 cup total liquid.

Green Ginger Smoothie

This nutrient-packed green smoothie gets a natural hit of sweetness from frozen pineapple and mango, while avocado adds creaminess. Feel free to swap out the chia seeds for hemp seeds or ground flaxseeds to switch up the flavors. Enjoy the full smoothie for breakfast, or have half as a snack. Leftovers will keep in the fridge for a day or so.

Active Time: 5 minutes
Total Time: 5 minutes
Makes 1 serving (about 1½ cups)

½ cup chopped kale

½ cup water

⅓ cup plain, pineapple-flavored, or mango-flavored coconut water

¼ cup frozen pineapple chunks

¼ cup frozen mango chunks

¼ medium avocado

1 tablespoon chia seeds, unsweetened shredded coconut, hemp seeds, or ground flaxseeds

½ teaspoon grated fresh ginger

In a blender or food processor, combine the kale, water, coconut water, pineapple, mango, avocado, seeds or coconut, and ginger. Blend or process until smooth.

Photo on page 230, *top left*

LUNCHES

Tuna and Cannellini Salad

Rich albacore tuna, creamy white beans, and crunchy vegetables in a bright lemon, parsley, and shallot dressing—this isn't your mom's tuna salad! Enjoy it on top of a simple green salad, with a simple piece of fruit, or by itself.

Remember, you can swap lunches for dinners, too!

Active Time: 15 minutes
Total Time: 20 minutes
Makes 2 servings

2 tablespoons diced shallot

2 tablespoons fresh lemon juice, plus 2 lemon wedges for serving

1 teaspoon Dijon mustard

$\frac{1}{8}$ teaspoon freshly ground black pepper

2 teaspoons extra-virgin olive oil

1 can or jar (5 ounces) clean tuna, drained and flaked

1 can (15 ounces) no-salt-added or low-sodium cannellini beans, rinsed and drained

$\frac{1}{2}$ cup peeled and chopped roasted red peppers (see Note on page 234)

$\frac{1}{3}$ cup peeled and diced carrot

$\frac{1}{4}$ cup coarsely chopped fresh flat-leaf parsley

1 whole wheat pita, split open

1. Heat the oven to 400°F.

2. In a medium bowl, combine the shallot, lemon juice, mustard, and black pepper. Let the mixture sit for 10 minutes to soften and mellow the shallot. Whisk in the oil and season to taste with additional black pepper (optional).

3. Fold in the tuna, beans, roasted red peppers, carrot, and parsley. Set aside to let the flavors meld.

4. Cut each pita half into 6 wedges. Place the wedges on a baking sheet and toast in the oven for about 5 minutes, or until crisp.

5. Divide the tuna salad between 2 plates and serve with the toasted pita wedges and lemon wedges.

(continued)

Change it up! Swap out the tuna for clean canned salmon or chicken. Or make a vegetarian version by subbing 2 chopped hard-boiled eggs.

Note: *To make homemade roasted red peppers:* Place whole fresh red bell peppers over an open flame on the stovetop or on a baking sheet under the broiler. Cook them for 3 to 5 minutes per side, or until they're charred all over. Transfer the peppers to a bowl and cover it with plastic wrap or an inverted plate for about 10 minutes, or until the peppers are cool enough to handle. (This steams them, making it easier to remove their skins.) Use your fingers to carefully peel off the charred pepper skins and remove the stems and seeds. Stored in an airtight container, roasted red peppers will keep for up to 1 week in the refrigerator or up to 1 month in the freezer.

Kale Quesadillas

Who needs bread when you've got greens? Sturdy kale leaves stand in for the usual tortillas in these bean and cheese–filled quesadillas—and the results are just as delicious.

Active Time: 20 minutes
Total Time: 30 minutes
Makes 2 servings

½ medium onion, sliced

1 small zucchini, cut into half-moons

1 cup no-salt-added or low-sodium canned black beans, rinsed and drained

1 cup fresh or thawed frozen corn kernels

8 large kale leaves, thick stems removed

1 cup shredded part-skim mozzarella cheese

2 tablespoons fresh cilantro leaves

¼ cup clean, store-bought tomato salsa

1. Coat a large skillet with cooking spray and place it over medium heat. Add the onion and cook for 5 minutes, or until softened. Add the zucchini and cook for about 2 minutes more, or until softened. Add the black beans and corn and cook for 5 minutes, or until heated through.

2. Heat a large nonstick or cast-iron skillet over medium heat. Place a kale leaf on a work surface and layer 2 tablespoons of mozzarella, ¼ of the zucchini mixture, and then another 2 tablespoons of the mozzarella on top of the leaf. Top with another kale leaf, carefully place the "quesadilla" in the pan, and cook for about 1 minute per side, or until the cheese is melted. Repeat with the remaining ingredients. Serve topped with the cilantro and salsa.

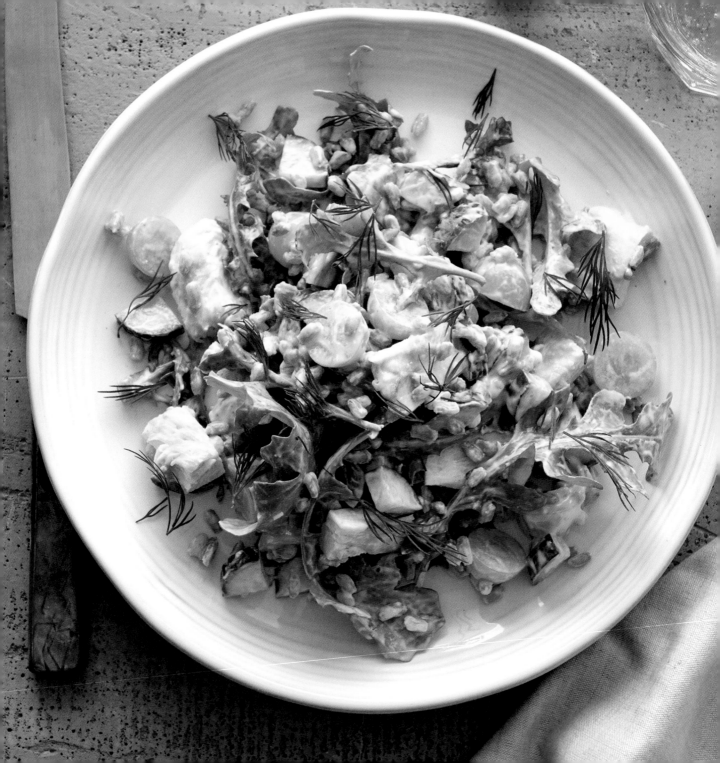

Creamy Chicken, Green Grape, and Farro Salad

Farro, an ancient Italian whole wheat, adds extra heft to this flavorful chicken salad. It's tasty warm, cold, or at room temperature—and the recipe is easy to double.

Active Time: 15 minutes
Total Time: 45 minutes
Makes 2 servings

¾ cup farro, rinsed and drained

1 boneless, skinless chicken breast (6 ounces), butterflied

¼ teaspoon sea salt

⅛ teaspoon freshly ground black pepper

¼ cup whole or low-fat plain Greek yogurt

2 tablespoons red wine vinegar

1 tablespoon extra-virgin olive oil

1 small garlic clove, mashed into a paste

¼ teaspoon ground cumin

1 cup arugula

¾ cup green grapes, halved

½ cup diced cucumber

1 tablespoon chopped fresh dill

1. Cook the farro according to the package directions. Let it cool slightly.

2. Season the chicken all over with the salt and pepper. Coat a cast-iron grill pan or skillet with cooking spray and place it over medium-high heat. Cook the chicken, flipping once, for about 8 minutes total, or until grill marks form and the chicken is cooked through to an internal temperature of 165°F. Chop into bite-size pieces.

3. In a large bowl, whisk together the yogurt, vinegar, oil, garlic, and cumin. Season to taste with additional salt and pepper, if necessary. Add the farro, chicken, arugula, grapes, cucumber, and dill, and toss to coat. Divide between 2 plates.

Change it up! To make this vegetarian, swap 1 cup of cooked chickpeas for the chicken. Want to experiment with another flavor profile? Substitute dried oregano for the ground cumin.

Turkey Cuban Wrap with Zesty Black Bean Salad

Savor the flavors of a traditional Cubano—without all of the not-so-clean extras. Add a side of black bean and veggie salad, and you've got a filling, flavorful meal.

Active Time: 25 minutes
Total Time: 25 minutes
Makes 2 servings

SALAD

2 tablespoons fresh lime juice

1 teaspoon extra-virgin olive oil

2 tablespoons diced red onion

½ teaspoon ground cumin

1 can (15 ounces) no-salt-added or low-sodium black beans, rinsed and drained

1 cup cherry or grape tomatoes, halved

1 head butter lettuce, torn into bite-size pieces

Pinch of kosher salt

Pinch of freshly ground black pepper

WRAPS

2 teaspoons coarse grain Dijon mustard

2 whole wheat tortillas (8" diameter)

1½ ounces thinly sliced Swiss cheese (about 2 slices)

5 ounces roast turkey breast, thinly sliced (about 6 slices)

8 dill pickle slices

1. *To make the salad:* In a medium bowl, whisk together the lime juice, oil, onion, and cumin. Add the beans and tomatoes and let sit for 10 minutes. Toss in the lettuce and season with the salt and pepper.

2. *To make the wraps:* Spread the mustard over the tortillas. Cut each of the cheese slices in half. Lay one of the half slices in the center of each of the tortillas. Top each tortilla with 3 slices of turkey breast and 4 dill pickle slices. Top with the remaining half-slice of cheese. Fold the sides of the tortillas in toward the center, then roll them up from the bottom to the top.

3. Place a griddle or skillet over medium heat and cook the wraps with their seam sides down. Press down with another pot or skillet to gently flatten the wraps. Cook for about 3 minutes per side, or until crisp and golden. Transfer to a cutting board and slice each wrap in half diagonally.

4. Serve the black bean salad with the warm wraps.

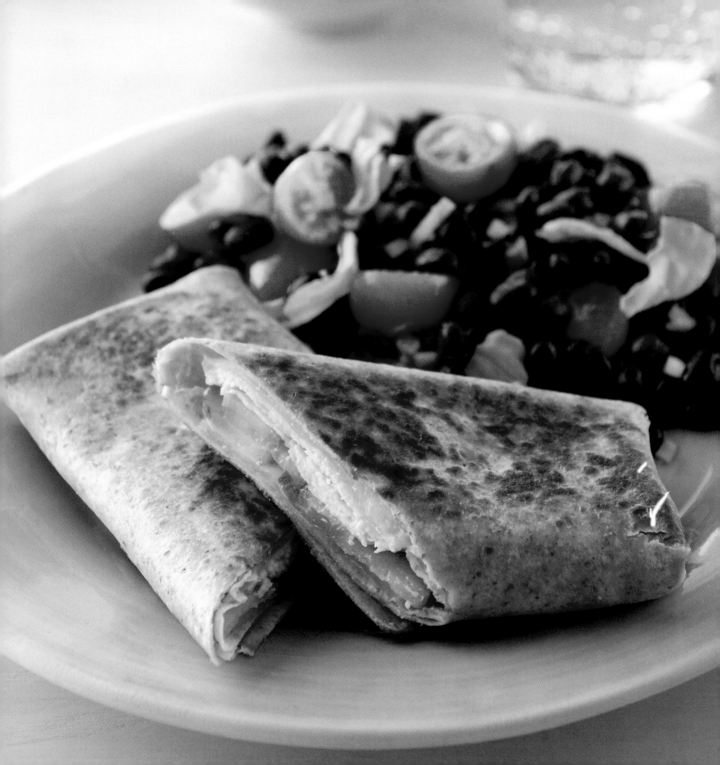

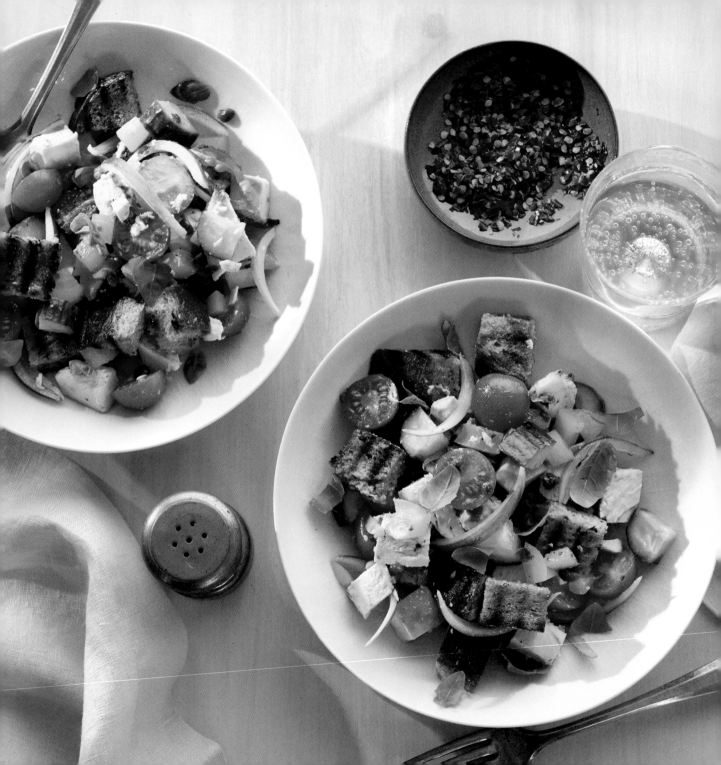

Hearty Chicken Panzanella

This hearty lunch salad brings together summer vegetables, a bright Dijon–caper vinaigrette, juicy grilled chicken, and chunks of toasted multigrain bread. Pack it for a picnic!

Active Time: 15 minutes
Total Time: 30 minutes
Makes 2 servings (about 2 cups each)

VINAIGRETTE

1 tablespoon avocado oil

1 tablespoon red wine vinegar

1 tablespoon capers, drained and chopped

½ teaspoon Dijon mustard

¼ teaspoon freshly ground black pepper

Pinch of sea salt

SALAD

2 slices multigrain or whole wheat bread

1 clove garlic, halved

1 cup cherry tomatoes, halved

1 small cucumber, peeled, seeded, and chopped

½ small red onion, halved and thinly sliced

1 yellow bell pepper, chopped

¼ cup fresh basil, chopped

8 ounces boneless, skinless chicken breast

1. *To make the vinaigrette:* In a large bowl, whisk together the oil, vinegar, capers, mustard, black pepper, and salt. Set aside.

2. *To make the salad:* Heat a grill or grill pan to medium-high, and brush and oil the grates. Grill the bread for 1 to 2 minutes, or until grill marks form and it's toasted. Remove the bread from the grill and rub each slice thoroughly with the garlic. Cube the bread and add it to the bowl with the vinaigrette, along with the tomatoes, cucumber, onion, bell pepper, and basil, and toss to coat. Set aside to let the flavors meld.

3. Grill the chicken for about 15 minutes, turning once, until an instant-read thermometer inserted in the thickest part of the chicken registers 165°F. Let it rest for 5 minutes, then cut it into cubes. Toss with the salad and serve.

Change it up! Low on time? Use the breast from an organic rotisserie chicken. Or to make a vegetarian version, swap out the chicken for one 15-ounce can of low-sodium white beans, rinsed and drained.

Beef Scallion Roll-Ups

Who needs greasy takeout when you have these sesame-, tamari-, and ginger-infused bites? These roll-ups aren't just full of savory goodness, they're fun to eat, too.

Active Time: 25 minutes
Total Time: 40 minutes
Makes 2 servings

3 tablespoons low-sodium tamari

2 tablespoons mirin

1 tablespoon water

4 cloves garlic, minced

2 teaspoons grated fresh ginger

8 ounces flank steak

1 cup baby spinach

16 scallions, green parts only, cut into 2" pieces

1 tablespoon sesame oil, divided

6 ounces baby bok choy

1 teaspoon sesame seeds

1. Heat the oven to 350°F. In a large, shallow dish, stir together the tamari, mirin, water, garlic, and ginger. Reserve half in a separate bowl. Slice the flank steak with the grain into 8 slices that are ¼" thick, then slice them in half crosswise into 16 strips that are about 5" long. Marinate the steak in half of the tamari mixture for 15 minutes.

2. Remove one strip of steak from the marinade and place a few spinach leaves and a few scallion pieces at the bottom. Roll up the strip and secure it with a toothpick. Repeat with the remaining strips until you have 16 rolls.

3. In a large, ovenproof skillet over medium heat, warm 2 teaspoons of the oil. Place the rolls in the pan and sear them for 1 to 2 minutes, turning as necessary to brown them on all sides. Cover and place the entire pan in the oven for about 3 minutes, or until they're cooked to your desired level of doneness.

4. Transfer the rolls to a serving dish. Add the reserved marinade to the pan and bring it to a boil over high heat, scraping up any browned bits on the bottom of the pan. Add the bok choy and toss, cooking for about 3 minutes, or until it's slightly wilted. Drizzle the beef roll-ups with the remaining oil and sprinkle them with sesame seeds. Serve with the bok choy.

Change it up! To make vegetarian roll-ups, swap out the beef and use 8 ounces of eggplant or zucchini sliced into strips and prepared as described above.

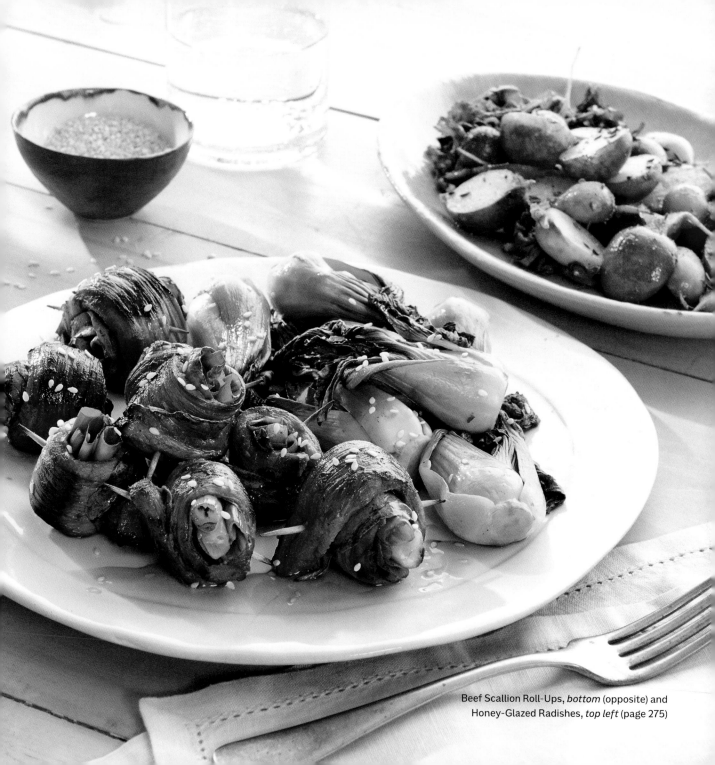

Beef Scallion Roll-Ups, *bottom* (opposite) and
Honey-Glazed Radishes, *top left* (page 275)

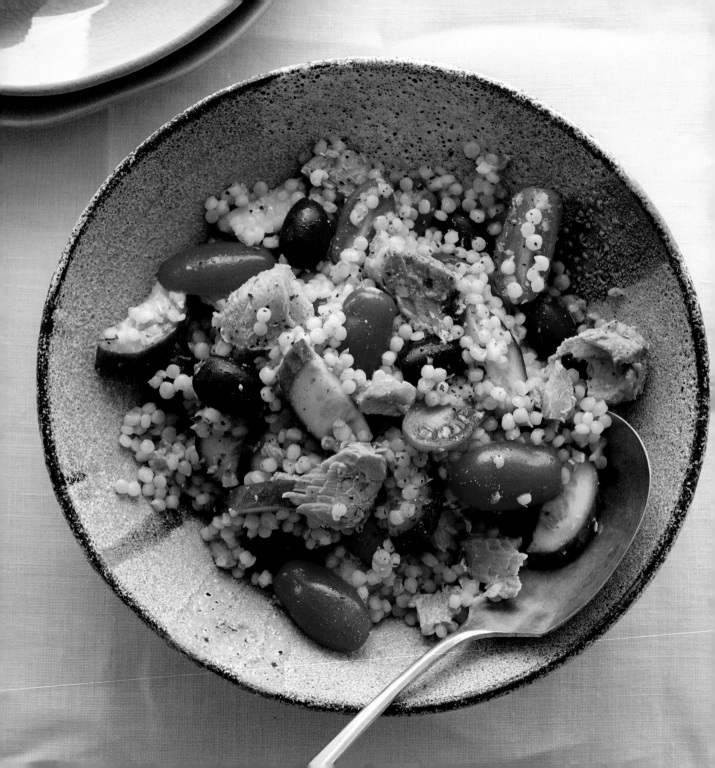

Israeli Couscous Salad with Salmon

The fresh, sunny combo of tomato, cucumber, feta, and oregano in this satisfying salmon salad just might transport you straight to the beaches of the Mediterranean. Find Israeli couscous, which is larger and chewier than regular couscous, in the pasta aisle.

Active Time: 10 minutes
Total Time: 30 minutes
Makes 2 servings

¾ cup Israeli couscous

Juice of ½ lemon

2 teaspoons olive oil

½ teaspoon dried oregano

I can (5 ounces) salmon, drained and flaked

½ cup grape tomatoes, halved

½ cucumber, peeled, seeded, and chopped

¼ cup feta cheese, crumbled

8 kalamata olives, pitted

Sea salt and freshly ground black pepper (optional)

I. Cook the couscous according to the package directions. In a jar with a tight-fitting lid, combine the lemon juice, oil, and oregano, and shake until combined.

2. In a large bowl, combine the couscous with the salmon, tomatoes, cucumber, feta, and olives. Pour the dressing over the top and toss to combine. Season lightly to taste with salt and pepper (if using), and serve.

DINNERS

Shrimp Scampi over Garlicky Greens

Swap the usual white pasta for a bed of garlicky greens and this classic seafood dish quickly transforms into a clean favorite.

Remember, you can swap dinners for lunches, too!

Active Time: 15 minutes
Total Time: 15 minutes
Makes 2 servings

¼ cup low-sodium chicken broth

4 cloves garlic, sliced

1 pound dandelion greens, coarsely chopped

2 tablespoons unsalted butter

1 tablespoon olive oil

12 large shrimp, peeled and deveined

2 tablespoons white wine

2 tablespoons lemon juice

1 teaspoon red pepper flakes

1 tablespoon chopped fresh parsley

1. In a large skillet over medium heat, heat the chicken broth. Add the garlic and cook for 1 minute. Add the dandelion greens, cover, and cook, tossing occasionally, for about 8 minutes, or until wilted. Remove the greens from the pan and set them aside.

2. Wipe out the skillet, place it over medium heat, and warm the butter and oil in it. Add the shrimp and cook for 1 minute, or until it starts to turn pink. Stir in the wine, lemon juice, and red pepper flakes. Cook for 30 seconds more, or until the shrimp is opaque. Serve over the greens, sprinkled with the parsley.

Change it up! You can swap in mustard greens, collard greens, kale, or spinach for the dandelion greens. Adjust the cooking time accordingly so the greens can wilt.

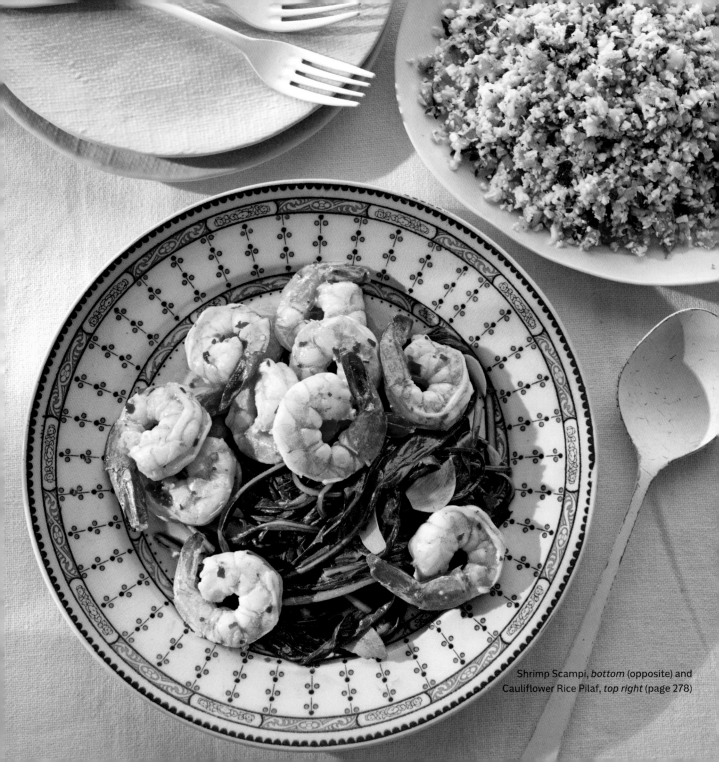

Shrimp Scampi, *bottom* (opposite) and
Cauliflower Rice Pilaf, *top right* (page 278)

Slow Cooker BBQ Pulled Chicken Flatbreads

Hectic day? Let the slow cooker do most of the dinner prep work for you by making these flavorful, open-faced BBQ chicken sandwiches. The coleslaw gets an extra kick—without the need for tons of mayo or cream—with a secret ingredient: pickle juice!

Active Time: 15 minutes
Total Time: 3 hours, 45 minutes
Makes 2 servings

¾ cup crushed tomatoes or tomato puree

2 tablespoons apple cider vinegar

1 tablespoon molasses

1 teaspoon smoked or sweet paprika

¼ teaspoon sea salt

¼ teaspoon freshly ground black pepper, divided

1 teaspoon Dijon mustard, divided

1 small red onion, thinly sliced, divided

8 ounces boneless, skinless chicken breast

1½ cups shredded green cabbage (about ¼ small head)

1 large carrot, grated

2 tablespoons dill pickle juice

1 tablespoon mayonnaise

4 corn tortillas, whole wheat flatbreads, or pita bread (6" diameter; use corn tortillas for gluten-free)

1. In a slow cooker, combine the tomatoes or puree, vinegar, molasses, paprika, salt, ⅛ teaspoon of the pepper, and ½ teaspoon of the mustard. Whisk until smooth. Add half of the onion. Add the chicken to the slow cooker, spooning some of the mixture over the top of it. Cover and cook on low for about 3½ hours, until the chicken is very tender and reaches an internal temperature of 165°F. (You should be able to pull the chicken apart with a fork.)

2. Meanwhile, in a large bowl, combine the cabbage, carrot, pickle juice, mayonnaise, the remaining ⅛ teaspoon pepper, the remaining ½ teaspoon mustard, and the remaining onion. Cover and refrigerate the coleslaw until ready to serve. (If you don't like the taste of raw onion, soak the onion slices in cold water for 10 minutes and then drain well before adding them to the slaw.)

3. Remove the chicken from the sauce and place it on a cutting board. Shred it with two forks and return it to the slow cooker. Mix until the chicken is evenly coated with the sauce.

(continued)

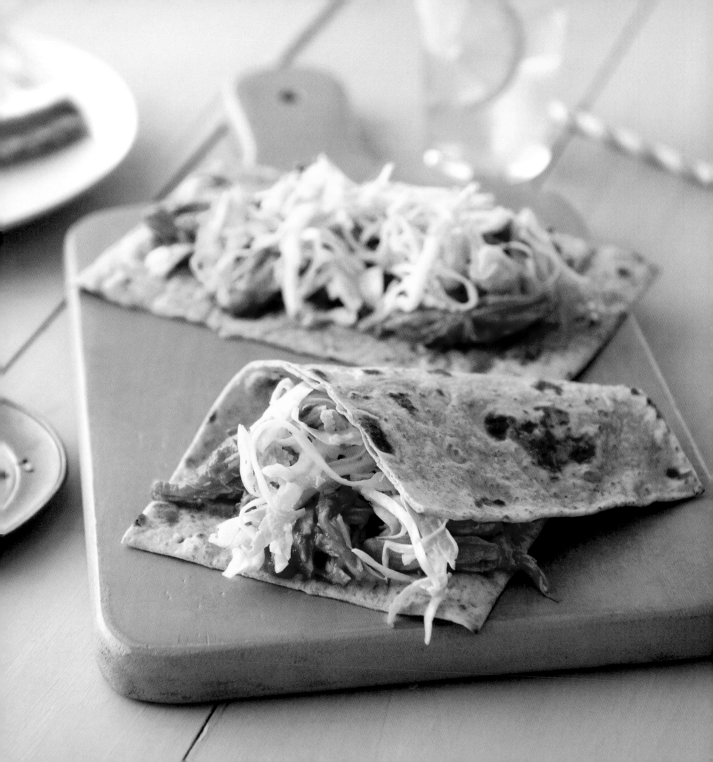

4. Divide the sauced chicken over the tortillas or flatbreads, and serve topped with the slaw.

Tip: If you don't have a slow cooker, combine the sauce ingredients in a medium saucepan with a lid. Whisk until smooth and bring to a simmer over medium heat. Add the chicken to the pan, spooning a bit of sauce over the top, then reduce the heat to the lowest setting and cover. Cook for about 1 hour, until the chicken is cooked through and very tender.

Make it ahead! Pulled chicken freezes well, and this recipe doubles easily. Make a big batch and freeze half for a fast weeknight dinner.

Change it up! To make vegetarian BBQ, omit the chicken, sub in 8 ounces of thinly sliced tempeh, and skip step 3.

Turkey Roulade

The tangy flavor combo of sun-dried tomatoes and basil makes your turkey cutlets anything but ordinary. This showstopper is impressive enough to serve to guests but easy enough to pull together on weeknights.

Active Time: 20 minutes
Total Time: 30 minutes
Makes 2 servings

½ cup canned no-salt-added or low-sodium white beans, rinsed and drained

½ cup sun-dried tomatoes in oil, drained and chopped

¼ cup pine nuts, chopped

1 tablespoon fresh basil leaves, chopped

¼ cup shredded Parmesan cheese

2 turkey breast cutlets, 4 ounces each

¼ teaspoon sea salt

¼ teaspoon freshly ground black pepper

1 cup baby spinach

1. In a medium bowl, mash the beans lightly. Add the tomatoes, pine nuts, basil, and Parmesan, and stir until combined. Set aside.

2. Divide the cutlets into four 2-ounce pieces. Place the cutlets between pieces of plastic wrap and pound them until they're ⅛" thick. Remove the plastic wrap and place one cutlet on a flat surface. Season it with salt and pepper, spread ¼ cup of the sun-dried tomato mixture on top, layer on ¼ cup of the spinach, and then roll up and secure with a toothpick. Repeat with the remaining cutlets.

3. Heat the oven to 350°F. Coat an ovenproof skillet with cooking spray and place it over medium heat. Sear the cutlets for about 2 minutes per side, or until browned. Cover the skillet and transfer it to the oven. Cook for about 10 minutes, or until the turkey is cooked through and no longer pink.

Florentine Chicken Meatballs with Spaghetti Squash and Salsa Cruda

Craving spaghetti and meatballs? Spaghetti squash has a taste and texture that's similar to that of whole wheat spaghetti—but with way more good-for-you nutrients. Pair it with a fresh no-cook tomato sauce and chicken-and-spinach meatballs, and get ready to break out the red-and-white checked tablecloth.

Active Time: 20 minutes
Total Time: 50 minutes
Makes 2 servings

8 ounces ground chicken

⅔ cup thawed frozen chopped spinach

2 tablespoons grated Parmigiano-Reggiano, plus more for serving (optional)

2 tablespoons whole wheat bread crumbs

I large egg white

¼ cup finely chopped yellow onion, divided

2 cloves garlic, minced, divided

¼ teaspoon sea salt, divided

¼ teaspoon freshly ground black pepper, divided

I small spaghetti squash, halved lengthwise and seeded

2 ripe tomatoes, coarsely chopped

2 tablespoons chopped fresh basil leaves

I. Position a rack in the center of the oven and heat the oven to 425°F. Line a large rimmed baking sheet with foil and coat it with cooking spray.

2. Combine the chicken, spinach, cheese, bread crumbs, egg white, half of the onion, half of the garlic, ⅛ teaspoon of the salt, and ⅛ teaspoon of the pepper. With wet hands, form 6 golf ball–size meatballs. Place the meatballs on the prepared sheet and coat them with a bit more cooking spray. Bake, turning the meatballs halfway through, for about 18 minutes, or until they're cooked through and lightly golden.

3. Meanwhile, place the spaghetti squash, cut side down, on a microwave-safe plate. Microwave on high for 8 to 12 minutes, or until the spaghetti squash is tender when pierced with a fork. Using a fork, comb through the flesh, releasing the strands of the squash. Transfer them to a colander to drain until the meatballs are ready.

4. In a medium bowl, toss the tomatoes, basil, the remaining onion, and the remaining garlic. Season with the remaining ⅛ teaspoon salt and ⅛ teaspoon pepper.

5. Divide the warm spaghetti squash between two plates and top each with half of the tomato sauce, 3 meatballs, and additional cheese, if desired.

Change it up! To make this dish vegetarian, swap the chicken with 8 ounces of crumbled firm tofu. Or use a full 10-ounce package of frozen spinach and top it with 2 tablespoons of grated Parmesan per serving to make spinach balls.

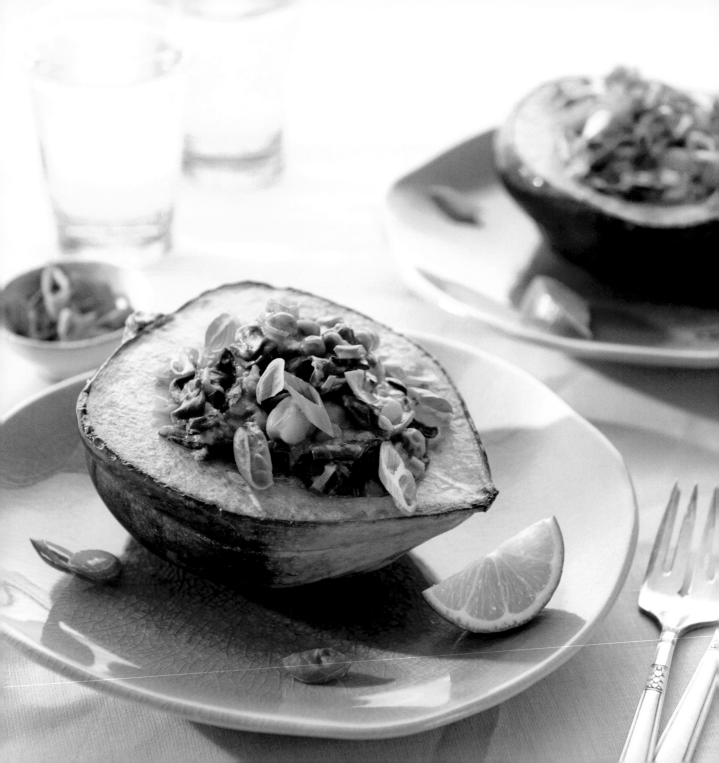

Chickpea Curry-Stuffed Squash

You've heard of an edible bread bowl, but how about an edible squash bowl? Nutty, earthy squash serves as a delicious—and nutrient-dense—serving vessel for this creamy, fragrant curry.

Active Time: 20 minutes
Total Time: 30 minutes
Makes 2 servings

I acorn squash or delicata, halved and seeded

2 teaspoons coconut oil, divided

2 scallions, thinly sliced (whites and greens kept separate)

I tablespoon chopped lemongrass

I teaspoon grated fresh ginger

½ cup light coconut milk

½ cup water

I teaspoon Thai red curry paste

½ teaspoon ground turmeric

¼ teaspoon sea salt

I cup canned no-salt-added or low-sodium chickpeas, rinsed and drained

4 cups baby spinach

I cup frozen green peas, thawed

2 teaspoons fresh lime juice, plus 2 lime wedges for serving

2 tablespoons chopped basil

I. Position a rack in the center of the oven, and heat the oven to 400°F. Rub the cut sides of the squash with I teaspoon of the oil and bake on a baking sheet, cut sides down, for 20 to 25 minutes, or until cooked through and tender.

2. In a medium saucepan, melt the remaining I teaspoon oil over medium heat. Add the scallion whites, lemongrass, and ginger, and sauté for about 3 minutes, or until tender. Stir in the coconut milk, water, curry paste, turmeric, and salt. Add the chickpeas and bring to a simmer. Cook for about 10 minutes, or until the chickpeas are heated through and have absorbed the other flavors.

3. Stir in the spinach, I cup at a time, and cook for about 5 minutes total, or until it's wilted. Add the peas and lime juice. Season to taste with additional salt, if desired.

4. Divide the chickpea curry between the squash halves. Sprinkle with the scallion greens and the basil. Serve with the lime wedges.

Maple Mustard Glazed Pork Tenderloin with Roasted Vegetables and Apples (GF)

What's for Sunday dinner? This hearty roast tenderloin with sweet roasted root vegetables and apples. It's your classic meat-and-potatoes meal—made deliciously clean and lean.

Active Time: 15 minutes
Total Time: 1 hour
Makes 2 servings

½ pound baby Yukon Gold potatoes, halved

½ pound carrots, peeled and cut into 1" chunks

2 leeks, trimmed, halved lengthwise, and cut into 1" chunks

1 teaspoon chopped fresh rosemary or ½ teaspoon dried

2 teaspoons olive oil, divided

¼ teaspoon sea salt, divided

½ teaspoon freshly ground black pepper, divided

1½ teaspoons Dijon mustard

1 teaspoon pure maple syrup

½ teaspoon chopped fresh sage or ¼ teaspoon dried

½ teaspoon chopped fresh thyme or ¼ teaspoon dried

1 small clove garlic, mashed into a paste

8 ounces pork tenderloin, trimmed of all visible fat

1 sweet, tart apple, such as Honeycrisp or Jonagold, cored and cut into ¾" wedges

1. Position a rack in the upper third of the oven and heat the oven to 425°F. In a 9" x 13" baking dish, toss the potatoes, carrots, leeks, rosemary, 1 teaspoon of the oil, ⅛ teaspoon of the salt, and ¼ teaspoon of the pepper. Roast for about 12 minutes, or until the vegetables begin to soften.

2. In a small bowl, combine the mustard, syrup, sage, thyme, garlic, and the remaining 1 teaspoon oil, ⅛ teaspoon salt, and ¼ teaspoon pepper. Rub this mixture on the pork, covering its entire surface.

3. Remove the vegetables from the oven, stir in the apple wedges, and place the pork on top. Roast, turning the tenderloin once halfway through cooking, for about 18 minutes, or until an instant-read thermometer registers 145°F when inserted into the thickest part of the tenderloin.

4. Transfer the pork to a cutting board and let it rest for a few minutes before slicing it into ½" slices. Divide the vegetables and pork between two plates.

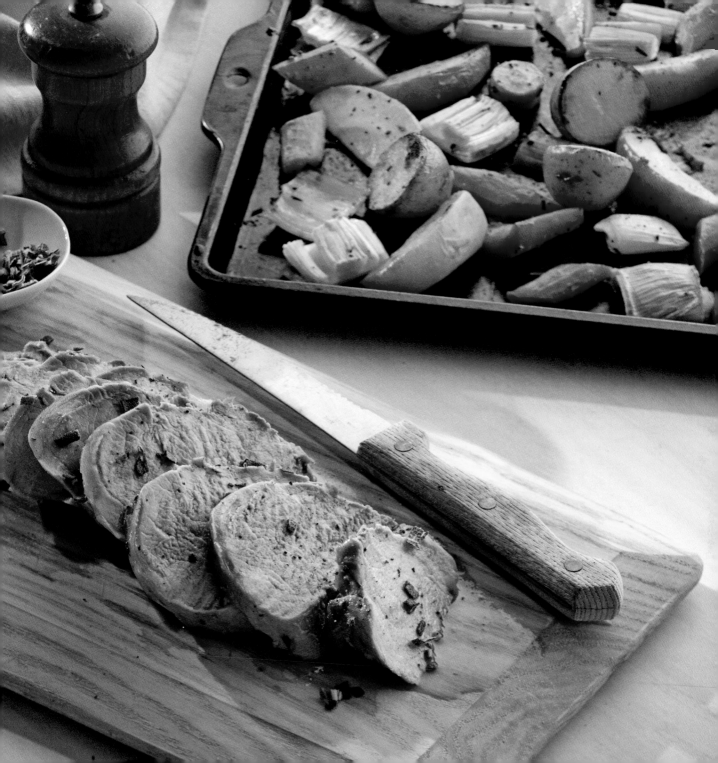

SOUPS

Create-Your-Own No-Cream Soups

What's the key to making a clean cream soup? Sweet, tender vegetables! Pureeing them with your favorite flavorful broth and a little bit of clean oil or butter yields a rich, velvety soup that rivals anything you'd find at a restaurant or deli. Best of all, the combinations are nearly endless. Follow this simple formula and get creative with your favorite flavors, or use one of our tried-and-true combos.

Active Time: 20 minutes
Total Time: I hour
Makes 6 servings

I tablespoon (total) *clean fat* (choose up to two)

- Unsalted butter, extra-virgin olive oil, avocado oil, grape-seed oil, canola oil, or coconut oil

I½ cups (total) *aromatics, chopped* (choose two to four)

- Onion, leek, shallot, celery (up to ¼ cup), grated ginger, or minced garlic (up to 1 tablespoon)

Pinch of salt in cooking water and optional salt and pepper to taste

I to 2 teaspoons *ground spice* (choose one)

- Curry powder, ground cumin, smoked paprika, mustard seeds, ground fennel seeds, garam masala, cinnamon, or up to ¼ teaspoon of ground red pepper or chili powder

2 pounds *vegetables, chopped* (choose one)

- Broccoli, cauliflower, carrots, butternut squash, mushrooms, asparagus, peas, or tomatoes (if using canned, use whole tomatoes in juice)

¼ cup *deglazing liquid* (optional; choose one)

- Dry white wine, red wine, beer, dry vermouth, cooking sherry, apple cider, or fresh orange juice

2½ cups *broth* (choose one)

- Low-sodium vegetable broth, chicken broth, beef broth, mushroom broth, or water

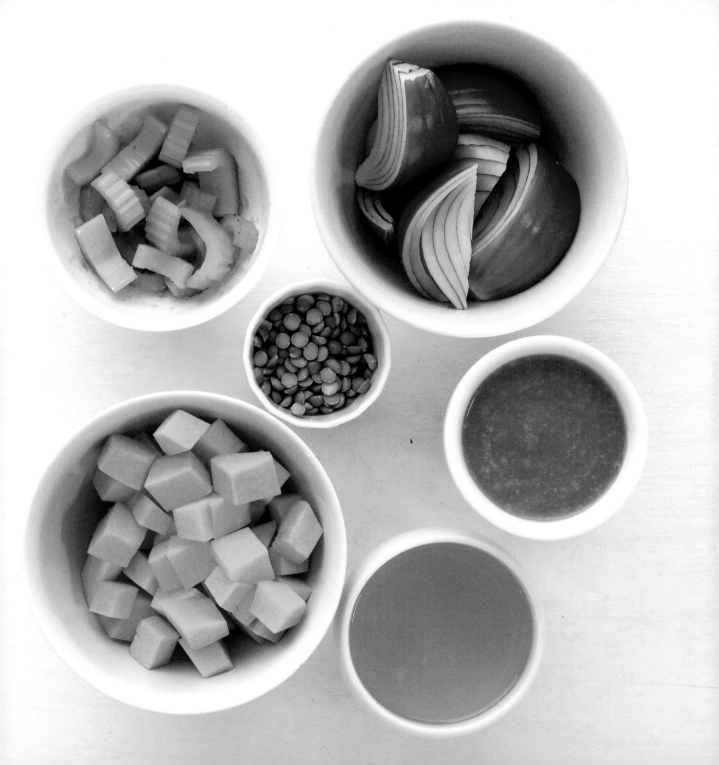

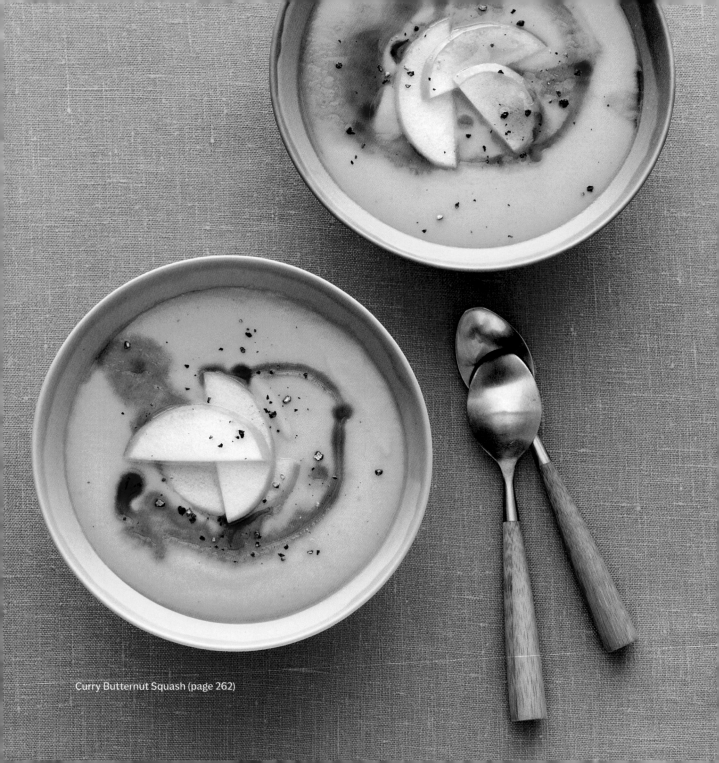

Curry Butternut Squash (page 262)

1 teaspoon *acid* (choose one)

- Fresh lemon or lime juice, red or white wine vinegar, sherry vinegar, balsamic vinegar, or rice vinegar

***Finishing touches* (optional; choose one)**

- Toasted sesame or extra-virgin olive oil ($1/2$ teaspoon), chopped toasted nuts or seeds (1 teaspoon), or chopped fresh herbs (1 to 2 tablespoons)

1. In a medium pot over medium-low heat, heat the fat until warm or melted. Add the aromatics with a pinch of salt and cook, stirring, for about 8 minutes, or until softened. Add the spice and stir to toast slightly for about 1 minute.

2. Add the vegetables and cook, stirring, for about 5 minutes to combine all of the flavors. (For mushrooms, cook for about 10 minutes, or until golden.)

3. Add the deglazing liquid (if using) and scrape the bottom of the pan. Cook for about 3 minutes, until the liquid has almost evaporated. Add the broth, plus an additional $2\frac{1}{2}$ cups of water, and bring the soup to a boil. Reduce to a simmer and cook for 10 to 25 minutes, until the vegetables are very tender and the soup has developed a deep flavor. (Harder vegetables, such as broccoli and butternut squash, will take longer to get tender than softer vegetables, such as tomatoes and mushrooms.)

4. Using an immersion blender, puree the soup until it's silky smooth. (If you're using a regular blender, puree the soup in batches and return it to the pan as you complete each batch.) If the soup is too thin, continue cooking until it reaches the consistency of heavy cream.

5. Stir in the acid and season to taste with salt and pepper. Top with a finishing touch of your choice, if desired.

Favorite Flavor Combos

Broccoli Leek: Butter, leek + garlic, pinch of ground red pepper, broccoli, dry white wine, chicken broth, lemon juice, extra-virgin olive oil garnish **GF**

Curry Butternut Squash: Coconut oil, onion + carrot + celery + ginger, curry powder, butternut squash, orange juice, vegetable broth, lime juice, toasted sunflower seed garnish **GF, LO, V** *[Photo on page 260]*

Sherry Mushroom: Grape-seed oil, shallot + garlic, cumin, mushrooms, sherry, mushroom broth, sherry vinegar, rosemary and thyme garnish **GF, LO, V**

Smoked Paprika Cauliflower: Avocado oil, onion + garlic, smoked paprika, cauliflower, chicken broth, white wine vinegar, toasted chopped pecan garnish **GF**

Tomato Basil: Extra-virgin olive oil, onion + carrot + garlic, fennel seed, tomatoes, red wine, water, balsamic vinegar, basil garnish **GF, LO, V**

Make it ahead! This soup will keep for up to 5 days in the refrigerator or 1 month in the freezer.

Tip: In a rush? Opt for frozen, chopped vegetables. Use them straight out of the freezer, increasing the cooking time by a few minutes.

Black Bean Sweet Potato Sherry Soup

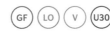

This black bean soup is sweet, savory, and hearty, thanks to the addition of unexpected ingredients like sweet potato and sherry. This entrée soup freezes well, so make a double batch and freeze individual servings for up to a month.

Active Time: 20 minutes
Total Time: 30 minutes
Makes 2 servings

I teaspoon extra-virgin olive oil

I cup chopped white onion

½ cup chopped red bell pepper

2 cloves garlic, minced

I medium sweet potato, peeled and cut into ½" cubes

½ teaspoon ground cumin

¼ teaspoon sea salt

¼ teaspoon freshly ground black pepper

¼ cup sherry, preferably amontillado

½ cup tomato puree

2½ cups water

I can (I5 ounces) no-salt-added or low-sodium black beans, rinsed and drained

2 tablespoons thinly sliced scallions or chopped cilantro

Lime wedges, for serving (optional)

I. In a medium saucepan set over medium heat, warm the oil. Add the onion, bell pepper, and garlic. Cook, stirring, for about 8 minutes, or until the onion is translucent. Stir in the sweet potato, cumin, salt, and black pepper.

2. Add the sherry and cook for about 3 minutes, or until the liquid is reduced by half. Stir in the tomato puree and bring to a boil. Add the water and beans, reduce to a simmer, and cook for about I5 minutes, or until the sweet potatoes are completely tender.

3. Using a potato masher, lightly mash some of the beans and vegetables until the soup is a thick, chunky texture. Divide between two bowls, top with the scallions or cilantro, and serve with the lime wedges.

White Gazpacho with Grapes and Almonds

When it's too hot to even think about standing over the stove, make gazpacho. This no-cook soup showcases summer's fresh produce—and best of all, it's served cold. Most gazpachos are thickened with white country bread, but this version uses more filling, high-protein white beans, instead. And this side soup can also be enjoyed as a snack!

Active Time: 15 minutes
Total Time: 1 hour
Makes 2 servings (about 1 cup each)

1 large English cucumber, peeled and roughly chopped

½ cup green grapes, half left whole, half cut in half

¼ cup canned no-salt-added or low-sodium navy or cannellini beans, rinsed and drained

¼ cup water

2 scallions, whites only, chopped (reserve greens, thinly sliced, for garnish if desired)

1 tablespoon white wine vinegar

¼ teaspoon sea salt

4 teaspoons sliced almonds

1 teaspoon avocado or extra-virgin olive oil

1. In a blender or food processor, combine the cucumber, whole grapes, beans, water, scallion whites, vinegar, and salt. Blend or process until the mixture reaches your desired consistency. (It can be slightly chunky or smooth.) Taste, and add more vinegar if desired. Refrigerate, covered, for about 1 hour, until the soup is well chilled and the flavors are blended.

2. In a small skillet over medium heat, toast the almonds for 5 to 8 minutes, until they're golden and fragrant.

3. Divide the soup between two bowls; top each with half of the halved grapes, half of the toasted almonds, and a ½ teaspoon drizzle of the oil. Sprinkle with the scallion greens, if desired.

Tip: For a faster gazpacho, have all of the ingredients already cold.

Hearty Lentil Mushroom Soup

Mushrooms are naturally rich in savory, meaty, umami flavor. To bump that up even more, substitute mushroom broth for the vegetable broth. Topping this entrée soup with crispy, roasted shiitake mushrooms adds an extra layer of richness.

Active Time: 25 minutes
Total Time: I hour
Makes 4 servings

½ ounce dried porcini mushrooms

8 ounces fresh shiitake mushrooms, stems removed

I tablespoon olive oil, divided

I medium yellow onion, diced

2 cloves garlic, minced

2 medium carrots, peeled and diced

½ teaspoon dried thyme

½ teaspoon sea salt

½ teaspoon freshly ground black pepper

I cup French lentils

4 cups unsalted vegetable stock

I teaspoon red wine vinegar

4 teaspoons Parmesan cheese, shaved

I. Soak the porcini mushrooms in I cup of hot water for I5 minutes. Drain, reserving the soaking liquid, and coarsely chop the mushrooms.

2. Heat the oven to 400°F. Coarsely chop half of the shiitake mushrooms and set them aside. Slice the remaining half of the shiitake mushrooms into ¼" pieces and toss them with 2 teaspoons of the oil. Spread the mushroom slices in one layer on a baking sheet and roast them for I0 to I5 minutes, until browned and crisp, flipping the mushrooms over once. Set aside.

3. In a medium pot over medium heat, heat the remaining I teaspoon oil. Add the onion and garlic and cook for 2 minutes, or until soft. Add the chopped porcini and shiitake mushrooms, carrots, thyme, salt, and pepper, and cook for 2 minutes. Add the lentils, stock, and mushroom-soaking liquid and bring to a boil. Reduce the heat and simmer for about 25 minutes, or until the lentils are soft. Stir in the vinegar.

4. Serve topped with the shaved Parmesan and the roasted mushrooms.

Shaved Salad

You've likely had plenty of chopped salads—but how about trying a shaved one as a tasty side dish? Peeling vegetables into thin strips makes for a pretty presentation and gives the veggies an unexpected texture that's the perfect vehicle for fresh dill dressing.

Active Time: 15 minutes
Total Time: 15 minutes
Makes 2 servings

- 2 teaspoons olive oil
- 1 teaspoon white wine vinegar
- 2 tablespoons fresh dill, chopped
- 1 teaspoon lemon zest
- ½ teaspoon sea salt
- ¼ teaspoon freshly ground black pepper
- 2 medium carrots, peeled
- 1 broccoli stalk (no florets)
- 6 to 8 asparagus spears
- 1 medium zucchini

1. In a large bowl, whisk together the oil, vinegar, dill, lemon zest, salt, and pepper.

2. Using a vegetable peeler, shave the carrots, broccoli stem, asparagus, and zucchini lengthwise into long ribbons. Add the vegetables to the bowl, toss with the dressing, and serve.

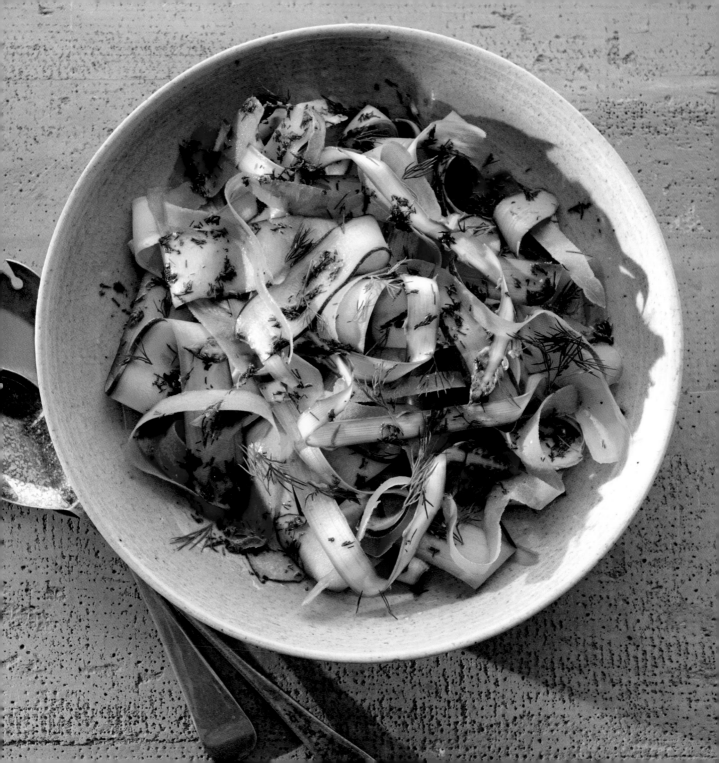

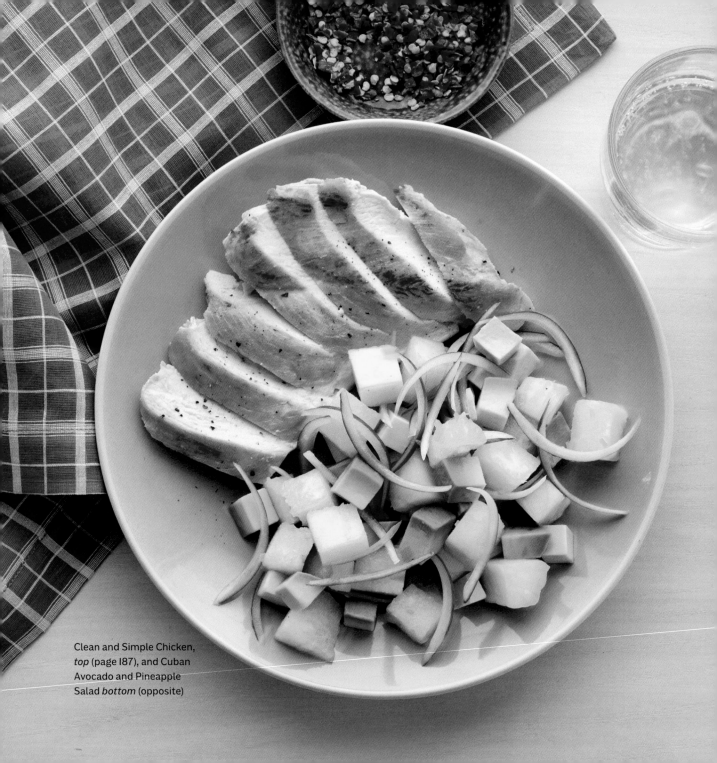

Clean and Simple Chicken, *top* (page 187), and Cuban Avocado and Pineapple Salad *bottom* (opposite)

Cuban Avocado and Pineapple Salad

Avocado and pineapple might seem like unusual ingredients for the base of a salad, but give this Caribbean-inspired combo one taste, and you're sure to be hooked. To preserve the avocado's vibrant green color, enjoy this salad right after you make it. Pair it with a soup or veggie side or enjoy it as a snack.

Active Time: 10 minutes
Total Time: 20 minutes
Makes 2 servings

2 tablespoons fresh lime juice

1 tablespoon extra-virgin olive oil

1 tablespoon fresh orange juice

Pinch of sea salt

Pinch of freshly ground black pepper

¼ cup thinly sliced red onion

¼ teaspoon minced habanero or Thai bird chiles

1 cup pineapple cut into ½"-thick chunks

½ medium avocado, seeded and cut into ½" pieces

1. In a medium bowl, whisk together the lime juice, oil, orange juice, and a pinch of salt and pepper. Add the onion and chile and toss to coat. Let the mixture sit for at least 10 minutes and up to 45 minutes.

2. Add the pineapple and avocado and toss gently. Serve immediately, or cover and refrigerate for up to 1 hour.

Summer Roll Salad
with Peanut Dipping Sauce

Pretty and refreshing, these crisp summer rolls are delicious dunked in a creamy Thai peanut dipping sauce. Feel free to use cooked chicken breast from a store-bought rotisserie chicken to save time. These summer rolls can be deliciously paired with a soup or veggie side.

Active Time: 50 minutes
Total Time: 50 minutes
Makes 2 servings

1½ ounces rice vermicelli

DIPPING SAUCE

2 tablespoons natural creamy peanut butter

1 tablespoon tamari

1 tablespoon fresh lime juice

1 tablespoon water

½ teaspoon Sriracha sauce

½ teaspoon dark brown sugar

½ teaspoon toasted sesame oil

ROLLS

16 mint leaves

16 basil leaves

6 small Bibb or leaf lettuce leaves, ribs removed

2 cups baby spinach

1 cup cooked and shredded chicken breast

½ small cucumber, seeded and cut into 3"- to 4"-long, ¼"-thick sticks

1 medium carrot, julienned (about 1 cup packed)

4 scallions, greens only, halved crosswise

8 rice paper rounds (8½" diameter)

1. Cook the vermicelli according to the package directions. Drain and run it under cold water until it's cool.

2. *To make the sauce:* In a small bowl, combine the peanut butter, tamari, lime juice, water, Sriracha, sugar, and oil. Stir until smooth. Set aside.

3. *To make the rolls:* Arrange the vermicelli, mint, basil, lettuce, spinach, chicken, cucumber, carrot, scallions, and rice paper rounds on a work surface. Fill a wide, shallow dish (such as a pie plate) with

(continued)

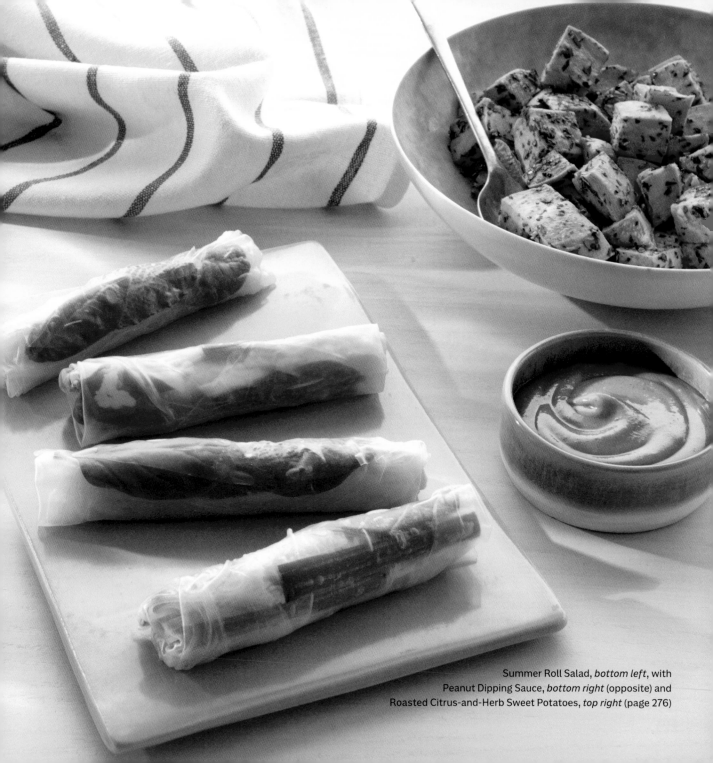

Summer Roll Salad, *bottom left*, with
Peanut Dipping Sauce, *bottom right* (opposite) and
Roasted Citrus-and-Herb Sweet Potatoes, *top right* (page 276)

warm water. Submerge a rice paper round in the water for about 15 seconds, or until it's pliable but still a bit stiff. Remove the round from the water, place it on the work surface, and pat it dry with a clean kitchen towel.

4. Layer ⅛ of each of the ingredients on the lower third of the round, leaving 1" of space along the sides and bottom. Keeping your fingers wet, fold in the sides and bottom over the filling. Hold the filling tightly as you roll up the wrapper. Place the roll on a plate and cover it with a damp towel. Do not let the rolls touch or they will stick and tear each other. Repeat with the remaining rolls.

5. Cut the rolls in half on a sharp diagonal and serve with the dipping sauce.

Change it up! To make these rolls vegetarian, substitute 8 ounces of cooked tempeh or tofu for the chicken.

Fiesta Quinoa with Shrimp

Packed with veggies and high-protein shrimp, this colorful quinoa salad is a meal in itself. Eat it hot, warm, or straight from the fridge. Not a huge shrimp fan? Sub in chicken, tuna, or steak!

Active Time: 15 minutes
Total Time: 30 minutes
Makes 2 servings

⅓ cup white quinoa, rinsed and drained

1 lime

1 clove garlic, mashed into a paste

¼ teaspoon dried oregano

Pinch of sea salt

⅛ teaspoon freshly ground black pepper

1½ tablespoons olive oil, divided

½ teaspoon ground cumin

1 cup canned no-salt-added or low-sodium black beans, rinsed and drained

½ cup thawed frozen corn kernels

½ cup finely diced red bell pepper

2 scallions, thinly sliced

½ pound jumbo shrimp, peeled and deveined

1 tablespoon chopped fresh cilantro

1. Cook the quinoa according to the package directions.

2. Zest the lime, reserving ½ teaspoon of zest, then juice the lime, reserving 2 tablespoons of juice.

3. In a jar with a lid, combine the lime juice, garlic, oregano, salt, black pepper, 1 tablespoon of the oil, and cumin. Shake until combined.

4. In a large bowl, combine the cooked quinoa, beans, corn, bell pepper, scallions, and dressing. Let the salad sit so the flavors can meld while you prepare the shrimp.

5. In a medium nonstick skillet over medium heat, warm the remaining ½ tablespoon oil. Add the shrimp and cook, tossing occasionally, for about 4 minutes, or until they're opaque and slightly curled. Toss in the lime zest and cilantro.

6. Divide the quinoa and shrimp between two plates and serve.

Change it up! To make this dish vegetarian, replace the shrimp with 8 ounces of cubed tempeh or tofu and increase the cooking time to about 10 minutes.

Clean Coleslaw

Most coleslaws are more mayo and cream than anything else. This one relies on a lighter dressing—made with zippy white vinegar, flavorful olive oil, and a touch of honey—to let the crunchy vegetables shine. This coleslaw can be paired with a soup or enjoyed as a snack.

Active Time: 10 minutes
Total Time: 30 minutes
Makes 2 servings

¼ cup white vinegar

2 tablespoons extra-virgin olive oil

1 teaspoon honey

½ teaspoon celery seed

½ teaspoon sea salt

¼ teaspoon freshly ground black pepper

½ head napa cabbage, finely shredded (about 2 cups)

1 medium carrot, shredded (about ½ cup)

½ red onion, shredded on a box grater

2 tablespoons fresh cilantro leaves, chopped

1. In a large bowl, whisk together the vinegar, oil, honey, celery seed, salt, and pepper.

2. Add the cabbage, carrot, and onion to the bowl, and toss to coat. Let it sit for ½ hour or longer. Sprinkle with the cilantro when you're ready to serve.

Honey-Glazed Radishes

Radishes are often overlooked for use in hot preparations, but they cook up beautifully. Adding the greens, which are often tossed, makes for a lovely side dish that's ideal with lamb, steak, or roasted fish. These tasty radishes can be paired with an entrée, or double the serving and enjoy them as a snack.

Active Time: 10 minutes
Total Time: 30 minutes
Makes 2 servings

I bunch radishes with greens (about ½ pound)

¼ cup water

I tablespoon honey

I teaspoon grape-seed or canola oil

½ teaspoon caraway seeds

Pinch of sea salt

⅛ teaspoon freshly ground black pepper

½ teaspoon champagne vinegar or white wine vinegar

1. Trim and wash the radishes, and cut them into quarters. Wash the greens but do not dry them. Set them aside to drain.

2. In a medium skillet set over low heat, warm the water, honey, and oil. When the honey has melted, add the radishes and stir to coat. Increase the heat to medium-low, cover, and cook, stirring often, for about 20 minutes, or until the radishes are crisp-tender and the glaze is clinging to them.

3. Stir in the caraway seeds, radish greens, a pinch of salt, and the pepper. Cook, stirring constantly, for about 3 minutes, or until the greens have wilted and the caraway is fragrant. Stir in the vinegar and serve.

Photo on page 243, *top left*

Roasted Citrus-and-Herb Sweet Potatoes

Zippy citrus zest and loads of fresh herbs turn simple sweet potatoes into a showstopping side dish that livens up any protein. Try these with chicken, pork, beef, or fish.

Active Time: 10 minutes
Total Time: 30 minutes
Makes 2 servings

I large sweet potato, peeled and cut into ¾" cubes

I teaspoon melted coconut oil

¼ teaspoon sea salt

¼ teaspoon freshly ground black pepper

2 tablespoons fresh mint leaves

2 tablespoons fresh cilantro leaves

I clove garlic

½ teaspoon orange zest

½ teaspoon lime zest

I. Heat the oven to 425°F. Line a large rimmed baking sheet with foil and coat it with cooking spray. Toss the sweet potato, oil, salt, and pepper on the sheet. Roast for about 20 minutes, turning halfway through, until the sweet potatoes are browned and tender.

2. Place the mint, cilantro, and garlic on a cutting board, and mince them together. Add the citrus zests, and toss together.

3. Transfer the sweet potatoes to a serving bowl and toss them with the citrus-and-herb mixture. Serve warm.

Photo on page 271, *top left*

Roasted Broccoli with Chile and Lemon

When roasted in a hot oven, broccoli turns creamy, golden, and irresistibly sweet. A hit of lemon and red pepper flakes adds extra zip and brightness. And don't forget those stalks! They're just as nutritious as broccoli crowns, and their texture softens when roasted. This side can be deliciously paired with a soup or enjoyed as a snack.

Active Time: 10 minutes
Total Time: 30 minutes
Makes 2 servings (about 2 cups each)

I head broccoli (12 ounces), chopped into bite-size florets and spears, stalks peeled

I tablespoon olive oil

¼ teaspoon crushed red pepper flakes

¼ teaspoon sea salt

I teaspoon lemon zest

Lemon wedges, to serve (optional)

1. Heat the oven to 425°F.

2. On a baking sheet, toss the broccoli, oil, red pepper flakes, and salt. Roast the broccoli, undisturbed, for 20 minutes, or until dark golden in most places. Remove from the oven and toss with the lemon zest before serving with additional lemon wedges, if desired.

Cauliflower Rice Pilaf

A quick blitz in the food processor makes cauliflower a flavorful, clean replacement for starch-heavy rice. Plus it's quicker to get on the dinner table than the usual pilaf.

Active Time: 15 minutes
Total Time: 25 minutes
Makes 2 servings (1 cup each)

- ½ small head cauliflower (about 1¾ pounds whole), trimmed and cored
- 1½ teaspoons coconut or olive oil
- ½ yellow onion, finely chopped
- 1 carrot, finely chopped
- ¼ teaspoon cumin seed
- ⅛ teaspoon ground cinnamon
- ¼ teaspoon freshly ground black pepper
- Pinch of ground cloves
- Pinch of sea salt
- ¼ cup water
- 2 tablespoons chopped fresh parsley
- 1 teaspoon orange zest
- 1 teaspoon fresh orange juice

1. Roughly chop the cauliflower. Transfer it to a food processor and pulse about 20 times, until it's finely chopped to roughly the size of rice grains. Do not overprocess. (Alternatively, grate the half head of cauliflower on the large holes of a box grater.) You should have about 2½ cups of cauliflower "rice" total.

2. In a large nonstick skillet over medium heat, warm the oil. Add the onion and carrot and cook, stirring, for about 8 minutes, or until they begin to brown and soften. Add the cumin, cinnamon, pepper, cloves, and salt, and toast for 1 minute. Add the water and stir. Add the cauliflower and cook, stirring, for about 5 minutes, or until tender. Sprinkle with the parsley, orange zest, and orange juice, and serve.

Make it ahead! Process or grate the entire head of cauliflower to make a double batch of "rice." Store half in a freezer-safe storage bag or container. Thaw before using it in this recipe. (If you're steaming the "rice," you can cook it straight from the freezer.)

Photo on page 247, *top right*

SNACKS

Gremolata Parmesan Popcorn

Surprise! Popcorn is a high-fiber whole grain that, like fruit, is rich in phytonutrients. Skip the usual buttery toppings in favor of a classic gremolata mixture featuring fresh lemon zest, parsley, and garlic, plus sprinkled Parmesan. It's clean—and delicious.

Active Time: 5 minutes
Total Time: 10 minutes
Makes 3 servings

½ cup popcorn kernels (or 10 cups clean, store-bought, plain air-popped popcorn)

¼ cup chopped fresh parsley

1 small clove garlic, minced

½ teaspoon lemon zest

1 tablespoon finely grated Parmesan cheese

Grape-seed oil in a mister

½ teaspoon sea salt

1. If you're popping your own popcorn with an air popper, pop the kernels per the machine instructions.

2. If you're popping your own popcorn in the microwave, place the kernels in a 2- to 3-quart microwave-safe bowl. Completely cover the bowl with a microwave-safe plate. Microwave on high for about 4 minutes, until the popping slows down to 3 to 4 seconds between each pop. Using a pot holder, carefully remove the top plate, avoiding the steam escaping from the bowl. Remove the bowl from the microwave and let it cool slightly.

3. On a cutting board, pile the parsley, garlic, lemon zest, and cheese on top of each other and finely chop them all together.

4. Toss the popcorn while spritzing it with the oil. Add the gremolata and salt, and toss until coated.

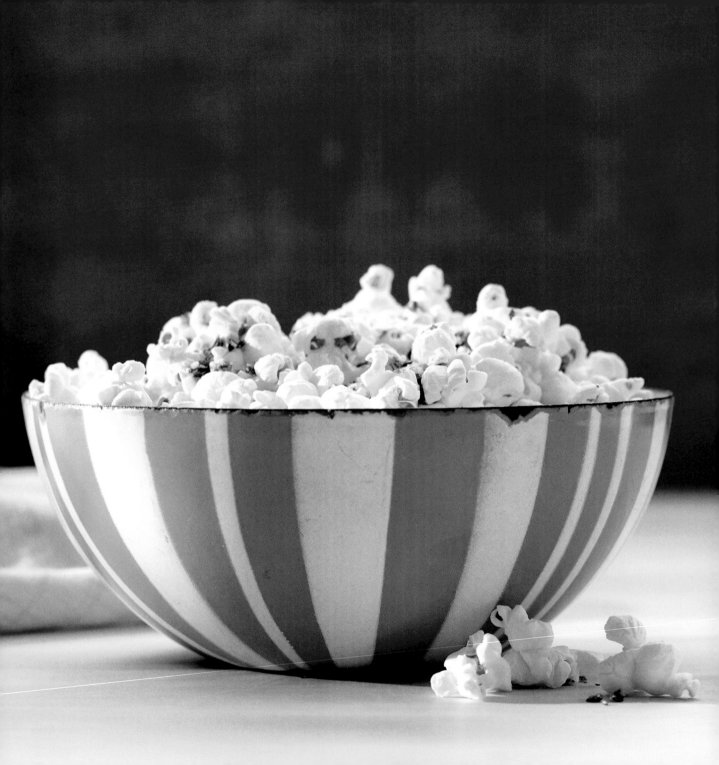

Savory Variations: Spritz with grape-seed oil and try one of the following flavor combinations for a tasty alternative:

1. Pizza Popcorn: Dried oregano, chopped-up sun-dried tomatoes (not packed in oil), grated Parmesan

2. Chive and Cheese: Snipped chives, garlic powder, Parmesan (or some other clean cheese)

3. Lemon-Dill: Dried dill, grated lemon zest

4. Chili Lime: Chili powder, lime zest

Sweet Variations

1. Sweet Popcorn: Either cocoa powder or cocoa nibs, drizzle of honey

2. Bombay Blend: Garam masala, toasted coconut flakes

3. Maple Cracker Jack: Peanuts, pumpkin pie spice, a drizzle of pure maple syrup

PB&J Granola

Once you make your own granola, you'll never go back to store-bought. This version is peanutty and sweet, with strawberries and dried cherries—but it's easy to customize: Switch out the nuts or dried fruit for whatever you have on hand. Just remember to limit yourself to a ¼-cup serving!

Active Time: 5 minutes
Total Time: 30 minutes
Makes 2½ cups, 10 servings

1½ cups old-fashioned rolled oats

½ cup puffed brown rice cereal

2 tablespoons flaxseeds

¼ cup peanuts

Pinch of sea salt

2 tablespoons extra-virgin olive oil

2 tablespoons strawberry all-fruit spread

2 tablespoons natural, unsalted, creamy peanut butter

1 teaspoon pure vanilla extract

¼ cup dried tart cherries or raisins

1. Heat the oven to 250°F. In a large bowl, combine the oats, rice cereal, flaxseeds, peanuts, and salt. Set aside.

2. In a small saucepan over medium heat, combine the oil, fruit spread, peanut butter, and vanilla. Stir until combined and smooth. Pour over the dry ingredients and toss together. Spread the mixture in an even layer on a baking sheet and bake for 30 minutes, stirring every 10 minutes. Let the granola cool to room temperature, and stir in the dried cherries or raisins.

Note: This granola is very versatile. It can be enjoyed as a snack, sprinkled on yogurt for breakfast, and use when making the apple "sandwich" on page 182.

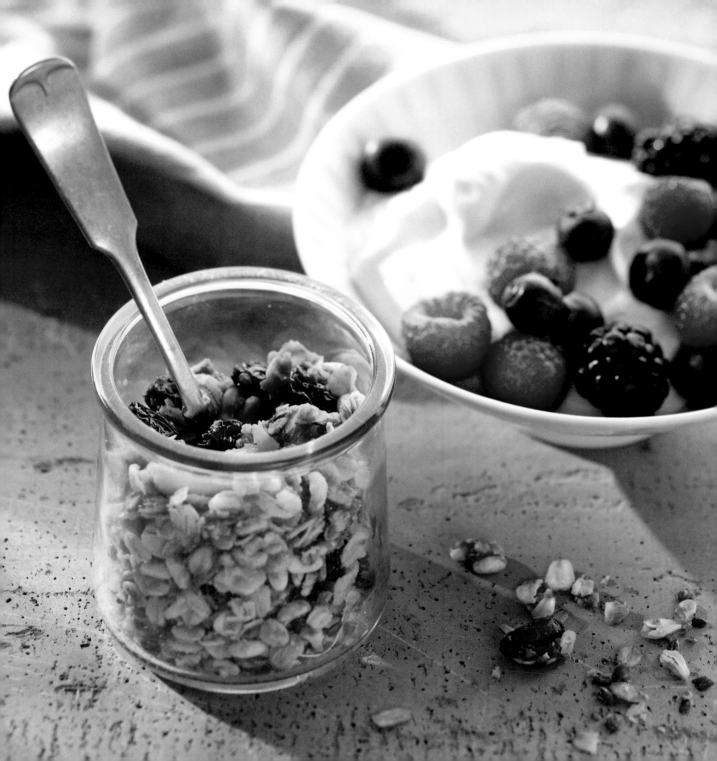

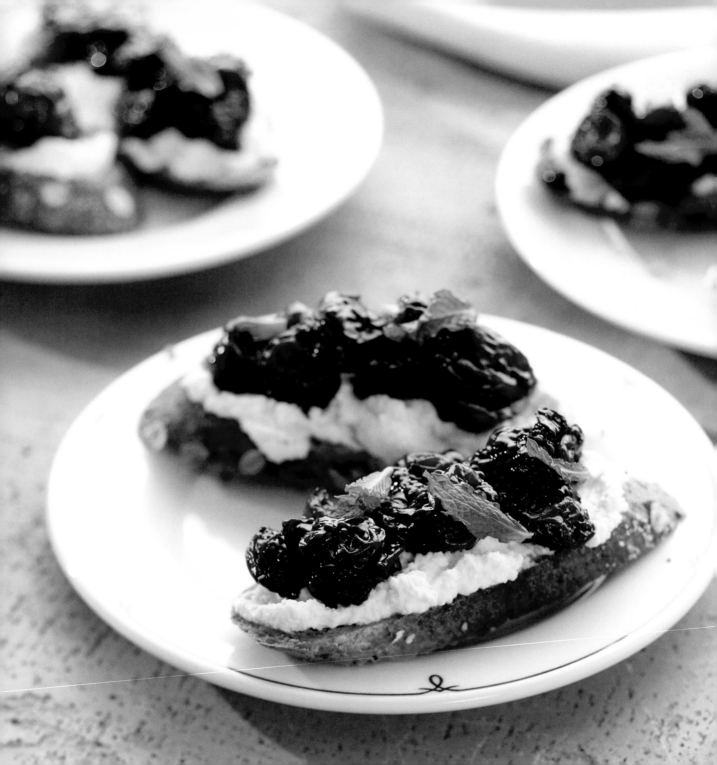

Dried Tart Cherry Chia Jam
and Ricotta on Toast

Take a simple jam made from phytonutrient-rich dried tart cherries and nutrient-dense chia seeds and pair it with creamy ricotta cheese and whole wheat toast. It's sweet, tart, creamy, and crunchy—in other words, everything you could want in a fast breakfast or anytime snack.

Active Time: 10 minutes
Total Time: 20 minutes
Makes 6 servings, 2 toasts per serving

¾ cup dry red wine

¾ cup dried tart cherries

1 tablespoon honey

1 tablespoon chia seeds

6 tablespoons part-skim ricotta cheese

2 tablespoons chopped fresh mint (optional)

12 slices, each ½"-thick, whole wheat or multigrain baguette, lightly toasted

1. In a small saucepan, combine the wine, cherries, and honey, and bring the mixture to a simmer over medium-low heat. Cook for about 6 minutes, until the cherries have softened and plumped and are beginning to break down. Stir in the chia seeds and let the jam cool to room temperature.

2. In a small bowl, combine the ricotta and mint, if using. Spread 1 tablespoon of ricotta on each piece of toast and add a 1-tablespoon dollop of cooled jam on top.

Make it ahead! The jam will keep in an airtight container in the refrigerator for up to 2 weeks.

Change it up! Use a gluten-free sandwich bread to make this snack gluten-free.

Lemony Rosemary White Bean Dip

Switch up your usual hummus with this creamy puree, seasoned with fresh rosemary, garlic, and lemon. Enjoy it with colorful sliced bell peppers, crunchy carrots or cucumbers, fresh broccoli florets, or whole wheat pita.

Active Time: 5 minutes
Total Time: 5 minutes
Makes 8 snack servings (about 2 tablespoons each)

I can (15 ounces) no-salt-added or low-sodium white beans, rinsed and drained

I clove garlic, roughly chopped

I tablespoon + ¼ teaspoon extra-virgin olive oil or walnut oil

I tablespoon water

2 teaspoons fresh lemon juice

I teaspoon lemon zest

¼ teaspoon sea salt

I teaspoon finely chopped fresh rosemary

1. In a food processor, combine the beans, garlic, 1 tablespoon of oil, water, lemon juice, lemon zest, and salt. Process until smooth. Pulse in the rosemary.

2. Transfer the dip to a serving dish and drizzle it with the remaining ¼ teaspoon of oil. Store leftovers in an airtight container in the refrigerator for up to 5 days.

Change it up! Use the dip as a sandwich spread, or thin it with water from cooking pasta and toss it with whole-grain pasta.

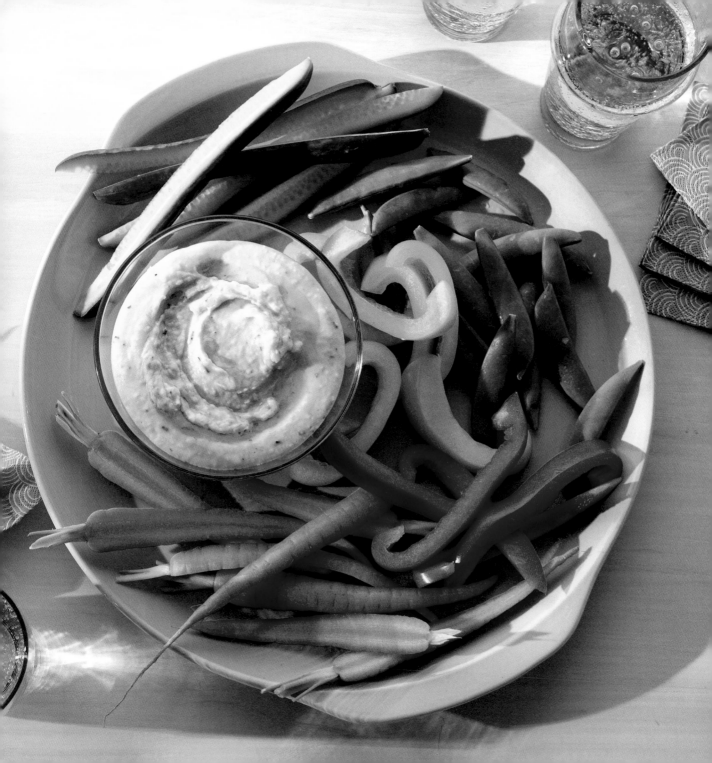

DESSERTS

Roasted Strawberries with Dark Chocolate Sauce

What's better than indulgent chocolate-covered strawberries? *Roasted* chocolate-covered strawberries! Roasting the berries in the oven intensifies their flavor, so you get more sweetness without tons of added sugar.

Active Time: 5 minutes
Total Time: 25 minutes
Makes 2 servings

I cup whole strawberries, hulled

2 teaspoons coconut oil

I tablespoon pure maple syrup

I tablespoon unsweetened cocoa powder

½ cup plain Greek yogurt

I tablespoon sliced almonds

1. Heat the oven to 350°F. Spread the strawberries on a small baking sheet and coat them lightly with cooking spray. Roast for about 20 minutes, or until softened.

2. Meanwhile, in a small microwave-safe bowl, combine the oil and syrup. Microwave on high for about 30 seconds, until the oil is melted. Add the cocoa powder and stir until smooth.

3. Serve the strawberries over the yogurt. Drizzle them with the chocolate sauce, and top them with the almonds.

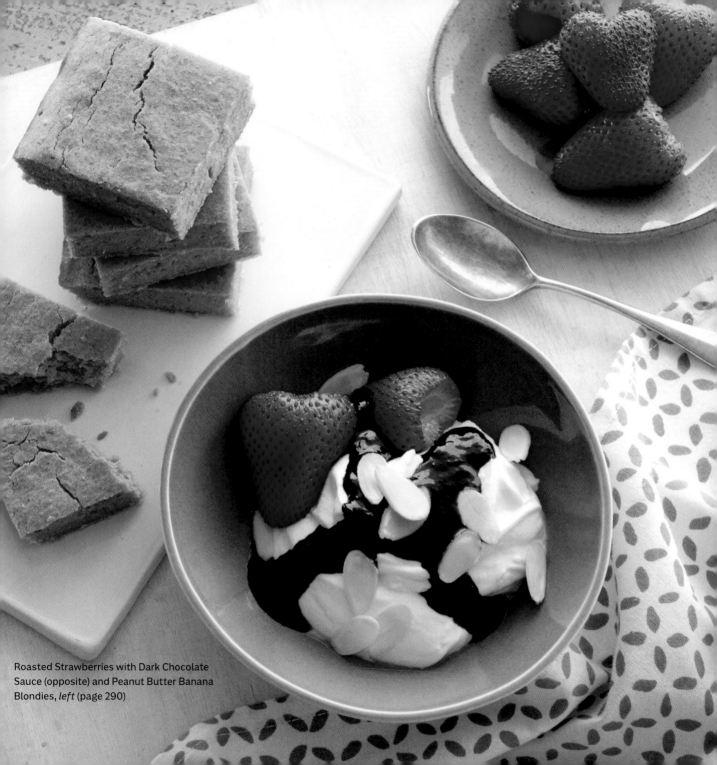

Roasted Strawberries with Dark Chocolate
Sauce (opposite) and Peanut Butter Banana
Blondies, *left* (page 290)

Peanut Butter Banana Blondies

Chickpeas don't just add extra protein and fiber to these blondies—they also lend a rich, fudgy texture. To make this dessert gluten-free, substitute almond flour or gluten-free oat flour for the whole wheat flour.

Active Time: 5 minutes
Total Time: 30 minutes
Makes 9 servings

¼ cup whole wheat flour

½ teaspoon baking powder

I can (I5 ounces) no-salt-added or low-sodium chickpeas, rinsed and drained

¼ cup all-natural creamy peanut butter, unsalted

¼ cup pure maple syrup

I medium ripe banana

I large egg

I teaspoon pure vanilla extract

I. Heat the oven to 350°F and coat an 8" x 8" baking pan with cooking spray.

2. In a small bowl, stir together the flour and baking powder.

3. In a food processor, combine the chickpeas, peanut butter, syrup, banana, egg, and vanilla. Process until the batter is smooth. Stir in the flour mixture until combined.

4. Spread the batter evenly in the prepared pan and bake for 20 to 25 minutes, or until a toothpick comes out clean and the edges of the blondies are golden. Cool completely before cutting into nine squares. Store covered in the refrigerator for up to I week.

Photo on page 289 *top left*.

Recipe Nutrition Stats

RECIPE	Pg.	CATEGORY	SERVINGS	I SERVING	CALORIES	PROTEIN (G)	CARBS (G)	FIBER (G)	SUGAR (G)	TOTAL FAT (G)	SAT FAT (G)	SODIUM (MG)	ADDED SUGARS (G)	ADDED SUGARS FROM
Avocado Tostadas with Huevos Rancheros	223	Breakfasts	2	I tostada	264	15	17	5	4	15	4	210	0	—
Beef Scallion Roll-Ups	244	Lunches	2	8 rolls	341	29	17	5	6	18	5	596	0	—
Black Bean Sweet Potato Sherry Soup	263	Soups	2	1½–2 cups	274	11	49	12	12	3	0.5	619	0	—
Cauliflower Rice Pilaf	278	Sides	2	I cup	95	4	14	5	6	4	3	119	0	—
Chickpea Curry–Stuffed Squash	255	Dinners	2	½ squash, stuffed	414	16	72	15	19	9	6	539	0	—
Clean Coleslaw	274	Sides	2	1¼ cups	177	2	11	3	7	14	2	429	3	Honey
Creamy Chicken, Green Grape, and Farro Salad	237	Lunches	2	I	471	32	63	6	11	10	2	639	0	—
Create-Your-Own No-Cream Soup: Broccoli Leek	262	Soups	6	I cup	102	6	14	4	4	3	I	101	0	—
Create-Your-Own No-Cream Soup: Curry Butternut Squash	262	Soups	6	I cup	160	4	25	5	6	7	2	93	0	—
Create-Your-Own No-Cream Soup: Sherry Mushroom	262	Soups	6	I cup	97	6	13	3	6	3	0	252	0	—
Create-Your-Own No-Cream Soup: Smoked Paprika Cauliflower	262	Soups	6	I cup	108	3	9	3	3	8	I	65	0	—
Create-Your-Own No-Cream Soup: Tomato Basil	262	Soups	6	I cup	77	2	11	3	6	3	0	41	0	
Cuban Avocado and Pineapple Salad	269	Salads	2	⅔ cup	171	I	17	4	10	12	15	65	0	—
Dried Tart Cherry Chia Jam	285	Breakfasts	8 servings (makes I cup)	2 tablespoons	95	I	17	I	13	I	0	2	3	Sweetened dried cherries

(continued)

Recipe Nutrition Stats *(cont.)*

RECIPE	Pg.	CATEGORY	SERVINGS	I SERVING	CALORIES	PROTEIN (G)	CARBS (G)	FIBER (G)	SUGAR (G)	TOTAL FAT (G)	SAT FAT (G)	SODIUM (MG)	ADDED SUGARS (G)	ADDED SUGARS FROM
Dried Tart Cherry Chia Jam and Ricotta on Toast	285	Snacks	6	2 toasts, 2 tablespoons ricotta, 2 tablespoons jam	192	5	34	2	15	2	1	212	3	Sweetened dried cherries
Easy Buckwheat Crepes	227	Breakfasts	6 servings (makes 12 crepes)	2 crepes	223	9	16	5	5	14	2.5	142	0	—
Easy Buckwheat Crepes, Savory: arugula, pear, cheddar	228	Breakfasts	2	2 crepes with filling	332	18	28	7	13	17	4	362	0	—
Easy Buckwheat Crepes, Savory: asparagus, mushroom, shallot	228	Breakfasts	2	2 crepes with filling	306	15	27	7	8	17	3	462	0	—
Easy Buckwheat Crepes, Savory: black bean, tomato, cumin	228	Breakfasts	2	2 crepes with filling	321	16	28	10	6	16	4	266	0	—
Easy Buckwheat Crepes, Savory: spinach, tomato, feta or olive	228	Breakfasts	2	2 crepes with filling	292	13	27	9	7	16	4	363	0	—
Easy Buckwheat Crepes, Sweet: grapefruit, banana, pistachio, cocoa	228	Breakfasts	2	2 crepes with filling	326	12	36	7	9	16	3	145	0	—
Easy Buckwheat Crepes, Sweet: strawberries, mint or cinnamon	228	Breakfasts	2	2 crepes with filling	316	15	25	6	9	18	5	202	0	—
Fiesta Quinoa with Shrimp	273	Salads	2	I cup	422	26	49	10	4	14	2	645	0	—
Florentine Chicken Meatballs with Spaghetti Squash and Salsa Cruda	252	Dinners	2	3 meatballs over squash	432	32	53	12	20	14	4	612	0	—

RECIPE	Pg.	CATEGORY	SERVINGS	I SERVING	CALORIES	PROTEIN (G)	CARBS (G)	FIBER (G)	SUGAR (G)	TOTAL FAT (G)	SAT FAT (G)	SODIUM (MG)	ADDED SUGARS (G)	ADDED SUGARS FROM
Green Ginger Smoothie	232	Smoothies	1	1½ cups	187	4	26	8	13	9	1	53	0	—
Gremolata Parmesan Popcorn	279	Snacks	3	3 cups	112	4	22	4	0	2	0.5	341	0	—
Hearty Lentil Mushroom Soup	265	Soups	4	1½ cups	274	14	43	11	7	6	1	538	0	—
Honey-Glazed Radishes	275	Sides	2	⅔ cup	78	2	14	3	11	3	0	106	3	Honey
Horchata Smoothie	231	Smoothies	2	1 cup	240	5	45	6	14	4	0	147	0	—
Israeli Couscous Salad with Salmon	245	Lunches	2 cups	1	420	23	47	3	4	15	4	671	0	—
Kale Quesadillas	235	Lunches	2	1	339	27	38	11	5	11	6	522	0	—
Lemony Rosemary White Bean Dip	286	Snacks	8	2 tablespoons	64	3	9	2	0	2	0	51	0	—
Maple Mustard Glazed Pork Tenderloin with Roasted Vegetables and Apples	256	Dinners	2	4 ounces pork with potatoes and apples	407	29	58	9	22	8	2	508	2	Maple syrup
Mini Spinach Mushroom Quiche	244	Breakfasts	4 (makes 12 mini quiches)	3 mini quiches	274	25	6	2	4	15	6	667	0	—
Overnight Steel-Cut Oatmeal	226	Breakfasts	2	1 cup	272	12	39	8	5	10	1	57	0	
Hearty Chicken Panzanella	243	Lunches	2 (makes 4 cups)	2 cups	365	29	33	4	11	12	2.5	559	0	
PB&J Granola	282	Snacks	10	¼ cup	147	4	16	2.4	4	8	1	22	0.6	Sweetened dried cherries
Peanut Butter Banana Blondies	290	Desserts	9	1 square	137	4	20	2	8	5	1	73	2.2	Maple syrup
Pumpkin-Cranberry-Cherry Breakfast Balls	229	Breakfasts	6	2 balls	325	11.5	33	6	12	17	15	86	1	Sweetened dried cherries

(continued)

Recipe Nutrition Stats *(cont.)*

RECIPE	Pg.	CATEGORY	SERVINGS	1 SERVING	CALORIES	PROTEIN (G)	CARBS (G)	FIBER (G)	SUGAR (G)	TOTAL FAT (G)	SAT FAT (G)	SODIUM (MG)	ADDED SUGARS (G)	ADDED SUGARS FROM
Roasted Broccoli with Chile and Lemon	277	Sides	2	2 cups	119	5	12	5	3	7	1	253	0	
Roasted Citrus-and-Herb Sweet Potatoes	276	Sides	2	⅔ cup	106	2	20	3	6	2	2	274	0	
Roasted Strawberries with Dark Chocolate Sauce	288	Desserts	2	4 strawberries with yogurt and chocolate	195	6	17	3	12	13	6	19	6	Maple syrup
Shaved Salad	266	Salads	2	2 cups	105	4	13	5	6	5	1	458	0	
Shrimp Scampi over Garlicky Greens	248	Dinners	2	6 shrimp over greens	286	13	26	8	2	16	8	424	0	
Slow Cooker BBQ Pulled Chicken Flatbreads	250	Dinners	2	2 flatbreads	420	30	53	8	18	11	1.5	581	3	Molasses
Summer Roll Salad with Peanut Dipping Sauce	270	Salads	2	4 rolls	382	29	33	5	6	16	2	662	15	Brown sugar
Tuna and Cannellini Salad	234	Lunches	2	1	382	26	45	10	6	11	1.5	492	0	
Turkey Cuban Wrap with Zesty Black Bean Salad	238	Lunches	2	1 wrap	404	36	42	11	5	10	4	651	0	
Turkey Roulade	251	Dinners	2	2 roulades	375	40	30	7	1	12	2	274	0	
White Gazpacho with Grapes and Almonds	264	Soups	2	1 cup	125	4	18	5	9	5	0.5	204	0	

Endnotes

Chapter 1

1   P. Møller, "Gastrophysics in the Brain and Body," *Flavour* 2, no. 8 (2013). Accessed July 11, 2016, doi: 10.1186/2044-7248-2-8.

2   S. Komatsu, "Rice and Sushi Cravings: A Preliminary Study of Food Craving among Japanese Females," *Appetite* 50, nos. 2–3 (2008): 353–58.

3   R. Just et al., "Lower Buffet Prices Lead to Less Taste Satisfaction," *Journal of Sensory Studies* 29, no. 5 (2014): 362–70.

4   H. Parretti et al., "Efficacy of Water Preloading before Main Meals as a Strategy for Weight Loss in Primary Care Patients with Obesity: RCT," *Obesity* 23, no. 9 (2015): 1785–91.

5   D. Weigle et al., "A High-Protein Diet Induces Sustained Reductions in Appetite, Ad Libitum Caloric Intake, and Body Weight despite Compensatory Changes in Diurnal Plasma Leptin and Ghrelin Concentrations," *American Journal of Clinical Nutrition* 82 (2005): 41–48.

6   H. Leidy et al., "Beneficial Effects of a Higher-Protein Breakfast on the Appetitive, Hormonal, and Neural Signals Controlling Energy Intake Regulation in Overweight/Obese, 'Breakfast-Skipping,' Late-Adolescent Girls," *American Journal of Clinical Nutrition* 97 (2013): 677–88.

7   J. Alcock et al., "Is Eating Behavior Manipulated by the Gastrointestinal Microbiota? Evolutionary Pressures and Potential Mechanisms," *BioEssays* 36 (2014): 940–49.

8   C. S. Johnston, "Strategies for Healthy Weight Loss: From Vitamin C to the Glycemic Response," *Journal of the American College of Nutrition* 24, no. 3 (2005): 158–65.

9   M. Bertoia et al., "Dietary Flavonoid Intake and Weight Maintenance: Three Prospective Cohorts of 124,086 US Men and Women Followed for up to 24 Years," *British Medical Journal* 352, no. 17 (2016). Accessed July 11, 2016, doi: http://dx.doi.org/10.1136/bmj.i17.

10   "Indole-3-Carbinol," Linus Pauling Institute, Oregon State University, accessed June 6, 2016, http://lpi.oregonstate.edu/mic/dietary-factors/phytochemicals/indole-3-carbinol.

11   H. Bjermo et al., "Effects of n26 PUFAs Compared with SFAs on Liver Fat, Lipoproteins, and Inflammation in Abdominal Obesity: A Randomized Controlled Trial," *American Journal of Clinical Nutrition* 95 (2012): 1003–12.

12   M. Lee et al., "Reduction of Body Weight by Dietary Garlic Is Associated with an Increase in Uncoupling Protein mRNA Expression and Activation of AMP-Activated Protein Kinase in Diet-Induced Obese Mice," *Journal of Nutrition* 141 (2011): 1947–53.

13 J. Higgins et al., "Resistant Starch Consumption Promotes Lipid Oxidation," *Nutrition & Metabolism* I, no. 8 (2004). Accessed July II, 2016, doi: 10.1186/1743-7075-1-8.

14 C. L. Bodinham et al., "Acute Ingestion of Resistant Starch Reduces Food Intake in Healthy Adults," *British Journal of Nutrition* 103, no. 6 (2010): 917–22.

15 "Does Caffeine Help with Weight Loss?" Mayo Clinic, accessed June 6, 2016, http://www.mayoclinic.org/healthy-lifestyle/weight -loss/expert-answers/caffeine/faq-20058459.

16 A. L. Brown et al., "Health Effects of Green Tea Catechins in Overweight and Obese Men: A Randomised Controlled Cross-Over Trial," *British Journal of Nutrition* 106 (2011): 1880–89.

17 D. Weiss et al., "Determination of Catechins in Matcha Green Tea by Micellar Electrokinetic Chromatography," *Journal of Chromatography A* 1011, nos. 1-2 (2003): 173–80.

18 R. Green et al., "Common Tea Formulations Modulate In Vitro Digestive Recovery of Green Tea Catechins," *Molecular Nutrition & Food Research* 51 (2007): 1152–62.

19 S. Fowler et al., "Diet Soda Intake Is Associated with Long-Term Increases in Waist Circumference in a Biethnic Cohort of Older Adults: The San Antonio Longitudinal Study of Aging," *Journal of the American Geriatrics Society* 63 (2015): 708–15.

20 S. Fowler et al., "Fueling the Obesity Epidemic? Artificially Sweetened Beverage Use and Long-Term Weight Gain," *Obesity* 16, no. 8 (2008): 1894–900.

21 J. Suez et al., "Artificial Sweeteners Induce Glucose Intolerance by Altering the Gut Microbiota," *Nature* 514 (2014): 181–86.

22 K. Betts, "Potential Obesogen Identified: Fungicide Triflumizole Is Associated with Increased Adipogenesis in Mice," *Environmental Health Perspectives* 120, no. 12 (2012): A474.

23 B. Chassaing et al., "Dietary Emulsifiers Impact the Mouse Gut Microbiota Promoting Colitis and Metabolic Syndrome," *Nature* 519 (2015): 92–96.

24 V. Barry et al., "Early Life Perfluorooctanoic Acid (PFOA) Exposure and Overweight and Obesity Risk in Adulthood in a Community with Elevated Exposure," *Environmental Research* 132 (2014): 62–69.

25 A. Calafat et al., "Exposure of the U.S. Population to Bisphenol A and 4-Tertiary-Octylphenol: 2003–2004," *Environmental Health Perspectives* 116, no. 1 (2008): 39–44.

Chapter 2

1 M. Karnani et al., "Activation of Central Orexin/Hypocretin Neurons by Dietary Amino Acids," *Neuron* 72, no. 4 (2011): 616–29.

2 K. Blum et al., "Dopamine and Glucose, Obesity, and Reward Deficiency Syndrome," *Frontiers in Psychology* 5, no. 919 (2014): 1–11.

3 R. Mujcic, "Are Fruit and Vegetables Good for Our Mental and Physical Health? Panel Data Evidence from Australia," *Munich Personal RePEc Archive* 59149, no. 8 (2014). Accessed July II, 2016, https://mpra.ub.uni-muenchen.de/59149/1/MPRA_paper_59149.pdf.

4 B. White et al., "Many Apples a Day Keep the Blues Away—Daily Experiences of Negative and Positive Affect and Food Consumption in Young Adults," *British Journal of Health Psychology* 18 (2013): 782–98.

5 F. Jacka et al., "Association of Western and Traditional Diets with Depression and Anxiety in Women," *American Journal of Psychiatry* 167 (2010): 1–7.

6   "Lack of Sleep Is Affecting Americans, Finds the National Sleep Foundation," National Sleep Foundation, accessed June 7 2016, https://sleepfoundation.org/media-center/press-release/lack-sleep-affecting-americans-finds-the-national-sleep-foundation.

7   P. Wirtz et al., "Dark Chocolate Intake Buffers Stress Reactivity in Humans," *Journal of the American College of Cardiology* 63 (2014): 2297–99.

8   D. Taubert et al., "Effects of Low Habitual Cocoa Intake on Blood Pressure and Bioactive Nitric Oxide: A Randomized Controlled Trial," *Journal of the American Medical Association* 298, no. 1 (2007): 49–60.

9   S. Patel et al., "Association between Reduced Sleep and Weight Gain in Women," *American Journal of Epidemiology* 164, no. 10 (2006): 947–54.

10   M. St-Onge et al., "Fiber and Saturated Fat Are Associated with Sleep Arousals and Slow Wave Sleep," *Journal of Clinical Sleep Medicine* 12, no. 1 (2016): 19–24.

11   E. Hanlon et al., "Sleep Restriction Enhances the Daily Rhythm of Circulating Levels of Endocannabinoid 2-Arachidonoylglycerol," *SLEEP* 39, no. 3 (2016): 653–64.

12   A. Liu et al., "Tart Cherry Juice Increases Sleep Time in Older Adults with Insomnia," *FASEB Journal* 28, no. 1, Supplement 830.9 (2014): 579–83.

13   R. J. Reiter et al., "Melatonin in Walnuts: Influence on Levels of Melatonin and Total Antioxidant Capacity of Blood," *Nutrition* 21, no. 9 (2005): 920–24.

14   A. M. Spaeth et al., "Resting Metabolic Rate Varies by Race and by Sleep Duration," *Obesity* 23, no. 12 (2015): 2349–56.

15   M. Beydoun et al., "Serum Nutritional Biomarkers and Their Associations with Sleep among US Adults in Recent National Surveys," *PLoS One* 9, no. 8 (2014): e103490. doi: 10.1371/journal.pone.0103490.

16   P. Montgomery et al., "Fatty Acids and Sleep in UK Children: Subjective and Pilot Objective Sleep Results from the DOLAB Study—A Randomized Controlled Trial," *Journal of Sleep Research* 23, no. 4 (2014): 364–88.

17   Paul Montgomery, interviewed by author, June 24, 2014.

18   St-Onge, "Fiber and Saturated Fat."

19   T. Satoh et al., "Effect of *Bifidobacterium breve* B-3 on skin photoaging induced by chronic UV irradiation in mice," *Beneficial Microbes* 6, no. 4 (2015): 497–504.

20   T. Levkovich et al., "Probiotic Bacteria Induce a 'Glow of Health,'" *PLoS One* 8, no. 1 (2013): e53867. doi:10.1371/journal.pone.0053867.

21   C. Leung et al., "Soda and Cell Aging: Associations between Sugar-Sweetened Beverage Consumption and Leukocyte Telomere Length in Healthy Adults from the National Health and Nutrition Examination Surveys," *American Journal of Public Health* 104, no. 12 (2014): 2425–31.

22   R. Whitehead et al., "You Are What You Eat: Within-Subject Increases in Fruit and Vegetable Consumption Confer Beneficial Skin-Color Changes," *PLoS One* 7, no. 3 (2012): e32988. doi:10.1371/journal.pone.0032988.

Chapter 3

1   M. Baranski et al., "Higher Antioxidant and Lower Cadmium Concentrations and Lower Incidence of Pesticide Residues in Organically Grown Crops: A Systematic Literature Review and Meta-Analyses," *British Journal of Nutrition* 112 (2014): 794–811.

2   M. Bertoia et al., "Changes in Intake of Fruits and Vegetables and Weight Change in United States Men and Women Followed for up to 24 Years: Analysis from Three Prospective Cohort Studies," *PLoS Medicine* 12, no. 9 (2015): e1001878. doi:10.1371/journal.pmed.1001878.

3   I. Cho et al., "Antibiotics in Early Life alter the Murine Colonic Microbiome and Adiposity," *Nature* 488, no. 7413 (2012): 621–26.

4   "PCBS in Farmed Salmon: Wild Versus Farmed," The Environmental Working Group, accessed June 7, 2016, http://www.ewg.org/research/pcbs-farmed-salmon/wild-versus-farmed.

5   "Buying Fish? What You Need to Know," Environmental Defense Fund, accessed June 7, 2016, http://seafood.edf.org/buying-fish-what-you-need-know.

6   "Oceana Reveals Mislabeling of America's Favorite Fish: Salmon," Oceana, accessed June 7, 2016, http://usa.oceana.org/press-releases/oceana-reveals-mislabeling-americas-favorite-fish-salmon.

7   L. Yanping et al., "Saturated Fats Compared with Unsaturated Fats and Sources of Carbohydrates in Relation to Risk of Coronary Heart Disease: A Prospective Cohort Study," *Journal of the American College of Cardiology* 66, no. 14 (2015): 1538–48.

8   M. Assuncao et al., "Effects of Dietary Coconut Oil on the Biochemical and Anthropometric Profiles of Women Presenting Abdominal Obesity," *Lipids* 44 (2009): 593–601.

9   A. Albertson et al., "Whole Grain Consumption Trends and Associations with Body Weight Measures in the United States: Results from the Cross Sectional National Health and Nutrition Examination Survey 2001–2012," *Nutrition Journal* 15, no. 8 (2016). doi: 10.1186/s12937-016-0126-4.

10   "CSPI Downgrades Sucralose from 'Caution' to 'Avoid,'" Center for Science in the Public Interest, accessed June 7, 2016, http://www.cspinet.org/new/201602081.html.

Chapter 4

1   E. Loucks et al., "Associations of Dispositional Mindfulness with Obesity and Central Adiposity: The New England Family Study," *International Journal of Behavioral Medicine* 23, no. 2 (2016): 224–33.

2   S. Fay et al., "Psychological Predictors of Opportunistic Snacking in the Absence of Hunger," *Eating Behaviors* 18 (2015): 156–59.

3   M. Shah et al., "Slower Eating Speed Lowers Energy Intake in Normal-Weight but Not Overweight/Obese Subjects," *Journal of the Academy of Nutrition and Dietetics* 114 (2014): 393–402.

4   B. Wansink et al., "Slim by Design: Kitchen Counter Correlates of Obesity," *Health Education & Behavior* (2015): pii: 1090198115610571.

5   B. Wansink et al., "The Clean Plate Club: About 92 Percent of Self-Served Food Is Eaten," *International Journal of Obesity* 39 (2015): 371–74.

6   L. Ledochowski et al., "Acute Effects of Brisk Walking on Sugary Snack Cravings in Overweight People, Affect and Responses to a Manipulated Stress Situation and to a Sugary Snack Cue: A Crossover Study," *PLoS One* 10, no. 3 (2015): e0119278. doi:10.1371/journal.pone.0119278.

7   C. Morewedge et al., "Thought for Food: Imagined Consumption Reduces Actual Consumption," *Science* 330 (2010): 1530–33.

8   E. Van Kleef et al., "Just a Bite: Considerably Smaller Snack Portions Satisfy Delayed Hunger and Craving," *Food Quality and Preference* 27 (2013): 96–100.

Chapter 5

1   "Facts & Statistics: Physical Activity," President's Council on Fitness, Sports & Nutrition, accessed June 7, 2016, http://www.fitness.gov/resource-center/facts-and-statistics/.

2   M. Case et al., "Accuracy of Smartphone Applications and Wearable Devices for Tracking Physical Activity Data," *Journal of the American Medical Association* 313, no. 6 (2015): 625–26.

3   J. Kulinski et al., "Association between Cardiorespiratory Fitness and Accelerometer-Derived Physical Activity and Sedentary Time in the General Population," *Mayo Clinic Proceedings* 89, no. 8 (2014): 1063–71.

4   A. Biswas et al., "Sedentary Time and Its Association with Risk for Disease Incidence, Mortality, and Hospitalization in Adults: A Systematic Review and Meta-Analysis," *Annals of Internal Medicine* 162, no. 2 (2015): 123–32.

5   "Fitness and Health Calculators by HealthStatus," HealthStatus, accessed June 7, 2016, https://www.healthstatus.com/perl/calculator.cgi. (Based on a 50-year old, 160-pound woman.)

6   C. Werle et al., "Is It Fun or Exercise? The Framing of Physical Activity Biases Subsequent Snacking," *Marketing Letters* 26 (2015): 691–702.

Chapter 6

1   "Top Tips for Safer Products," EWG's Skin Deep Cosmetics Database, accessed June 7, 2016, http://www.ewg.org/skindeep/top-tips-for-safer-products/.

2   "Lipstick & Lead: Questions & Answers," US Food and Drug Administration, accessed June 7, 2016, http://www.fda.gov/cosmetics/productsingredients/products/ucm137224.htm.

3   H. S. Brown et al., "The Role of Skin Absorption as a Route of Exposure for Volatile Organic Compounds (VOCs) in Drinking Water," *American Journal of Public Health* 74, no. 5 (1984): 479–84.

4   M. Robinson et al., "The Importance of Exposure Estimation in the Assessment of Skin Sensitization Risk," *Contact Dermatitis* 42 (2000): 251–59.

5   "Volatile Organic Compounds (VOCs)," NIH Tox Town, accessed June 7, 2016, https://toxtown.nlm.nih.gov/text_version/chemicals.php?id=31.

6   J. L. Tang-Peronard et al., "Endocrine-Disrupting Chemicals and Obesity Development in Humans: A Review," *Obesity Reviews* 12, no. 8 (2011): 622–36.

7   J. Legler et al., "Obesity, Diabetes, and Associated Costs of Exposure to Endocrine-Disrupting Chemicals in the European Union," *Journal of Clinical Endocrinology & Metabolism* 1000, no. 4 (2015): 1278–88.

8   "Cleaning Supplies: Secret Ingredients, Hidden Hazards," Environmental Working Group, accessed June 7, 2016, http://www.ewg.org/guides/cleaners/content/weak_regulation.

9   E. Clayton et al., "The Impact of Bisphenol A and Triclosan on Immune Parameters in the U.S. Population, NHANES 2003–2006," *Environmental Health Perspectives* 119, no. 3 (2011): 390–96.

10   "Ingredients," IFRA International Fragrance Association, accessed June 7, 2016, http://www.ifraorg.org/en-us/ingredients#.VIaqhzY4lAY.

11   M. Silva et al., "Urinary Levels of Seven Phthalate Metabolites in the US Population from the National Health and Nutrition Examination Survey (NHANES) 1999–2000," *Environmental Health Perspectives* 112, no. 3 (2004): 331–38.

12   L. Parlett et al., "Women's Exposure to Phthalates in Relation to Use of Personal Care Products," *Journal of Exposure Science & Environmental Epidemiology* 23, no. 2 (2013): 197–206.

13   R. Brown et al., "Secular Differences in the Association between Caloric Intake, Macronutrient Intake, and Physical Activity with Obesity," *Obesity Research & Clinical Practice* (2015): pii: S1871-403X(15)00121-0, doi: 10.1016/j.orcp.2015.08.007.

14   Ibid.

15   "Top Tips for Safer Products," EWG's Skin Deep Cosmetics Database.

16   Y. Song et al., "Urinary Concentrations of Bisphenol A and Phthalate Metabolites and Weight Change: A Prospective Investigation in US Women," *International Journal of Obesity* 38, no. 12 (2014): 1532–37; T. James-Todd et al., "Urinary Phthalate Metabolite Concentrations and Diabetes among Women in the National Health and Nutrition Examination Survey (NHANES) 2001–2008," *Environmental Health Perspectives* 120, no. 9 (2012): 1307–13; L. Lopez-Carrillo et al., "Exposure to Phthalates and Breast Cancer Risk in Northern Mexico," *Environmental Health Perspectives* 118 (2010): 539-44.

17   "Parabens," Campaign for Safe Cosmetics, accessed June 7, 2016, http://www.safecosmetics.org/get-the-facts/chemicals-of -concern/parabens/.

18   "Draft Toxicological Profile for Toluene," US Department of Health and Human Services Public Health Service Agency for Toxic Substances and Disease Registry, September 2015.

19   US Congress, House of Representatives, Committee on Energy and Commerce, "Cleaning Product Right to Know Act of 2014." 113th Cong., 2nd sess., April 10, 2014.

20   US Congress, Senate, Committee on Environment and Public Works, "Safe Chemicals Act of 2014." 113th Cong., 2013–2014.

21   J. Lankester et al., "Urinary Triclosan Is Associated with Elevated Body Mass Index in NHANES," *PLoS One* 8, no. 11 (2013): e80057, doi: 10.1371/journal.pone.0080057.

22   "Triclosan: What Consumers Should Know," US Food and Drug Administration, accessed June 7, 2016, http://www.fda.gov /ForConsumers/ConsumerUpdates/ucm205999.htm.

Chapter 7

1   J. A. Wolfson et al., "Is Cooking at Home Associated with Better Diet Quality or Weight-Loss Intention?" *Public Health Nutrition* 18, no. 8 (2015): 1397–406.

2   "Larger Portion Sizes Contribute to US Obesity Problem," National Institutes of Health, accessed June 7, 2016, http://www.nhlbi.nih .gov/health/educational/wecan/news-events/mattel.htm.

3   R. R. Wing et al., "Benefits of Recruiting Participants with Friends and Increasing Social Support for Weight Loss and Maintenance," *Journal of Consulting and Clinical Psychology* 67, no. 1 (1999): 132–38.

Chapter 9

1   H. Leidy et al., "Beneficial Effects of a Higher-Protein Breakfast on the Appetitive, Hormonal, and Neural Signals Controlling Energy Intake Regulation in Overweight/Obese, 'Breakfast-Skipping,' Late-Adolescent Girls," *American Journal of Clinical Nutrition* 97 (2013): 677–88.

2   "NWCR Facts," The National Weight Control Registry, accessed June 12 2016, http://nwcr.ws/research/default.htm.

Chapter 11

1   R. Sebastian et al., "Snacking Patterns of US Adults: What We Eat In America, NHANES 2007-2008," *Food Surveys Research Group Dietary Data Brief No. 4,* June 2011.

2   "Overweight and Obesity Statistics," NIH Publication No. 04-4158.

3   "Snack Attack: What Consumers Are Reaching for around the World," Nielsen Global Snacking Report, September 2014.

Chapter 12

1   A. V. Nedeltcheva et al., "Insufficient Sleep Undermines Dietary Efforts to Reduce Adiposity," *Annals of Internal Medicine* 153, no. 7 (2010): 453–41.

2   S. Racette et al., "Influence of Weekend Lifestyle Patterns on Body Weight," *Obesity* 16, no. 8 (2008): 1826–30.

3   G. A. O'Reilly et al., "Mindfulness-Based Interventions for Obesity-Related Eating Behaviours: A Literature Review," *Obesity Reviews* 15, no. 6 (2014): 453–61.

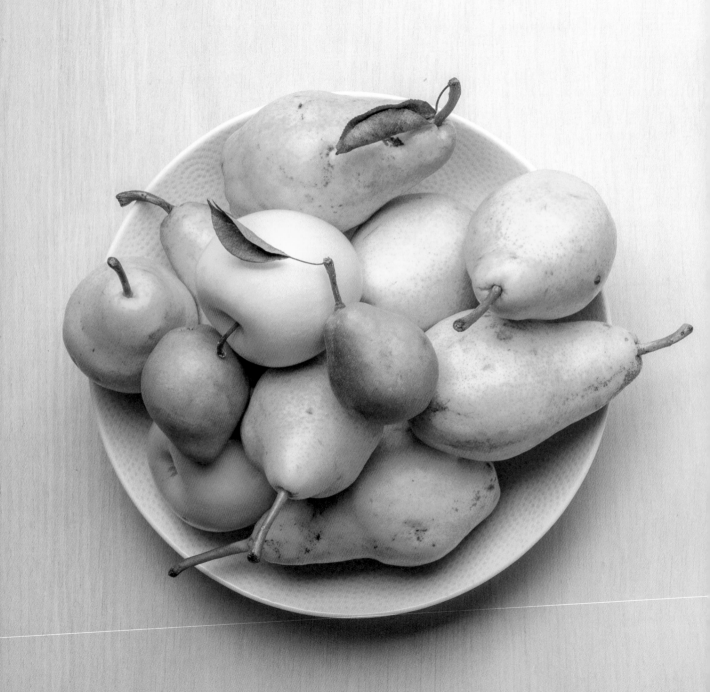

Photo Credits

Pages i-2, 4, 16, 18, 20, 28 (candy bar, chocolate, chips, cashews), 34, 36, 44, 45, 48, 60-61, 62, 76, 82, 94, 101, 103 (olive oil), 106, 110 (lemon oil, lemon juice, olive oil), 113, 114, 116, 135, 136-137, 138, 159, 160, 162, 164 (scrambled eggs), 166, 167, 168, 174, 179 (fruit salad), 180, 183 (hummus), 185 (salad), 187, 188 (rice, broccoli), 194, 202, 204, 207, 219, 302, 318
Photographer: Ryan Hulvat
Food stylist: Paul Grimes
Prop stylist: Paola Andrea

Pages 8-9, 24-25, 30-31, 54-55, 66-67, 78-79, 109 (essential oil), 118-119, 126-127, 144-145, 190, 210-211
Photographer: Matt Rainey
Hair and makeup (after): Claudia/Halley Resources
Wardrobe stylist (after): Kathlie Young/Ennis

Pages 11, 15, 28 (cookies, banana), 33, 38, 39, 40, 43, 46-47, 52, 53, 70, 71, 74, 77 (celery), 80, 96, 102 (chia, avocado, yogurt, wheatgrass), 103 (blueberries, almonds, oats, milk), 105 (milk, sugar, vanilla, cilantro, buttermilk), 109 (vinegar, baking soda), 140, 164 (orange), 165 (strawberries), 169 (walnuts, mushroom, asparagus, pistachios), 170 (berries), 177, 178, 179 (crackers), 181 (orange), 182 (apple), 184, 189 (rice), 191, 213, 259
Photographer: Mitch Mandel/Rodale Images

Pages 222, 225, 230, 236, 239, 240, 243, 244, 247, 249, 255, 257, 267, 269, 271, 280, 283, 284, 287, 289,
Photographer: Mitch Mandel/Rodale Images
Food stylist: Khalil Hymore
Prop Stylist: Courtney DeWet/Big Leo

Pages 64, 97, 104 (tea), 109 (water), 171 (cereal), 172
Getty Images

Page 75
Photodisk

Pages 77 (Fizzy water), 98, 112 (group shot)
Istockphoto

Pages 86, 110 (kettle)
Stockbyte

Page 102 (green apple)
PhotoAlto

Pages 102, 103 (honey)
BrandX

Page 104 (beer and mouthwash),
Alamy

Page 259
Andrew Purcell

Index

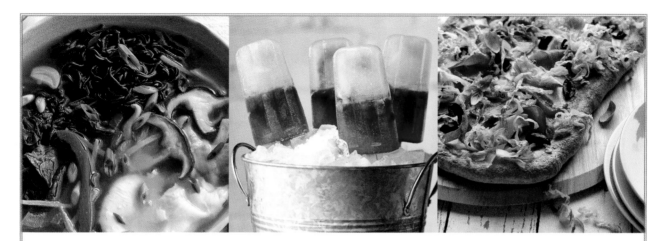

Real Food for Real Weight Loss— Real Fast!

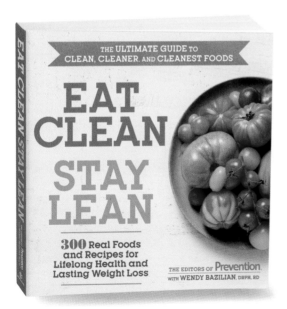

EATING HEALTHY REALLY MEANS EATING CLEAN, or choosing whole foods with the least amount of processing and fewest ingredients. And to help you eat better, the editors of *Prevention* have created *Eat Clean, Stay Lean*—your easy-to-use, visual guidebook to better health, delicious food, and a slimmer you. This guide shows you how to make 50 smarter choices in the supermarket and 150 cleaner fast meals at home so you can enjoy real, worry-free food that tastes great.

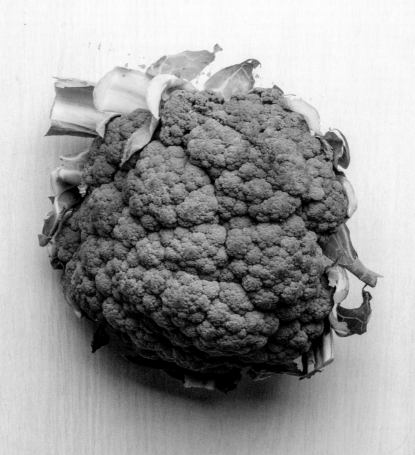